CW00797849

European Paediatric Advanced Life Support

5th Edition, May 2021

Reprinted October 2021

Reprinted June 2022

Reprinted January 2023

Reprinted May 2023

Reprinted October 2023

EPALS

European Paediatric Advanced Life Support
5th Edition, May 2021

Reprinted October 2021
Reprinted June 2022
Reprinted January 2023
Reprinted May 2023
Reprinted October 2023

ISBN 978-1-903812-37-2

Published by © Resuscitation Council UK 2021
1st Floor, 60-62 Margaret Street, London, W1W 8TF
Tel: 020 7388 4678 email: enquiries@resus.org.uk www.resus.org.uk

Printed by All About Print.
Tel: 020 7205 4022 email: hello@allaboutprint.co.uk www.allaboutprint.co.uk
Printed on responsibly sourced environmentally friendly paper made with elemental chlorine free fibre from legal and sustainably managed forests.

Photographs © Resuscitation Council UK

Photography by Ed Tyler, Mark Sedge and Ashley Prytherch
ECGs © Oliver Meyer
Electrical conduction of the heart (Figure 6.1) © LifeART image (1989–2001)
Wolters Kluwer Health, Inc. Lippincott Williams & Wilkins. All rights reserved.
Intraosseous space and relationship with circulation (Figure 5.2)
with permission from EZ-IO.
The Chain of Prevention (Figure 8.1) © reproduced with permission of
Professor Gary B Smith

Design and artwork by Fruition London
www.fruitionlondon.com

The Resuscitation Council UK guidelines are adapted from the European Resuscitation Council guidelines and have been developed using a process accredited by The National Institute for Health and Care Excellence. The UK guidelines are consistent with the European guidelines but include minor modifications to reflect the needs of the National Health Service.

This European Paediatric Advanced Life Support (EPALS) manual is written by the Resuscitation Council UK EPALS Subcommittee and forms part of the resources for the Resuscitation Council UK EPALS course, which is delivered in accredited course centres throughout the UK.

Acknowledgements

We thank and acknowledge the members of the ERC 2021 Guidelines Writing Group who have contributed directly or indirectly to this EPALS manual.

We thank the Nuffield Hospital, Guildford, for the use of their facilities, the Royal Surrey NHS Foundation Trust, specifically the Resuscitation Department for their assistance with photography, Lifecast Body Simulation for the loan of manikins and all the Instructors who gave up their time to take part in the photography shoot

We thank Oliver Meyer for the digital preparation of the rhythm strips.

We thank Ed Tyler, Ashley Prytherch and Mark Sedge for the photography taken and for being digitally prepared for the manual.

Previous contributors

Souhail Alouni
Dominique Biarent
Paolo Biban
Keith Brownlee
Gudrun Burda
Gerard Cheron
Karen Cooper
Serena Cottrell
Fotini Danou
Jo Draaisma
Christoph Eich
Christine Fonteyne
Miguel Felix
Mojca Groselj-Grenc
Sylvia Hunyadi-Anticevic
Ben Lakin
Torsten Lauritsen
Francis Leclerc
Anselmi Luciano
Jesus Lopez-Herce
Ralph Mackinnon
David Mason
Thomas Rajka
Sam Richmond
Antonio Rodriguez-Nunez
Sheila Simpson
Ruchi Sinha
Frederic Tits
Felicity Todd
John Trounce
Nigel Turner
Patrick Van de Voorde
Burkhard Wermter
Mark Woolcock
Jonathan Wyllie
David Zideman

Authors

Marion De Almeida Santos
Sean Ainsworth
Liesje Andre
Adam Benson Clarke
Robert Bingham
Mandy Brailsford
Fiona Clements
Mike Coren
Jane Davies
Isabelle Hamilton-Bower
Sue Hampshire
Mae Johnson
Ralph Mackinnon
Ian Maconochie
Ian McDougall
Liz Norris
Michael Page
Sophie Skellett
Denise Welsby
Mark Worrall
Deborah Zeitlin

Editors

Sophie Skellett
Adam Benson Clarke
Robert Bingham
Isabelle Hamilton-Bower
Sue Hampshire
Ian Maconochie

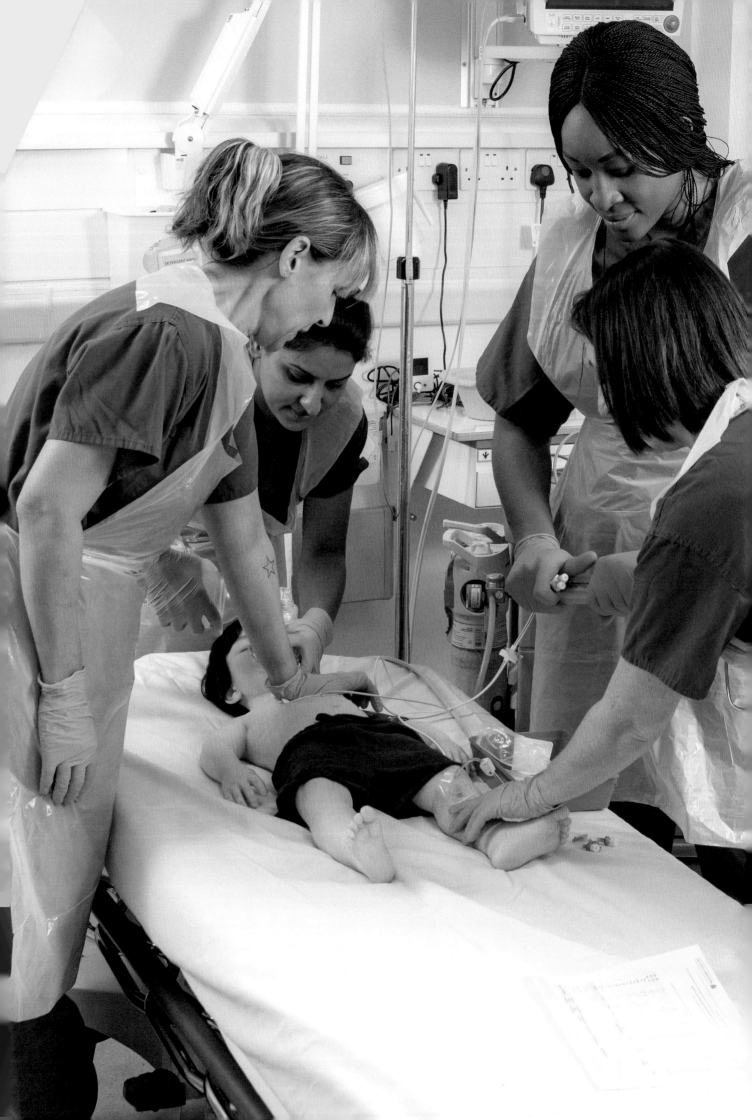

Foreword

The European Paediatric Advanced Life Support (EPALS) provider course is a pan-European project developed under the auspices of the European Resuscitation Council. It provides training for multidisciplinary healthcare professionals in the early recognition of the child in respiratory or circulatory failure and the development of the knowledge and core skills required to prevent further deterioration towards a respiratory or cardiorespiratory arrest.

The course comprises the manual, lectures, workshops, skill stations, teaching simulations and assessments. It now also encompasses many paediatric specific illnesses that those caring for children will encounter. We hope you find the manual to be informative as it contains not only information covered in the course but additional information which will be useful to your practice. Candidate interaction and participation is a key element of the face-to-face element of the course.

Instructors on the course teach voluntarily, giving their time and expertise without financial gain. Their enthusiasm and commitment to the subject helps to maintain the courses' high standards and ensure its availability to healthcare professionals who would be expected to apply the skills taught as part of their clinical duties.

We very much hope you enjoy the course.

Dr Sophie Skellett
Chairman, EPALS course Subcommittee, Resuscitation Council UK

Contents

Contents

Notes

Glossary

Abbreviation	In full
ABG	arterial blood gas
AED	automated external defibrillator
BLS	basic life support
BP	blood pressure
CRT	capillary refill time
CO_2	carbon dioxide
CO	cardiac output
CPR	cardiopulmonary resuscitation
DNACPR	do not attempt cardiopulmonary resuscitation
$ETCO_2$	end-tidal carbon dioxide
ECG	electrocardiogram
FiO_2	fraction of inspired oxygen
HR	heart rate
h	hour
IM	intramuscular
IO	intraosseous
IV	intravenous
LMA	laryngeal mask airway
Mg^{2+}	magnesium
Min	minute
Na^+	sodium
O_2	oxygen
PEA	pulseless electrical activity
PEF	peak expiratory flow
PICU	paediatric intensive care unit
$PaCO_2$	partial pressure of arterial carbon dioxide
PaO_2	partial pressure of arterial oxygen
PEEP	positive end expiratory pressure
pMDI	pressurised metred dose inhaler
K^+	potassium
RR	respiratory rate
SaO_2	arterial oxygen saturation
s	second
SGA	supraglottic airway
SpO_2	peripheral oxygen saturation (pulse oximetry)
SV	stroke volume
SVT	supraventricular tachycardia
SVR	systemic vascular resistance
TT	tracheal tube
VF	ventricular fibrillation
VT	ventricular tachycardia
pVT	pulseless ventricular tachycardia

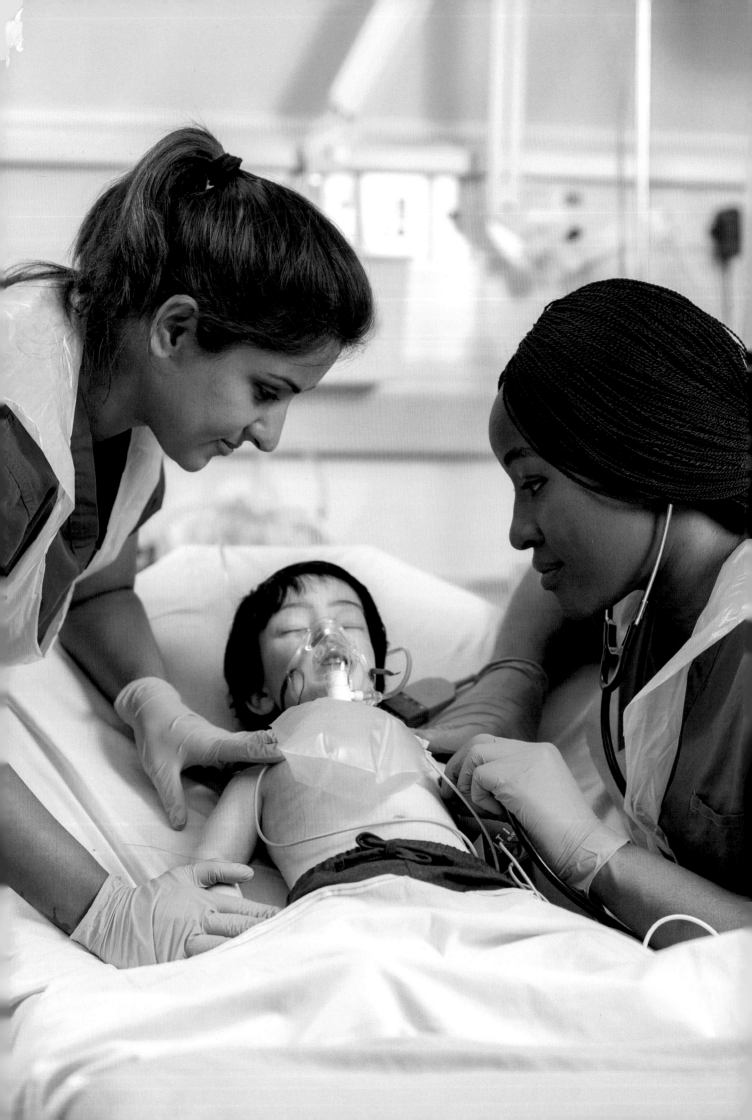

Introduction to Paediatric Advanced Life Support

Aetiologies of cardiorespiratory arrest

The aetiology of cardiorespiratory arrest in children differs from adults. This is due to anatomical, physiological and pathological differences, which alter throughout childhood.

Primary cardiorespiratory arrest is a sudden acute event, which occurs without warning. It is commonly due to a cardiac arrhythmia reflecting intrinsic heart disease. A successful outcome is generally dependent on rapid defibrillation, as the commonest arrhythmias encountered in primary cardiorespiratory arrests are ventricular fibrillation (VF) or pulseless ventricular tachycardia (pVT) Every minute of delay until defibrillation results in the number of successful cases with a return of spontaneous circulation (ROSC) decreasing by approximately 10%.

A primary cardiac arrest is most common in adults but can occur in older children or children with congenital heart disease. Overall, however, the most common cause of cardiorespiratory arrest in children is secondary to other intercurrent illnesses.

A secondary cardiorespiratory arrest is usually due to hypoxia and reflects the limit of the body's ability to compensate for the effects of underlying illness or injury. Severe tissue hypoxia causes myocardial dysfunction, resulting in profound bradycardia, which typically deteriorates to asystole or pulseless electrical activity (PEA). Both PEA and asystole are associated with a poor outcome.

A secondary cardiorespiratory arrest is rarely a sudden event but follows a progressive deterioration. As respiratory and circulatory failure worsen (Figure 1.1), the body initially activates adaptive physiological responses compensating for the effects of the deterioration on vital organs (compensated respiratory or circulatory failure). These adaptive responses result in signs and symptoms that can be recognised, thereby providing an opportunity to intervene before further deterioration to cardiorespiratory arrest.

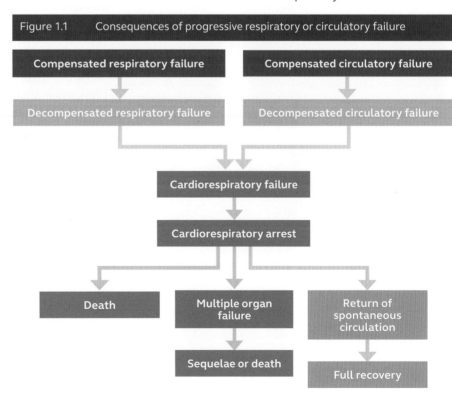

Figure 1.1   Consequences of progressive respiratory or circulatory failure

Outcome from secondary cardiorespiratory arrest

The outcome from secondary cardiorespiratory arrest is poor. Severe tissue hypoxia occurring before the heart stops means that all the vital organs are potentially seriously compromised; the heart finally arrests as a result of severe myocardial hypoxia.

Even if ROSC is achieved, morbidity and mortality remain high. Rates of successful resuscitation from out-of-hospital cardiorespiratory arrest (OHCA) are low (4–12% survival); less than 5% of children will survive without neurological sequelae. In-hospital cardiac arrest (IHCA) results are better with a 60-80% ROSC rate, but many children succumb to severe organ injury (e.g. brain, kidney) or multi-system organ failure 48–72 h post-arrest. Data from the National Cardiac Arrest Audit (NCAA) in the UK between 2012–2018 indicated that 69% of patients achieve ROSC, but only 54% of children survived to hospital discharge following IHCA in this time period.

Resuscitation from respiratory arrest, when there is still a cardiac output, is associated with better (80–90%) good quality, long-term survival.

Anatomical and physiological considerations

The underlying anatomical and physiological differences between infants, young children and adults largely account for the difference in aetiology of cardiorespiratory arrest.

The key differences will be considered in order of management priority based on the ABCDE approach.

A	Airway
B	Breathing
C	Circulation
D	Disability (mental status)
E	Exposure

A Airway

The infant/young child has an airway that is proportionately narrower and more susceptible to oedema and swelling than the adult. The absolute diameter of the airway is also smaller, and therefore respiratory infections account for a significantly higher level of morbidity and mortality in young children.

The effect of oedema and swelling can be seen in Poiseuille's law, which relates the resistance of the gas flowing through a tube (R) to its length (l), the viscosity of the gas (v) and the radius of the tube (r).

$$R = \frac{8l\,v}{\pi r^4}$$

Thus, a small decrease in the airway radius (r) results in a huge increase (to the power of 4) of resistance to flow of gases throughout the respiratory passages.

Relationship between head and neck

The infant's head is large in relation to the rest of their body. Since the occiput is protuberant, the head tends to flex on the neck when the infant is placed in a supine position. This leads to potential obstruction of the airway when the conscious level is reduced. With increasing age, the child's head becomes smaller in relation to their thorax, the neck lengthens, and the larynx becomes more resistant to external pressure as tissues become less compliant. This explains why airway opening positions are different at different ages.

Face and mouth

The infant's face is small, and therefore the sizing of face masks needs to be accurate; otherwise, it is difficult to achieve an effective seal. Additionally, pressure to the eyes can lead to damage and reflex bradycardia and must be avoided.

Inside the small mouth, the tongue is relatively large. This combination means that airway obstruction is more likely in the unconscious infant/young child. The floor of the mouth is easily compressible; care is required to avoid compressing the soft tissues under the mandible to prevent airway obstruction when performing airway manoeuvres.

Nose and pharynx

The infant is a preferential nasal breather for the first six months or so of life. As a result, anything that causes nasal obstruction (e.g. anatomical abnormalities such as choanal atresia, copious secretions, nasogastric tubes or tapes) can lead to increased work of breathing and respiratory compromise. The epiglottis in infants is larger and floppier than in adults. This means that it is vulnerable to damage by airway devices and manoeuvres; additionally, manipulation of the epiglottis can lead to vagal stimulation.

The larynx

The larynx is higher in the infant compared to the older child and adult (where it is level with C5–6). It was previously thought that the younger child's larynx was funnel-shaped, with its narrowest segment at the level of the cricoid cartilage; however, this was based on cadaver examinations. Recent studies using MRI examination of the laryngeal structures under deep sedation (when laryngeal muscles are tonically active) suggest children and infants have mainly ellipsoid shaped airways, cylindrical in the antero-posterior diameter but cone-shaped in the transverse diameter with the vocal cords at the apex of the cone. The anatomical variations have the following practical implications:

- Blind finger sweeps to remove a foreign body must not be performed in young children with partial airway obstruction as these may convert a partial into a complete obstruction. The foreign body can become impacted into the narrowest part of the larynx.

- The relatively large tongue may create airway obstruction as the epiglottis and larynx are higher in the neck.

- Control of the large tongue with a laryngoscope blade may be difficult.

- The high position of the larynx in an infant creates a sharp angle between the oropharynx and the glottis. Direct visualisation of the glottis with the laryngoscope is therefore difficult. It may be easier to use a straight blade rather than a curved blade to obtain a view, particularly in infants up to three months of age (this does, however, result in more vagal stimulation).

B Breathing

Physiological considerations

The air-alveolar surface area for gas exchange in the lungs at birth is 3 m² compared with 70 m² in the adult. There is also a 10-fold increase in the number of small airways from birth to adulthood.

Normal respiratory function requires the movement of gas in and out of the lungs and the exchange of oxygen (O_2) for carbon dioxide (CO_2) across the alveolar-capillary interface. Minute ventilation (the main determinant of CO_2 removal) depends upon the tidal volume (volume of gas with each breath) and the respiratory rate.

Minute ventilation = tidal volume x respiratory rate

Spontaneous tidal volume stays constant throughout life at 4–6 mL kg⁻¹. It can be qualitatively assessed by auscultation of the chest, listening to air entry in the upper and lower zones of both sides of the chest.

Infants and small children have a relatively small resting lung volume and hence a low oxygen reserve. In addition, they have a high rate of oxygen consumption. This combination results in rapid falls in blood oxygen levels when respiration is compromised.

Mechanics of breathing

As they age, the mechanics of children's breathing changes. The infant has cartilaginous and pliable ribs, while their intercostal muscles are weak and relatively ineffective. The main muscle of respiration is the diaphragm. During inspiration, the diaphragm descends towards the abdomen, generating a negative pressure, which draws air into the upper airway and the lungs.

Mechanical impedance to the contraction of the diaphragm (e.g. gastric distension, intestinal obstruction) will result in ineffective ventilation, as will any obstruction of the airway (e.g. bronchiolitis, asthma or foreign body aspiration).

In older children, the more developed intercostal muscles contribute significantly to the mechanics of breathing. The ribs ossify and act as a secure anchor for the muscles, as well as forming a more rigid structure that is less likely to collapse in respiratory distress. In children above five years, the presence of significant intercostal recession should therefore be considered as an ominous sign and indicative of serious respiratory compromise.

Respiratory rate

Normal respiration requires minimal effort, and the resting respiratory rate varies with age. The infant has a relatively high metabolic rate, O_2 consumption and CO_2 production, which is the main reason for their increased respiratory rates (Table 1.1). The respiratory rate also increases with agitation, anxiety and the presence of fever; therefore, a record of respiratory rate as it changes over time is more useful than a single value.

Table 1.1   Respiratory rate ranges by age

Age (years)	Respiratory rate (breaths min⁻¹)
< 1	30–40 min⁻¹
1–2	26–34 min⁻¹
2–5	24–30 min⁻¹
5–12	20–24 min⁻¹
> 12	12–20 min⁻¹

C Circulation (and oxygen delivery)

The circulating volume of the newborn is 80 mL kg^{-1} and decreases with age to 60–70 mL kg^{-1} in adulthood. This means that the total circulating volume of an infant is very small (e.g. 240 mL in a newborn of 3 kg and 480 mL in a six-month-old with a weight of 6 kg). Relatively small losses can be a significantly high percentage of their total circulating volume; this is why apparently minor diarrhoeal illnesses can result in considerable morbidity and even mortality in infants and young children.

Oxygen delivery (DO_2) to cells in the body's tissues is determined by arterial oxygen content and cardiac output. Arterial O_2 content (CaO_2) is determined by circulating haemoglobin concentration and O_2 saturation and, to a small extent, the dissolved O_2 in the plasma.

> **Oxygen delivery to the body tissues**
> $$DO_2 = CaO_2 \times CO$$
>
> DO_2 = oxygen delivery (mL min^{-1})
> CaO_2 = arterial O_2 content (mL L^{-1})
> CO = cardiac output (L min^{-1})

> **Arterial oxygen content**
> $$CaO_2 = Hb \times 1.34 \times SaO_2$$
>
> Hb = haemoglobin concentration (g L^{-1})

The constant 1.34 is the O_2 carrying capacity of 1 g of haemoglobin (mL O_2 g Hb^{-1}).

SaO_2 = oxygen saturation of haemoglobin (between 0 and 1 converted from percentage saturation value).

(SpO_2 is the peripheral oxygen saturation of blood which is, for practical purposes, almost identical to SaO_2).

If either of the parameters of DO_2 (CaO_2 and CO) decreases and is not compensated for by an increase in the other parameter, tissue O_2 delivery decreases.

In respiratory failure, the fall in arterial oxygen content (CaO_2) can be compensated by increasing cardiac output (CO).

A decrease in CO, as in circulatory failure, cannot be compensated by a rise in O_2 content. It is accompanied immediately by a decrease in tissue O_2 delivery. It is also important to compare DO_2 with O_2 demand, which may be higher than normal (as in septic shock).

Heart rate

Stroke volume (i.e. the amount of blood ejected with each contraction of the heart) is relatively small in infancy (1.5 mL kg^{-1} at birth) and increases along with heart size. However, the cardiac output relative to body weight is higher than at any other stage of life (300 mL kg^{-1} min^{-1}, decreasing to 100 mL kg^{-1} min^{-1} in adolescence and 70–80 mL kg^{-1} min^{-1} in adults).

Cardiac output is the product of stroke volume and heart rate, and so the high cardiac outputs in infants and young children are primarily achieved by rapid heart rates (Table 1.2).

Since cardiac output is directly related to the heart rate, bradycardia is a serious event and should be treated vigorously. Systemic vascular resistance increases as the child ages, and this is reflected in the changes seen in blood pressure (BP) ranges (Table 1.3).

In sick children and infants, it is useful to consider the mean arterial blood pressure as an indicator of blood flow, and it is believed to be a better indicator of tissue perfusion than systolic BP (as it accounts for the fact that two thirds of the cardiac cycle is spent in diastole). Mean arterial pressure (MAP) is derived from a patient's systolic blood pressure (SBP) and diastolic blood pressure (DBP). Since MAP is a product of cardiac output (CO) and systemic vascular resistance (SVR) (MAP = CO x SVR), variations in SVR make the relationship between MAP and CO often unreliable (e.g. a patient with a poor CO but high SVR such as a patient in cardiogenic shock may have an acceptable MAP but a CO that is too low to provide adequate perfusion to tissues). The MAP should be calculated in acute conditions by the method below and compared to MAP expected (Table 1.3).

> $$((2 \times \text{diastolic}) + \text{systolic}) / 3 = \text{MAP (mmHg)}$$

Table 1.2 Heart rate ranges (beats min^{-1})

Age	Mean	Awake	Deep sleep
Newborn – 3 months	140	85–205	80–140
3 months – 2 years	130	100–180	75–160
2–10 years	80	60–140	60–90
> 10 years	75	60–100	50–90

Table 1.3 Blood pressure ranges by age systolic and mean

Blood pressure for age	1 month	1 year	5 years	10 years	15 years
50th centile for Systolic BP	75 mmHg	95 mmHg	100 mmHg	110 mmHg	120 mmHg
5th centile for Systolic BP	50 mmHg	70 mmHg	75 mmHg	80 mmHg	90 mmHg
50th centile for mean arterial pressure (MAP)	55 mmHg	70 mmHg	75 mmHg	75 mmHg	80 mmHg
5th centile for mean arterial blood pressure (MAP)	40 mmHg	50 mmHg	55 mmHg	55 mmHg	65 mmHg

D Disability

The limited communication skills of infants and children have to be considered when attempting to assess neurological status. There is a tendency for ill children to regress to behaviour more befitting a younger child, especially if they are anxious or in pain. Therefore, effective pain control, empathy, and appropriate language are all essential factors when dealing with children. The presence of parents or other significant adults may help alleviate many communication difficulties, as well as helping to ease fear and anxiety and is to be encouraged.

A rapid assessment of the child's conscious level can be obtained by determining the AVPU score (Chapter 2) or by the Glasgow Coma Scale score if doctors and nurses are familiar with its use; there is a modified scale for children under five years of age. Additionally, assessing pupil size and reaction, and the child's posture, muscle tone, and any focal signs should be noted to determine neurological status.

E Exposure

To ensure that no significant clinical information is missed, examine the child fully by exposing their body. Appropriate measures to minimise heat loss (especially in infants) and respect dignity must be adopted at all times. The core body temperature should also be recorded, and appropriate measures to normalise it initiated if necessary.

Medications are prescribed based on a child's body weight. In an emergency situation, it is often impractical to weigh the child; therefore, an alternative method of estimating weight as accurately as possible is required. In order of preference:

1. use the child/infant's body weight for drug calculations if known
2. use a body length tape with pre-calculated drug doses
3. use a paediatric emergency drug chart (Appendix A)
4. use an age-based weight calculation formula. For the age group between one and ten years, the following formula provides an approximation of weight:
   - Weight (kg) = (Age in years + 4) x 2
   - An infant weighs approximately 3 kg at birth and 10 kg at one year of age.

The simplicity of this formula facilitates recollection under pressure, and although the actual weight of overweight children will be underestimated, drug dosage is usually based on lean body mass rather than actual mass. For obese patients, use ideal body weight and do not use actual weight to avoid drug toxicity. **Beware of exceeding the adult doses of drugs and fluids in older children (see Appendix A).**

Whatever method is used to establish a child's body weight, all healthcare professionals must be prepared and sufficiently familiar in its use to be able to utilise it quickly and accurately.

Causes of death and prevention

In the neonatal period, the most common aetiology of death is congenital anomaly, followed by adverse perinatal events and sudden infant death syndrome.

In infancy, congenital anomaly is still the leading cause of death, followed by respiratory and cardiovascular illness, infectious disease and trauma.

The most common causes of mortality in pre-school children (ages 1–4 years) are malignancy and trauma followed by congenital anomalies, central nervous system disease (including epilepsy) and respiratory disease. For school-aged children between 5–9 years old, malignancy and trauma are the major causes of death, followed by central nervous system disease. Trauma is the second highest cause of death in children from 10–14 years old and the highest cause of death in 15–19 year olds, along with death caused by suicides and risk-taking behaviour (e.g. drug use). Accident and mental health prevention/intervention schemes need to be tailored to the different age groups. Such schemes depend on a combination of three elements:

- **primary prevention** – prevention of the accident (e.g. by using safe material in playgrounds, stair gates etc.), education on risks from drug taking
- **secondary prevention** – reducing the severity of an accident (e.g. by promoting the wearing of bicycle helmets), adequate mental health access for children in need
- **tertiary prevention** – diminishing the consequence of the event by improving the effectiveness of emergency services after injury (e.g. the establishment of major trauma centres in the UK).

Expected and unexpected death

The death of a child is emotionally distressing for parents, relatives and the healthcare professionals involved.

This latter group may include pre-hospital staff as well as those based at the hospital. An opportunity to hold a debriefing session for all staff after the death is important to allow them to process any concerns, feelings or emotions that arise from having delivered care to the child. It is also an important learning tool that has been shown to improve performance. Any member of the healthcare team should feel able to seek help and advice from colleagues, their general practitioner (GP), bereavement counsellors or occupational health department if they feel they require it.

In any case of an unexpected death, particularly when the cause is not clear, staff have a duty to make a referral to the coroner or procurator fiscal in Scotland and consider any safeguarding issues.

In October 2018, NHS England published new statutory and operational guidance for child death review (CDR). The guidance sets out the key stages:

a) the immediate actions that take place after all children's deaths

b) the investigations that follow some deaths

c) the local review by those who looked after the child

d) the independent multiagency review by a child death overview panel (CDOP)

e) the actions professionals should take in certain circumstances.

The GP, health visitor (for children under five years) and school nurse (for children over five years) must be informed about any paediatric deaths. In the UK, it is common practice to invite the parents approximately 4–6 weeks after the child's death to meet with the consultant in charge. This enables the parents to ask questions and to receive information about the results of investigations that have taken place.

A child may have a condition for which it is agreed that resuscitation would not be beneficial. Looking after such a child and their family requires compassionate and considered management (palliative care) and is beyond the scope of the EPALS course.

In these circumstances, advance care planning is advocated, and RCUK supports the use of the ReSPECT (Recommended Summary Plan for Emergency Care and Treatment) process and form. This process is increasingly being adopted in hospitals throughout the UK, and all providers should be familiar with it.

It is important to feel that the best possible care has been delivered as not all resuscitation attempts are successful. Early intervention based on the ABCDE approach will reduce the number of unexpected deaths. The EPALS course aims to provide this structured approach for the optimal care of children.

Figure 1.2	Child death review process

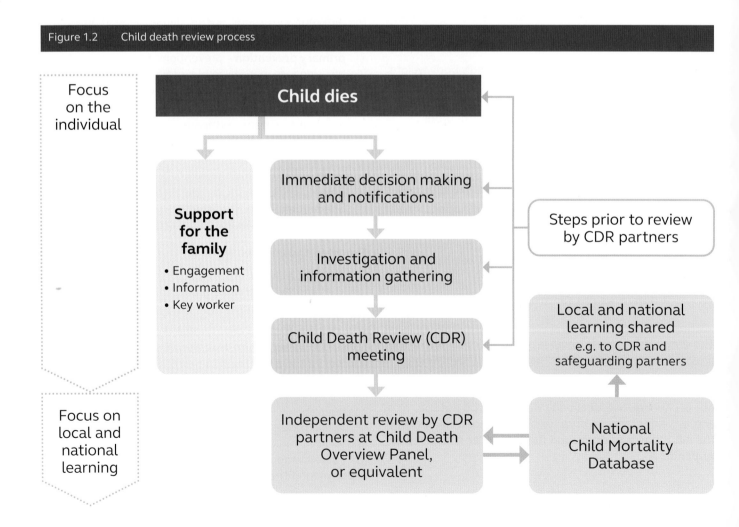

01: Summary learning

Children are more likely to suffer a secondary rather than a primary cardiorespiratory arrest.

Successful resuscitation from respiratory arrest, where there is still a cardiac output, is associated with 80–90% good quality, long-term survival.

Survival from full secondary cardiorespiratory arrest without neurological sequelae is considerably less likely (< 5% out-of-hospital and approximately 54% in hospital).

Infants and young children's respiratory and circulatory anatomy and physiology, influence both the aetiology and management of their illnesses/injuries.

The ABCDE approach is the basis of both the assessment and the management of seriously ill and/or injured children.

My key take-home messages from this chapter are:

Further reading

Atkins DL, Everson-Stewart S, Sears GK, Daya M, Osmond MH, Warden CR, Berg RA; Resuscitation Outcomes Consortium Investigators. Epidemiology and outcomes from out-of-hospital cardiac arrest in children: the Resuscitation Outcomes Consortium Epistry-Cardiac Arrest. Circulation 2009; 24;119:1484-91.

Berg MD, Nadkarni VM, Berg RA. Cardiopulmonary Resuscitation in Children. Curr Opin Crit Care. 2008;14:254-60.

Deasy C, Bernard SA, Cameron P et al. Epidemiology of paediatric out-of- hospital cardiac arrest in Melbourne, Resuscitation 2010; 81: 1095-1100.

Donoghue AJ, Nadkarni V, Berg RA, Osmond MH, Wells G, Nesbitt L, Stiell IG. Out-of-Hospital Pediatric Cardiac Arrest: An Epidemiologic Review and Assessment of Current Knowledge Ann Emerg Med. 2005;46:512-522.

Dudley NC, Hansen KW, Furnival RA, Donaldson AE, Van Wagenen KL, Scaife ER. The effect of family presence on the efficiency of pediatric trauma resuscitation. Ann Emerg Med 2009; 53: 777-784, e3.

Gupta P, Tang X, Gall CM, Lauer C, Rice TB, Wetzel RC. Epidemiology and outcomes of in-hospital cardiac arrest in critically ill children across hospitals of varied center volume: A multi-center analysis. Resuscitation 2014;85:1473-9.

Kuisma M, Suominen P, Korpela R. Paediatric out-of-hospital cardiac arrests: epidemiology and outcome. Resuscitation 1995;30:141-50.

Lopez-Herce J, Garcia C, Rodriguez-Nunez A, Dominguez P, Carillo A, Calvo C, Delgado MA. Long term outcome of paediatric cardiorespiratory arrest in Spain. Resuscitation 2005: 64:79-85.

Nadkarni VM, Larkin GL, Peberdy MA, Carey SM, Kaye W, Mancini ME, et al. First documented rhythm and clinical outcome from in-hospital cardiac arrest among children and adults. JAMA. 2006; 4;295:50-7.

Tibballs J, Kinney S. A prospective study of outcome of in-patient paediatric cardiopulmonary arrest. Resuscitation 2006;71;310-8.

Topjian AA, Nadkarni VM, Berg RA. Cardiopulmonary resuscitation in children. Curr Opin Crit Care. 2009; 15:203-8.

Safranek DJ, Eisenberg MS, Larsen MP. The epidemiology of cardiac arrest in young adults. Annals of emergency medicine 1992;21:1102-6.

Sirbaugh PE, Pepe PE, Shook JE, et al. A prospective, population based study of the demographics, epidemiology, management, and outcome of out-of- hospital pediatric cardiopulmonary arrest. Annals of emergency medicine 1999;33:174-84.

Go AS, Mozaffarian D, Roger VL et al (2014) Heart disease and stroke statistics-2014 update: a report from the American Heart Association. Circulation 129:e28-e292.

Naim MY, Burke RV, McNally BF et al. Association of Bystander Cardiopulmonary Resuscitation with Overall and Neurologically Favorable Survival after Pediatric Out-of-Hospital Cardiac Arrest in the United States; a report from the Cardiac Arrest Registry to Enhance Survival Surveillance Registry (CARES). JAMA Pediatr 2017;17(2):133-141.

Nitta M, Iwami T, Kitamura T, Nadkarni VM, Berg RA, Shimizu N, Ohta K, Nishiuchi T, Hayashi Y, Hiraide A, Tamai H, Kobayashi M, Morita H (2011) Age-specific differences in outcomes after out-of-hospital cardiac arrests. Pediatrics 128:e812-820.

Girotra S, Spertus JA, Li Y, Berg RA, Nadkarni VM, Chan PS; American Heart Association Get With the Guidelines–Resuscitation Investigators (2013) Survival trends in pediatric in hospital cardiac arrests: an analysis from Get With the Guidelines-Resuscitation. Circ Cardiovasc Qual Outcomes 6:42-49.

Haque IU, Zaritsky AL. Analysis for evidence for lower limit of systolic and mean arterial pressure in children, Paediatric critical care Medicine. 2007; 8, 2,138-122.

The Children's Action Prevention Trust www.capt.org.uk

Office for National Statistics. Child and infant mortality in England and Wales (2018) (published February 2020) www.ons.gov.uk

www.respectprocess.org.uk

Litman RS, Weissend EE, Shibata D, Westesson PL. Developmental changes of laryngeal dimensions in unparalysed sedated children. Anesthesiology 2003:98:41-5.

Skellett S, Orzechowska I, Thomas K, Fortune PM. The landscape of paediatric in-hospital cardiac arrest in the United Kingdom National Cardia Arrest Audit. Resuscitation 2020;155:165-171.

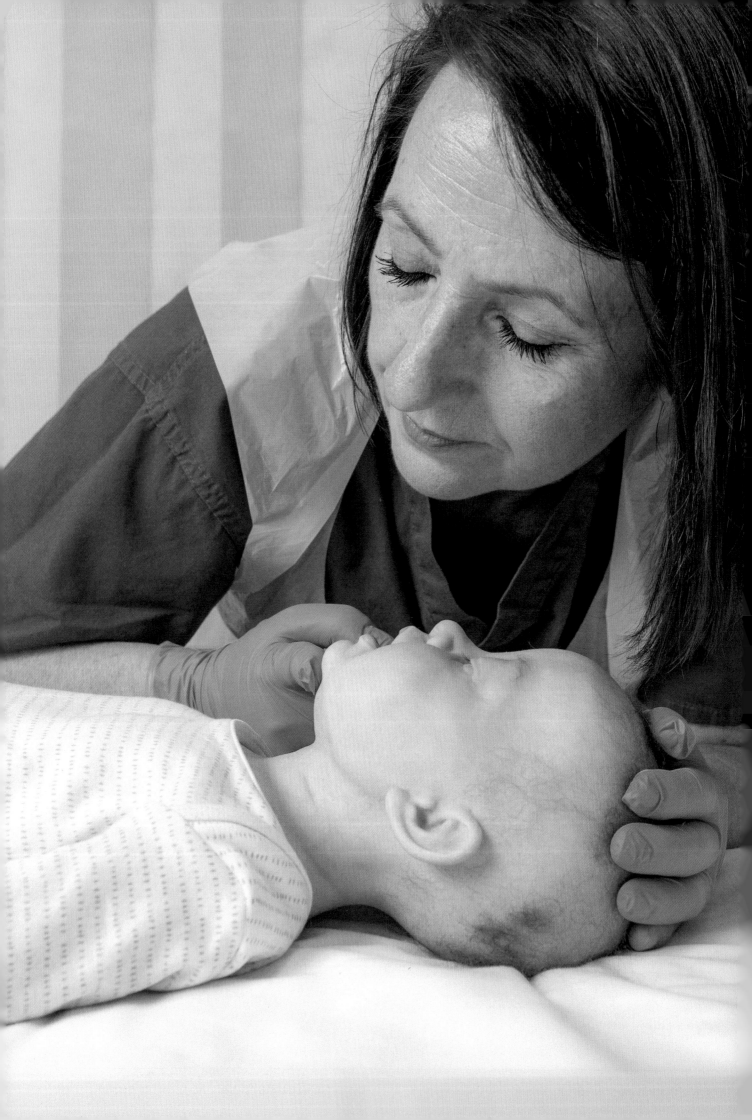

Recognition and initial management of the seriously ill child

02

In this chapter

Signs and symptoms of respiratory, circulatory and cardiorespiratory failure

Parameters assessed during the ABCDE approach

The ABCDE approach to the initial management of airway, breathing and circulation

The learning outcomes will enable you to:

Understand the importance of early recognition of the seriously ill child

Describe the importance of the structured ABCDE approach to rapidly identify potential respiratory, circulatory and/or central neurological failure in the seriously ill child

Consider the importance of the structured ABCDE approach to prioritise and assess the effectiveness of initial management strategies

Early recognition of the seriously ill child

In children, a cardiorespiratory arrest is usually due to hypoxia, reflecting the end of the body's ability to compensate for the effects of underlying illness or injury. The initial problem may originate from the airway, breathing or circulation. Irrespective of the primary aetiology, cardiorespiratory arrest in children is rarely a sudden event but a progressive deterioration from combined respiratory and circulatory failure. Early recognition and effective management of respiratory and/or circulatory failure will prevent the majority of paediatric cardiorespiratory arrests and thus reduce morbidity and mortality. It can also help identify children for whom attempted cardiopulmonary resuscitation may be inappropriate, helping facilitate suitable end-of-life care.

The principles outlined in this chapter apply to the seriously ill child in all environments (i.e. the acute hospital setting or out-of-hospital). For some clinical settings, it is less common to see a critically ill child, and those responsible for the initial management might have limited experience. For all healthcare workers looking after the critically ill child, using the structured ABCDE approach helps to ensure that potentially life-threatening problems are identified and managed in order of their priority.

Using the structured ABCDE approach helps to ensure that potentially life-threatening problems are identified and managed in order of their priority

The A B C D E approach: general principles

1. Ensure personal safety and appropriate level of personal protective equipment.

2. Observe the child to determine the overall level of illness (i.e. do they look seriously unwell, are they interacting with parents/care providers). Speak to the child and assess the appropriateness of their response; ask the parents about the child's 'usual' behaviour and any concerns they have.

3. If they are unresponsive to your voice, administer tactile stimulation. If they respond by speaking or crying, this indicates they have a patent airway, are breathing and have cerebral perfusion. Appropriate high-flow oxygen delivery should be commenced immediately.

4. Vital sign monitoring should be requested early (ECG, SpO_2 and non-invasive BP monitoring).

5. Circulatory access should be achieved as soon as possible. Blood test investigations and a bedside glucose estimation should be obtained.

6. Communicate findings of the A–E assessment to your team and to other clinical and medical professionals called to help with the management of the patient. Outside of the intensive care unit, many hospitals employ an early warning score (EWS) system to aid in the detection of deteriorating children; this information should also be highlighted (see Chapter 8). Structured communication tools such as SBAR (see Chapter 15) will aid the handover of important clinical information between teams.

7. Document your assessment and interventions as soon as possible.

A Airway problems

A review of practical airway management procedures is provided in Chapter 3.

Causes of upper airway obstruction

Airway obstruction can be partial or complete, sudden or insidious, progressive or recurrent. Respiratory rate and work of breathing generally increase in airway obstruction. When assessing airway patency, chest movement does not guarantee that the airway is clear. Air entry needs to be assessed by looking, listening and feeling for air movement and by chest auscultation.

Initially, airway obstruction is often partial but can lead to respiratory failure, exhaustion, secondary apnoea and eventually hypoxic brain damage. Additionally, partial airway obstruction can rapidly become total and result in cardiorespiratory arrest.

Congenital abnormalities such as choanal atresia or Pierre-Robin syndrome can be initially managed using an appropriate airway adjunct to open the airway and buy time before definitive treatment.

Depression of the central nervous system can cause loss of airway control as protective upper airway reflexes and muscle tone are lost. This may be compounded in the infant due to the age-related anatomical features. In an unconscious infant, the pronounced occiput and short neck causes head flexion in the supine position and, together with the proportionately large tongue, this can quickly lead to airway obstruction.

Causes of central nervous system depression include hypoxia following decompensated respiratory or circulatory failure, head trauma, metabolic disorders (e.g. hypoglycaemia, inborn errors of metabolism), hypercapnia, alcohol and medications (e.g. opiates, benzodiazepines).

Airway obstruction due to these causes may not be accompanied by tachypnoea or increased work of breathing.

Recognition of upper airway obstruction

Airway obstruction may be demonstrated by difficulty in breathing and/or increased respiratory effort. In a conscious child, there may be visible distress. There may be additional respiratory noises, such as inspiratory stridor if the obstruction is partial. Causes are seen in Table 2.1.

Management of upper airway obstruction

The treatment of partial airway obstruction is to maintain airway patency and ensure that it does not become completely occluded. This may be achieved by head positioning, clearance of any secretions or foreign bodies, and summoning further assistance as indicated.

In patients with airway obstruction, delivery of supplemental oxygen is advised as early as possible to minimise the potential effects of hypoxia.

The conscious child will usually adopt a position that optimises airway patency. If the child is stable and deterioration is considered unlikely, they should be left with their parents/carers who can help administer oxygen and minimise stress and anxiety. Feeding should be avoided, and any fever treated to reduce increased metabolic demand. **If there is a decreased level of consciousness, airway compromise must be assumed.** The management priorities are to get more help whilst safeguarding the airway and preventing complications such as aspiration of gastric contents by placing the child in the recovery position or supporting the head-up position.

Basic airway opening manoeuvres (e.g. head tilt and chin lift or jaw thrust) should be used. Adjuncts such as oro/nasopharyngeal airways can also be used until more experienced help is available. Advanced emergency airway management may involve the insertion of a tracheal tube (TT), supraglottic airway (e.g. i-gel, laryngeal mask airway (LMA)) or cricothyroidotomy, although the latter will only provide temporary oxygenation until a definitive airway can be achieved.

Table 2.1   Causes of airway obstruction

Causes of airway obstruction
Congenital abnormality (e.g. choanal atresia, Pierre-Robin syndrome)
Secretions (e.g. vomit, blood)
Respiratory tract infections (swelling or mucus secretions)
Pharyngeal swelling (e.g. oedema, infection)
Epiglottitis
Laryngotracheobronchitis (croup)
Nasal feeding tubes
Oxygen delivery devices (e.g. nasal cannulae)
Foreign body (e.g. food, toy, orthodontic appliances)
Central nervous system depression (loss of muscle tone)
Trauma (facial or throat)

B Breathing problems

In all seriously ill or injured children, the priority is for the appropriate management of the airway and ventilation (breathing).

Causes of breathing (respiratory) problems

Respiratory failure can result from acute or chronic breathing inadequacy; where the movement of air into and out of the lungs (ventilation) and/or gas exchange at the alveolar-capillary interface is compromised. The underlying problem may be due to lung pathology (i.e. congenital or acquired diseases or trauma) or have a non-respiratory origin (e.g. circulatory failure, metabolic disorder, neurological problem).

Failure of ventilation results in CO_2 accumulation and reduced oxygen levels. Reduced gas exchange across the alveolar-capillary interface is often a result of fluid accumulation within the alveoli (pulmonary oedema or infection) and results in a fall in arterial O_2 levels and increased lung stiffness (i.e. decreased lung compliance). Other common causes of gas exchange failure include bronchospasm and atelectasis, which are also associated with stiff lungs. The arterial O_2 levels fall, which stimulate breathing via peripheral chemoreceptors (the aortic and carotid bodies).

Arterial CO_2 levels may initially be normal or even low due to an increased respiratory rate, although they will rise, stimulating the respiratory centre to increase the respiratory rate further as failure worsens. The work of breathing then increases not only due to the increased respiratory rate but also due to the increased lung stiffness.

Increased arterial CO_2 levels may also result in tachycardia, vasodilatation and bounding pulses, but these are unreliable findings.

The respiratory rate can be classified as abnormal if it is too rapid (tachypnoea), too slow (bradypnoea), or absent (apnoea). Respiratory distress is a clinical syndrome, which reflects increased work of breathing, often associated with attempts to increase tidal volume and can be associated with either tachypnoea or bradypnoea.

As the work of breathing increases, an increased proportion of the cardiac output is diverted to the respiratory muscles with a consequent increase in the amount of CO_2 produced.

Ultimately, if decompensation occurs, the respiratory system is unable to provide sufficient oxygen for tissue requirements, anaerobic metabolism occurs, and respiratory acidosis is complicated by metabolic acidosis.

Recognition of respiratory failure

From a physiological viewpoint, respiratory failure is usually defined as the failure of the respiratory system to maintain an arterial oxygen level (PaO_2) > 9 kPa with 21% inspired O_2 (room air) and/or arterial carbon dioxide level of ($PaCO_2$) < 6.5 kPa. This definition requires arterial blood gas analysis.

PaO_2 of 9 kPa corresponds approximately to a peripheral oxygen saturation (SpO_2) of approximately 90%.

A child with respiratory distress may be able to maintain their arterial blood gas values within relatively normal limits by increasing their respiratory effort. Therefore, it is important to evaluate whether the child's situation is stable or if decompensation to respiratory failure is imminent. This evaluation requires knowledge of the signs and symptoms of respiratory distress and/or respiratory failure. When the compensatory mechanisms fail, deterioration is rapid and imminent cardiorespiratory arrest must be anticipated.

Warning signs are:

- decreased level of consciousness
- hypotonia (floppiness)
- decreased respiratory effort
- cyanosis or extreme pallor (despite oxygen being given)
- sweating
- bradycardia.

In children, recognition of respiratory failure is based on the full assessment of respiratory effort and efficacy, and the identification of evidence of respiratory inadequacy on major organs.

Work of breathing

Evidence of increased work of breathing is based on observation of the following:

- increased respiratory rate
- intercostal recession
- sternal recession
- subcostal recession
- use of accessory muscles (e.g. head bobbing)
- nasal flaring.

Respiratory rate

Tachypnoea is frequently the first indication of respiratory insufficiency. Normal respiratory rates vary with age, and this must be considered when determining the presence of tachypnoea (Table 2.2). When referring to any chart with paediatric 'normal physiological values', be aware that none of these values taken in isolation have sufficient test performance and should always be considered in relation to other signs and symptoms.

Trends are more informative than single readings.

Changes in the respiratory rate over time are very important. An increasing respiratory rate represents increasing physiological compensation to offset the deterioration in respiratory function. A sudden reduction in the respiratory rate in an acutely ill child is an ominous sign and maybe a pre-terminal event. Causes may include exhaustion, central nervous system depression or hypothermia. Fatigue is always an important consideration in children; an infant with a respiratory rate of 80 min^{-1} will tire quickly.

Table 2.2 Respiratory rate ranges by age

Age (years)	Respiratory rate (breaths min^{-1})
< 1	30–40 min^{-1}
1–2	26–34 min^{-1}
2–5	24–30 min^{-1}
5–12	20–24 min^{-1}
> 12	12–20 min^{-1}

Recession

Recession (or retractions) may be sternal, subcostal or intercostal. The degree of recession gives an indication of the severity of respiratory disorder. Infants and young children can exhibit significant recession with relatively mild to moderate respiratory compromise, owing to their highly compliant chest wall. However, in children over approximately five years (by which age the chest wall is less compliant), recession is a sign of significant respiratory compromise.

Use of accessory muscles

When the work of breathing is increased, the sternocleidomastoid muscles in the neck are often used as accessory respiratory muscles. In infants, this may cause the head to bob up and down with each breath. This 'head bobbing' actually reduces the efficiency of each breath.

'See-saw' respiration

A breathing pattern, described as 'see-saw' respiration, is sometimes observed in severe respiratory compromise. It is the paradoxical movement of the abdomen during inspiration (i.e. the abdomen expands and the thorax retracts as the diaphragm contracts). This is inefficient respiration because the tidal volume is reduced, despite the increased muscular effort.

Inspiratory and expiratory noises

Normally, the airway above the thoracic inlet (extrathoracic) narrows and the airway below (intrathoracic) widens during the inspiratory phase of breathing. This pattern reverses on expiration. Observing the timing of an abnormal noise can indicate the site of airway obstruction. The presence of a high-pitched inspiratory noise (stridor) is characteristic of an upper airway (extrathoracic) obstruction and is due to rapid, turbulent flow through a narrowed portion of the upper tracheal airway. In severe obstruction, the stridor may also occur on expiration (biphasic stridor) but is usually less pronounced than it is during inspiration.

Wheezing is generally an expiratory noise. It is indicative of lower (intrathoracic) airway narrowing, usually at bronchiolar level, and maybe audible with the ear, or only on chest auscultation with a stethoscope.

The volume of airway noises is not indicative of the severity of respiratory compromise; diminishing noises may be indicative of increasing airway obstruction or exhaustion of the child.

Grunting

Grunting is mainly heard in neonates and small infants but can also occur in young children. It is the result of exhaling against a partially closed glottis and is an attempt to generate a positive end-expiratory pressure, thus preventing airway collapse at the end of expiration. Grunting is generally associated with 'stiff' lungs (e.g. respiratory distress syndrome, pulmonary oedema, atelectasis). Regardless of the underlying condition, grunting is an indication of severe respiratory compromise.

Nostril flaring

Flaring of the nostrils is often seen in infants and young children with increased respiratory effort.

Position

Children in respiratory distress will usually adopt a position to maximise their respiratory capacity. In upper airway obstruction, they often adopt a 'sniffing the morning air' position to optimise their upper airway patency. In generalised or lower respiratory problems, children often sit forward, supporting their weight on their arms, and holding on to (or wrapping their arms around) their knees. This position results in a degree of shoulder girdle 'splinting', which enhances accessory muscle use. The child should be supported in a position of optimal airway maximisation/comfort for them and have oxygen therapy given accordingly.

The degree of respiratory distress generally provides clinical evidence of the severity of respiratory insufficiency. However, there are three general exceptions to this.

Table 2.3   Exceptions to increased work of breathing in respiratory failure

1. Exhaustion
Children who have had severe respiratory compromise for some time may have progressed to decompensation and no longer show signs of increased work of breathing. **Exhaustion is a pre-terminal event.**
2. Neuromuscular diseases
e.g. muscular dystrophy
3. Central respiratory depression
Reduced respiratory drive results in respiratory inadequacy (e.g. encephalopathy, medications such as morphine).

Efficacy of breathing

The infant's relatively higher metabolic rate and oxygen consumption accounts for their increased respiratory rates (Table 2.2). Thus, the effectiveness of breathing can be assessed by respiratory rate together with tidal volume, which in turn is evaluated by observation of chest movement, quality of crying, palpation, auscultation and percussion.

Additional information can be easily obtained by non-invasive pulse oximetry.

Chest movement, palpation and percussion

Observation of chest movement demonstrates the extent and symmetry of chest expansion. As well as revealing increased work of breathing, observing the movement of the chest wall can help identify diminished or asymmetrical respiratory effort.

Palpation of the chest wall may identify deformities, surgical emphysema or crepitus.

Percussion of the chest wall can demonstrate areas of collapse (dullness) or hyperresonance (e.g. in pneumothorax).

Chest auscultation

When listening with a stethoscope, air entry should be heard in all areas of the lungs. The volume of air movement occurring with inspiration and expiration can be estimated by auscultation. It is useful to compare the areas on one side of the chest with the other.

A very quiet or near-silent chest indicates a dangerously reduced tidal volume and is an ominous sign.

Pulse oximetry

A pulse oximeter should be used on any child with potential respiratory failure to provide an assessment of the patient's arterial oxygen saturation.

Without pulse oximetry, it is not always clinically possible to detect that the child has a decreased arterial oxygen saturation of haemoglobin (SaO_2) until the saturation is between 80–85%. Pulse oximetry is simple to use, relatively cheap, non-invasive and provides an immediate, objective measure of arterial blood oxygen saturation.

Start oxygen therapy if SpO_2 <94% (or for infants or children with chronic conditions at a SpO_2 3% below known baseline). The goal is to keep SpO_2 between 94–98% with as little supplemental oxygen as possible. When giving supplemental oxygen, sustained SpO_2 readings of 100% should generally be avoided (except in specific circumstances such as carbon monoxide poisoning). Do not give pre-emptive oxygen therapy to children and infants without signs of, or immediate risk of hypoxaemia or shock.

Pulse oximeter readings must not be used in isolation; it is vital to interpret them in light of the clinical picture, alongside other investigations and potential sources of error. Pulse oximetry only provides a measure of oxygen saturation, not content, and gives no reliable indication of actual tissue oxygenation. Furthermore, it provides no information on the adequacy of ventilation. A patient, particularly if on oxygen therapy, may be breathing inadequately and have a high carbon dioxide level despite a normal oxygen saturation. Arterial blood gases are needed in critically ill patients to assess oxygenation and ventilation.

Pulse oximetry has four main uses:
- detection of/screening for hypoxaemia
- targeting oxygen therapy
- routine monitoring during anaesthesia
- diagnostic (e.g. sleep apnoea).

There are several acknowledged sources of error with pulse oximetry:
- presence of other haemoglobins: carboxyhaemoglobin (carbon monoxide poisoning) and methaemoglobin (congenital or acquired)
- surgical and imaging dyes: methylene blue, indocyanine green and indigo carmine cause falsely low saturation readings
- nail varnish (especially blue, black and green)
- high-ambient light levels (fluorescent and xenon lamps)
- motion artefact

- reduced pulse volume:
  - hypotension
  - low cardiac output
  - vasoconstriction
  - hypothermia.

Pulse oximeters are not affected by:
- anaemia (reduced haemoglobin concentration)
- jaundice (hyperbilirubinaemia).

Skin pigmentation:
- darker skin may lead to an overestimation of the oxygen saturation value, so consider relative changes in an individual patient's readings as well as the numerical result.

Pulse oximetry does not provide a reliable signal during CPR.

Central cyanosis

Central cyanosis appears when the SpO_2 is < 80% (it indicates that desaturated haemoglobin is > 5 g dL^{-1}). The absence of cyanosis, particularly in anaemic patients, does not imply that the blood oxygen levels are normal.

Cyanosis is an inconsistent sign of respiratory failure. It is most apparent on the mucosae of the mouth and in the nail beds. Cyanosis limited to the extremities is usually due to circulatory failure (peripheral cyanosis) rather than respiratory failure (central cyanosis). Hypoxia may also cause vasoconstriction and skin pallor, which will mask cyanosis. However, in a child with acute respiratory compromise, the development of central cyanosis is a late indication of severe hypoxia and is a pre-terminal sign.

Effects of respiratory inadequacy on other body organs

Ongoing respiratory compromise rapidly affects other body organs/systems.

Heart rate

Hypoxia initially causes tachycardia. As this is a non-specific sign, it needs to be considered alongside other clinical signs. Severe or prolonged hypoxia ultimately leads to bradycardia, and therefore it is important to observe for trends rather than absolute values in heart rate. In a severely hypoxic child, bradycardia is a pre-terminal sign.

Skin perfusion

Hypoxia produces vasoconstriction and pallor of the skin. As their clinical condition deteriorates, the child's colour may become mottled before cyanosis appears centrally (lips and mouth).

Conscious level

Hypoxia and/or hypercapnia initially lead to agitation and/or drowsiness. Ongoing cerebral hypoxia ultimately results in loss of consciousness. In infants and young children, initial cerebral hypoxia may be difficult to detect, but their parents/carers frequently report that the baby/child is not responding to them as usual. This information is important and should not be ignored. The level of consciousness should be assessed using the AVPU score (Table 2.4).

Generalised hypotonia also accompanies cerebral hypoxia.

Table 2.4   The level of consciousness

A	Alert
V	responds to **V**oice
P	responds to **P**ain
U	**U**nresponsive to painful stimuli

The management of respiratory compromise

The initial treatment of breathing problems is dependent on achieving and maintaining a patent airway and effective delivery of oxygen. The method of oxygen administration will vary according to the child's clinical condition and age. Children who have adequate breathing should have high-flow oxygen delivered in a non-threatening manner and delivered in a way which is best tolerated by them (e.g. from a free-flow device held by their parents, a non-rebreathing face mask or nasal cannulae). When agitated, the child's airflow will become turbulent and resistance to flow will increase.

When breathing is inadequate (or absent), high-flow oxygen should be delivered by ventilation with a bag and mask system. In situations where the child is exhausted and is likely to need ongoing respiratory support, tracheal intubation may be indicated.

Targeted oxygen therapy

In critically ill patients, those presenting with acute hypoxaemia or in the peri-arrest situation give high-concentration oxygen immediately. Give this initially with an oxygen mask with reservoir bag (non-rebreathing mask) using an oxygen flow of 12–15 L min^{-1}. During cardiorespiratory arrest, use 100% oxygen to maximise arterial oxygen content and delivery to the tissues.

When the oxygen saturation can be monitored reliably, adjust the inspired oxygen concentration to maintain a SpO$_2$ of 94–98%. If pulse oximetry (with a reliable reading) is unavailable, continue to give oxygen with a non-rebreathing face mask with reservoir until definitive monitoring or assessment of oxygenation is available.

Evidence suggests hyperoxaemia and, particularly in newborns, hyperoxaemia (PaO$_2$ > 20 kPa) in the post-resuscitation phase may lead to worse outcomes than those in whom normoxaemia is maintained.

C Circulatory problems

The appropriate management of the airway and ventilation (breathing) is the priority in all seriously ill children and should be addressed before considering their circulatory status.

Circulatory failure and shock

Shock is a clinical state where the delivery of oxygenated blood and associated nutrients (e.g. glucose) to the body tissues is inadequate for metabolic demand. Additionally, the removal of cellular waste (e.g. CO$_2$, lactic acid) may also be impaired.

> Circulatory failure refers to insufficient blood being delivered to the body's tissues.

Shock may occur with increased, normal or decreased cardiac output (CO) or blood pressure (BP). Initially, the child's body can physiologically compensate for reduced tissue perfusion. However, when blood pressure starts to fall, as seen in circulatory failure, perfusion of the vital organs (e.g. brain, myocardium, kidneys) becomes increasingly compromised. Inadequate tissue blood flow results in tissue hypoxia and anaerobic metabolism with lactic acid accumulation. The resultant cell damage may be irreversible. Therefore, it is essential to promptly recognise and treat any child with compensated circulatory failure to prevent deterioration to a decompensated state.

Compensated circulatory failure may present with a normal blood pressure, but signs of abnormal perfusion will be present: tachycardia, poor skin perfusion (prolonged capillary refill time), weak peripheral pulse, tachypnoea and reduced urine output.

Decompensated circulatory failure is present when hypotension develops, and vital organ perfusion is compromised. The clinical signs of inadequate tissue perfusion are much more apparent.

Aetiology of shock

Shock can arise from circulatory or respiratory failure. Most children with sustained shock, whatever its aetiology, have some degree of cardiovascular dysfunction requiring more than one type of treatment (i.e. managing the airway, breathing and circulation).

Although CO is usually decreased in circulatory failure, it may also be increased (e.g. septic, anaphylactic shock) In this case, the systemic vascular resistance (SVR) is low, and although the child appears to be well perfused (so-called 'warm shock') with bounding peripheral pulses and increased pulse pressure (the difference between the systolic and diastolic BP), the metabolic requirements of the tissues are not being met due to a mismatch between blood flow and metabolic demand.

The most common causes of circulatory failure in children are hypovolaemia, sepsis or anaphylaxis.

There are 5 main categories of shock

- **Hypovolaemic shock:** characterised by a decreased circulating volume (preload). It may result from severe fluid loss (as in dehydration) or haemorrhage.
- **Distributive shock:** typified by an inadequate distribution of blood, so that the blood flow is insufficient for the metabolic demand of the tissues (e.g. anaphylaxis, sepsis or neurogenic).
- **Cardiogenic shock:** circulatory failure is less commonly the result of a primary cardiac problem due to congenital or acquired heart disease (e.g. cardiomyopathy, myocarditis or following cardiac surgery).
- **Obstructive shock:** an uncommon cause of circulatory failure due to obstruction of blood flow to/from the heart (e.g. tension pneumothorax, cardiac tamponade or constrictive pericarditis).
- **Dissociative shock:** characterised by insufficient oxygen-carrying capacity of the blood (e.g. anaemia or carbon monoxide poisoning).

Evaluation of the circulatory system

Oxygen delivery to the tissues is dependent on the arterial oxygen content and the CO. CO is the product of the blood volume ejected from the left ventricle with each contraction and the heart rate.

Cardiac output
CO = HR x SV

CO = cardiac output

HR = Heart rate

SV (stroke volume) = blood volume ejected with each contraction

Blood pressure
BP = CO x SVR

BP = blood pressure

SVR = systemic vascular resistance

Of the variables affecting or affected by CO (Figure 2.1), some can be easily measured (HR and BP), and others (SV and SVR) must be indirectly assessed by examining the amplitude and quality of pulses and the adequacy of end-organ perfusion (mental status, capillary refill time, skin temperature and, when available, urine output).

A low SVR or CO should be suspected if the systolic BP is below the normal range for the child's age.

Recognition of circulatory failure

In children, the recognition of circulatory failure is based on a complete cardiovascular assessment, looking for the effects of any circulatory insufficiency on major organs.

Parameters evaluated include:
- heart rate
- pulse volume
- capillary refill time
- blood pressure
- filling pressure (liver size in infants or jugular vein filling in older children)
- end-organ perfusion status.

Heart rate

The heart rate initially rises to maintain cardiac output.

Sinus tachycardia is a common response to many situations (e.g. pain, anxiety, fever), but it is also seen in hypoxia, hypercapnia and hypovolaemia. When tachycardia is accompanied by other signs of circulatory insufficiency, it is evidence of the body's attempts at physiological compensation. Neonates have a limited cardiac reserve; they increase their CO primarily by increasing their heart rate rather than stroke volume (SV). They develop tachycardia as the first response to hypoxia. When the increased heart rate cannot maintain adequate tissue perfusion, the subsequent tissue hypoxia and acidosis result in bradycardia. The presence of bradycardia is a pre-terminal sign, indicating that cardiorespiratory arrest is imminent.

Pulse volume

Feeling for the volume (or amplitude) of central pulses (e.g. femoral, carotid, brachial) gives a subjective indication of SV; as SV decreases, so does the pulse amplitude. In progressive circulatory failure, the pulse amplitude diminishes, becomes weak and thready before finally, it is impalpable. Simultaneous palpation and comparison of central and peripheral pulses (e.g. radial and carotid) may be useful. Peripheral pulses decrease in amplitude earlier than central ones. Note that caution is required in their interpretation when vasoconstriction is present (e.g. ambient temperature is low, or in an anxious or pyrexial child).

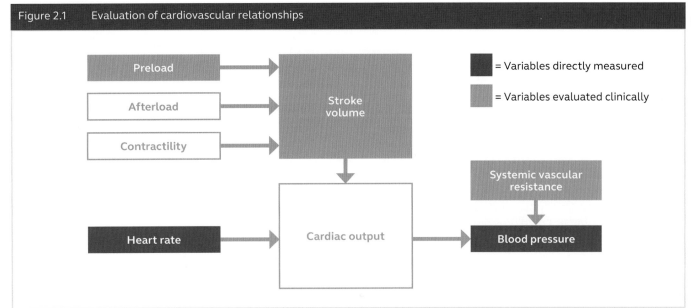

Figure 2.1   Evaluation of cardiovascular relationships

The presence or absence of peripheral pulses is neither a specific nor a sensitive indicator of circulatory compromise but is useful in conjunction with other clinical signs.

However, diminishing central pulses are a pre-terminal sign, indicating that cardiorespiratory arrest is imminent.

Capillary refill and skin colour

The skin of a healthy child is warm to touch unless the ambient temperature is low. Their capillary refill time (CRT) is normally < 2 s, but when there is decreased skin perfusion, the CRT is prolonged. Be aware that CRT, although simple and quick to assess, is not very sensitive, and like all observations, must not be assessed as a stand-alone observation.

Evaluation of CRT is best performed by applying cutaneous pressure on the centre of the sternum for 5 s. Following removal of the pressure, the blanching of the skin should disappear within 2 s. A slower refill time (i.e. prolonged CRT) is indicative of poor skin perfusion. A pyrexial child with hypovolaemia will have a prolonged CRT, despite having a raised body temperature. A low ambient temperature or poor local lighting conditions reduces the accuracy of CRT. The CRT should be considered in the context of the accompanying cardiovascular signs.

Initially, hypoxia produces vasoconstriction, and hence the child appears pale. As their clinical condition deteriorates, the child's colour becomes mottled and ultimately cyanosed. Cyanosis due to circulatory failure is initially peripheral, whereas hypoxaemia due to respiratory failure results in central cyanosis.

Peripheral vasoconstriction and decreased perfusion may also be indicated by a demarcation line between warm and cold skin. This can be detected by running the back of your hand up the child's limb. The demarcation line will travel towards the trunk over time if the child's condition is deteriorating, and vice versa if it is improving.

Blood pressure

In most forms of shock, the BP is initially maintained within the normal range (Table 2.5) for the child as a result of the body's compensatory mechanisms (e.g. tachycardia, vasoconstriction, increased myocardial contractility). Only when compensation is no longer possible does hypotension (BP less than 5th centile for age) occur, and a decompensated state results.

In hypovolaemia, approximately 40% of the child's total circulating volume can be lost before hypotension occurs. This means that BP only drops at a late stage in hypovolaemia (e.g. trauma, diarrhoeal illness, gut necrosis). Therefore, it is important that compensated circulatory failure is detected and managed at an early stage (i.e. before BP drops and decompensation occurs).

Table 2.5 shows the 5th and 50th centiles for systolic and mean BP for children. In full-term neonates, the lower limit for systolic BP (5th centile) is 50 mmHg. For infants from 1–12 months, it is 70 mmHg.

Table 2.5   Blood pressure ranges by age systolic and mean

Blood pressure for age	1 month	1 year	5 years	10 years	15 years
50th centile for Systolic BP	75 mmHg	95 mmHg	100 mmHg	110 mmHg	120 mmHg
5th centile for Systolic BP	50 mmHg	70 mmHg	75 mmHg	80 mmHg	90 mmHg
50th centile for mean arterial pressure (MAP)	55 mmHg	70 mmHg	75 mmHg	75 mmHg	80 mmHg
5th centile for mean arterial blood pressure (MAP)	40 mmHg	50 mmHg	55 mmHg	55 mmHg	65 mmHg

Regardless of the method used to obtain the BP (auscultatory or oscillometric), it is important that the appropriate cuff size is used. The cuff width should be > 80% of the child's upper arm length, and the bladder should cover more than 40% of the circumference of their arm. The same size cuff should be used on each occasion that the BP is measured.

Hypotension is a sign of physiological decompensation and indicates imminent cardiorespiratory arrest.

Filling pressure (preload)

If the heart is unable to effectively pump the blood returned to it, either because there is fluid overload or because the heart is failing, the pressure in the veins supplying the heart is raised. This is manifested by crackles at the lung bases, distention of the jugular veins in older children or enlargement of the liver in infants. Observation of these signs forms part of the reassessment following a fluid bolus.

Effects of circulatory inadequacy on other body organs

Ongoing circulatory compromise rapidly affects other body organs/systems:

Respiratory system

The metabolic acidosis that results from circulatory compromise leads to tachypnoea. However, there will not initially be other signs of increased work of breathing.

Conscious level

Hypoxia and/or hypercapnia initially lead to agitation and/or drowsiness. Progressive cerebral hypoxia ultimately results in loss of consciousness.

In infants and young children, initial cerebral hypoxia may be difficult to detect, but their parents/carers frequently report that the baby/child is not responding to them as usual and, as in respiratory failure, this information should not be ignored. The level of consciousness should be assessed using the AVPU score.

Generalised hypotonia also accompanies cerebral hypoxia.

Urine output

Information regarding the degree of reduced renal perfusion can be obtained by measuring the output of urine. A urinary output of < 2 mL kg^{-1} h^{-1} in infants or < 1 mL kg^{-1} h^{-1} in children older than one year is an indication of inadequate renal perfusion. Asking parents/carers about the child's urine output (e.g. the number of wet nappies; normal would be at least six wet nappies per day) may reveal a history of oliguria or anuria.

Management of circulatory compromise

The treatment of circulatory problems is dependent on achieving a patent airway and effectively managing ventilation with appropriate delivery of high-flow oxygen before turning attention to circulatory procedures.

Of course when there are immediately life-threatening causes of circulatory failure, such as massive or continuing haemorrhage, these must be managed simultaneously to managing A and B.

Insertion of at least one large-bore vascular cannula should be performed rapidly. This can be achieved by either intravenous or intraosseous routes.

In children with recognised shock, give volume replacement with bolus therapy 10 mL kg^{-1} of balanced isotonic crystalloid solution (e.g. Plasma-Lyte or Ringer's Lactate or 0.9% sodium chloride). Glucose containing fluids with low sodium levels should NEVER be used for resuscitation, only to correct low blood glucose levels.

The use of vasoactive medications may be needed in fluid resistant shock (circulatory access procedures, fluids and medications are in Chapter 5).

Cardiorespiratory failure

Signs of cardiorespiratory failure include alteration of consciousness, hypotonia, tachycardia, decreased central pulses and absent peripheral pulses. Bradycardia, hypotension, bradypnoea, gasping and apnoea are terminal events preceding imminent cardiorespiratory arrest.

If any of the following signs are present, immediate intervention should be undertaken:

- coma or alteration of consciousness
- exhaustion
- cyanosis
- tachypnoea (RR > 60 min^{-1})
- HR < 100 min^{-1} for newborn
- HR > 180 min^{-1} or < 80 min^{-1} before one year (note: chest compressions in all ages should be started if HR < 60 min^{-1} with signs of inadequate perfusion)
- HR > 160 min^{-1} after one year
- seizures.

A rapid assessment must be made of every child whom respiratory, circulatory or cardiorespiratory failure is expected.

D Disability – central neurological assessment

Following the appropriate management of the child's airway, ventilation and circulation, their neurological status should be evaluated.

Whilst both respiratory and circulatory failure can have central neurological effects, some neurological conditions may affect the respiratory and circulatory systems.

Table 2.6   Causes of altered conscious level

Cause
Respiratory failure
Circulatory failure
Neurological disorders (e.g. status epilepticus, meningitis, encephalitis)
Hypoglycaemia
Head injury
Raised intracranial pressure
Drugs (e.g. opiates, alcohol)
Metabolic disorders

Neurological function

Conscious level

A rapid assessment of the child's conscious level can be determined by the AVPU score.

If required, a painful stimulus should be delivered either by applying pressure to the supraorbital ridge or rubbing the sternum. A child who is only responsive to painful (P) stimuli has a significant degree of neurological derangement equivalent to a Glasgow Coma Scale score of approximately 8.

Pupils

The size and reactivity of pupils can be affected by a number of things, including medications, intracranial pressure and cerebral lesions. Important signs to look for are dilatation, inequality and non-reactivity of the child's pupils. These features potentially indicate serious brain dysfunction.

Posture

Seriously ill children become hypotonic and floppy. However, if there is serious brain dysfunction, stiff posturing may be demonstrated. This posturing (which may only be evident when a painful stimulus is applied) can be decorticate (flexed arms and extended legs) or decerebrate (extended arms and legs); both indicate serious brain dysfunction and maybe signs of raised intracranial pressure.

Blood glucose

Point of care blood sugar estimation should be performed in all seriously ill children. The increased metabolic rate associated with acute illness leads to increased use of glucose. Infants and small children do not have large glycogen liver stores, which can be broken down to generate more glucose. Therefore, they may become hypoglycaemic with any acute illness, particularly when oral intake is reduced.

Effects on other systems of central neurological failure

Central neurological dysfunction may affect other body systems.

Respiratory system

Comatose children with brain dysfunction may exhibit abnormal respiratory patterns (e.g. hyperventilation, Cheyne-Stoke respiratory pattern (alternate periods of hyperventilation and apnoea) or complete apnoea).

Circulatory system

Raised intracranial pressure causes the Cushing's triad (i.e. abnormal breathing pattern with bradycardia and hypertension). This is a late and pre-terminal sign of neurological failure.

Management of neurological compromise

The initial steps in managing any child with a reduced conscious level must always be to maintain an open airway, ensure adequate ventilation and oxygenation, and support circulation to maintain cerebral oxygenation and perfusion.

Other causes of neurological compromise must then be considered, and specific investigations and treatments given as indicated (e.g. glucose for hypoglycaemia, CT scanning if head injury or cerebral infections are suspected).

E Exposure

To ensure that no additional significant clinical information (e.g. rashes) is missed, examine the child fully by exposing their body. Appropriate measures to minimise heat loss (especially in infants) and respect dignity must be adopted at all times.

The ABCDE approach should be employed when assessing any critically unwell child and there will be some additional factors to assess when dealing with some paediatric emergencies and trauma (Chapter 10–11); however, the underlying principles remain the same.

Specific assessments and actions in initial ABCDE approach

Assessment		Information sought	Possible resultant actions
On approaching the child		Note: • General appearance (colour, posture, activity) • Interaction with parent/caregiver	
A	Airway patency	Is the airway: • Patent (i.e. conscious, vocalising) • At risk • Obstructed	Suction if indicated Head positioning Oropharyngeal airway Reassess Summon expert help
B	Breathing adequacy	Note/observe/perform: • Conscious level • Air movement (look, listen, feel) • Respiratory rate • Chest expansion • Use of accessory muscles/recessions • Palpation • Percussion • Auscultation • SpO_2 and FiO_2	Administer high-flow oxygen appropriately Support breathing with bag-mask ventilation (BMV) as necessary Reassess Summon expert help
C	Circulation adequacy	Note/observe/perform: • Evidence of haemorrhage/fluid loss • Conscious level • Heart rate • Capillary refill time • Presence of distal/central pulses • Pulse volume features • Skin temperature and colour • Blood pressure • Urine output	Control any external bleeding Attach monitoring (as appropriate to setting) Obtain circulatory access (IV or IO) Estimate weight Blood samples for laboratory testing and bedside glucose estimation Fluid bolus (10 mL kg^{-1}) Reassess Summon expert help
D	Disability (conscious level)	Note: • AVPU score • Interaction with parent and surroundings • Posture and muscle tone • Pupil size and reactivity	Reconsider A, B and C management as conscious level dictates Establish bedside glucose estimation Establish if any medications have been given/possibly ingested Reassess Summon expert help
E	Exposure	Note/observe: • Evidence of any blood loss/skin lesions/wounds/drains/rashes etc. • Core temperature	Reconsider specific management e.g. antibiotics in sepsis Consider appropriate temperature control measures Reassess Summon expert help

02: **Summary learning**

Early recognition of the seriously ill child prevents the majority of cardiorespiratory arrests, thus reducing morbidity and mortality.

The structured ABCDE approach helps ensure that potentially life-threatening problems are identified and dealt with in order of priority.

My key take-home messages from this chapter are:

Further reading

Fleming S, Thompson M, Stevens R, et al. Normal ranges of heart rate and respiratory rate in children from birth to 18 years of age: a systematic review of observational studies. Lancet 2011;377:1011-8.

Parshuram CS, Hutchison J, Middaugh K. Development and initial validation of the bedside Paediatric Early Warning System and score. Critical Care 2009;13:R135.

Plum F, PosnerJB. The diagnostic of stupor and coma, 3rd edition. FA Davis Co, Philadelphia, USA, 1982.

Seguin P, Le Rouzo A, Tanguy M, Guillou YM, Feuillu A, Malledant Y. Evidence for the need of bedside accuracy of pulse oximetry in an intensive care unit. Critical care medicine 2000;28:703-6.

Van de Louw A, Cracco C, Cerf C, et al. Accuracy of pulse oximetry in the intensive care unit. Intensive care medicine 2001;27:1606-13.

Brady PW, Muething S, Kotagal U, Ashby M, Gallagher R, Hall D, Goodfriend M, White C, Bracke TM, DeCastro V, Geiser M, Simon J, Tucker KM, Olivea J, Conway PH, Wheeler DS. Improving situation awareness to reduce unrecognised clinical deterioration and serious safety events. Pediatrics. 2013 Jan;131(1):e298-308. doi: 10.1542/peds.2012-1364. Epub 2012 Dec 10. PMID: 23230078; PMCID: PMC4528338.

Fleming S, Gill P, Jones C, et al. The diagnostic value of capillary refill time for detecting serious illness in children: a systematic review and meta-analysis. PLOS ONE 2015;10:e0138155, doi:http://dx.doi.org/ 10.1371/journal.pone.0138155.

Blacklock C, Mayon- White R, Coad N, Thompson M. Which symptoms and clinical features correctly identify serious respiratory infection in children attending a paediatric assessment unit? Arch Dis Child 2011;96:708 14, doi:http://dx.doi.org/10.1136/adc.2010.206243. 41.

Daw WJ, Kingshott RN, Elphick HE. Poor inter-observer agreement in the measurement of respiratory rate in children: a prospective observational study. BMJ Paediatr Open 2017;1:e000173, doi:http:// dx.doi.org/10.1136/bmjpo-2017-000173.

de Groot MG, de Neef M, Otten MH, van Woensel JBM, Bem RA. Interobserver agreement on clinical judgment of work of breathing in spontaneously breathing children in the pediatric intensive care unit. J Pediatr Intensive Care 2020;9:34 9, doi:http://dx.doi.org/10.1055/ s-0039-1697679

Weiss SL, Peters MJ, Alhazzani W, et al. Surviving sepsis campaign international guidelines for the management of septic shock and sepsis-associated organ dysfunction in children. Pediatr Crit Care Med 2020;21:e52 e106, doi:http://dx.doi.org/10.1097/PCC.0000000000002198.

Hagedoorn NN, Zachariasse JM, Moll HA. A comparison of clinical paediatric guidelines for hypotension with population-based lower centiles: a systematic review. Crit Care 2019;23:380, doi:http://dx.doi.org/10.1186/s13054-019-2653-9.

Haque IU, Zaritsky AL. Analysis of the evidence for the lower limit of systolic and mean arterial pressure in children. Pediatr Crit Care Med 2007;8:138 44, doi:http://dx.doi.org/10.1097/01.PCC.00002 57039.32593.

Kobayashi M, Fukuda S, Takano KI, Kamizono J, Ichikawa K. Can a pulse oxygen saturation of 95% to 96% help predict further vital sign destabilization in school-aged children? A retrospective observational study. Medicine (Baltimore) 2018;97:e11135.

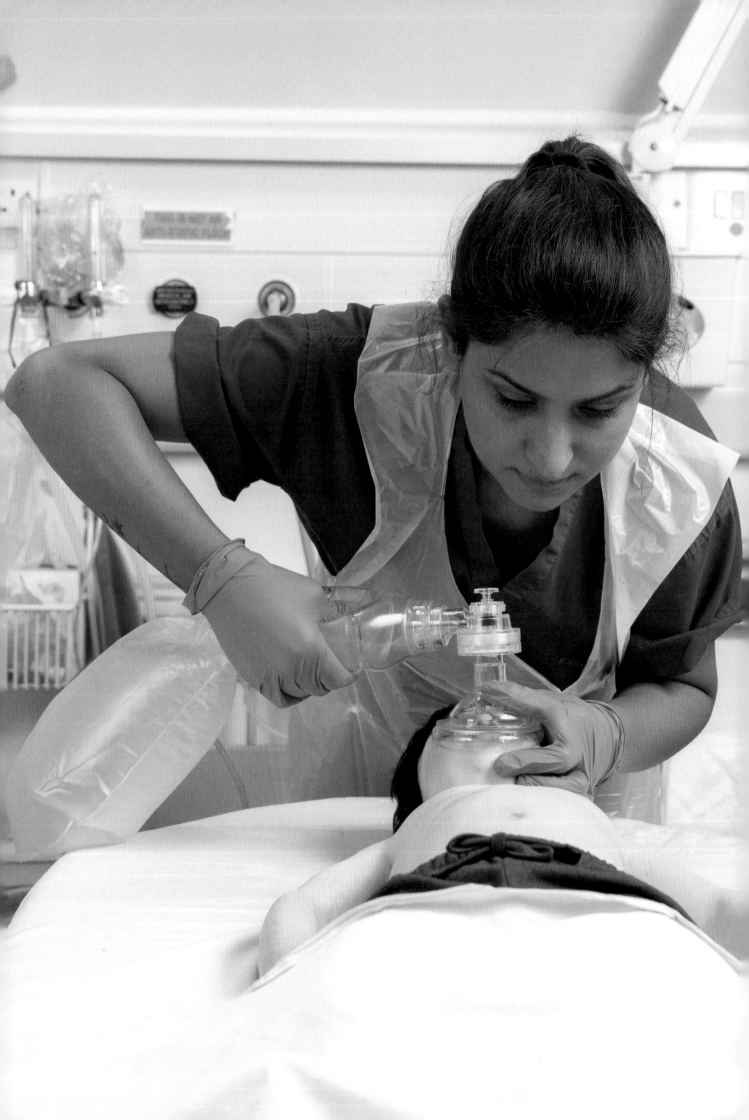

Advanced management of the airway and ventilation

03

Causes of upper airway obstruction

As previously described, the most common cause of cardiorespiratory arrest in children is secondary to respiratory failure resulting in hypoxia and acidosis. The outcome following hypoxic induced cardiorespiratory arrest is poor. Therefore, the management of the airway and ventilation (breathing) is the first priority in dealing with the seriously ill child regardless of the underlying cause.

Early recognition and adequate management of compensated respiratory failure are essential. This chapter describes the initial advanced management of the airway and ventilation based on the child's physiological dysfunction.

Airway obstruction

Airway obstruction is a common occurrence in the seriously ill child. It may be the primary cause of the cardiorespiratory arrest (e.g. choking) or a consequence of the underlying disease process (e.g. seizures, head trauma), which leads to loss of consciousness. In the unconscious child, the tongue can fall backwards and occlude their airway (Figure 3.1). Regardless of the cause, airway obstruction must be rapidly recognised and managed to prevent secondary hypoxic damage to the vital organs.

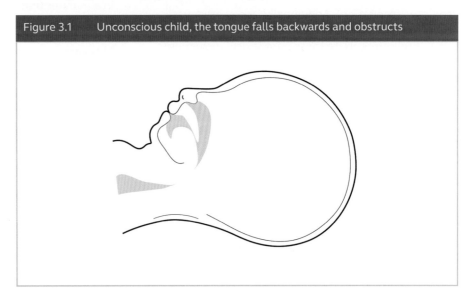

Figure 3.1   Unconscious child, the tongue falls backwards and obstructs

Management of the airway and ventilation (breathing) is the first priority in dealing with the seriously ill child regardless of the underlying cause

Recognition of airway obstruction

In a conscious child, airway obstruction may be demonstrated by difficulty in breathing and/or increased respiratory effort. In both conscious and unconscious children, there may be additional respiratory noises if the obstruction is partial, whereas respiration will be silent if there is complete obstruction.

The most effective way to detect airway obstruction in all children is to look, listen and feel.

LOOK for chest (and abdominal) movements.

LISTEN for airflow at the mouth and nose (+/- additional noises).

FEEL for airflow at the mouth and nose.

LOOKING for breathing

During normal breathing, the chest wall expands, and the abdomen is pushed slightly outwards as the diaphragm contracts. However, when the airway is obstructed, the abdomen protrudes markedly, and the chest is drawn inwards when the diaphragm contracts during inspiration ('see-saw' respiration). Additionally, accessory muscle usage and recession are likely to be observed. It can be difficult to differentiate these paradoxical movements from normal breathing; the rescuer must also listen for the presence or absence of breath sounds and feel for air movement. If a clear face mask is being used, misting of the mask may be observed.

LISTENING for breathing

Normal respiration is quiet. Partially obstructed breathing is noisy, whilst completely obstructed breathing will be silent.

FEELING for breathing

The movement of air on inspiration and expiration can be felt at the mouth and nose (or tracheostomy) during normal breathing. If there is airway obstruction, this will be limited or absent.

Partial airway obstruction can quickly deteriorate to complete obstruction and therefore must always be considered as an emergency. Complete airway obstruction will lead to profound hypoxia, vital organ failure and cardiorespiratory arrest if the obstruction is not relieved very rapidly. Immediate action must be taken to relieve the obstruction and clear the airway.

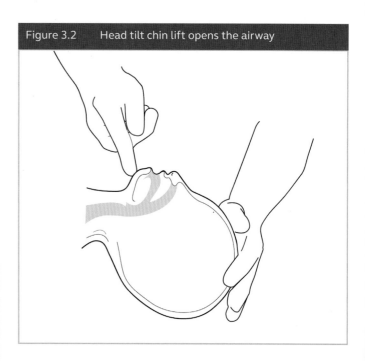

Figure 3.2   Head tilt chin lift opens the airway

Basic techniques to optimise the airway

Conscious children

If the child is making adequate spontaneous respiratory effort, they should be supported in a comfortable position (preferably the one they naturally assume themselves to optimise their airway). High-flow oxygen should be given in a manner that the child will tolerate whilst experienced help is sought.

Unconscious children

Whether or not the child is making spontaneous respiratory effort, the patency of the airway needs to be optimised immediately. This initially means positioning their head by performing either a head tilt and chin lift or a jaw thrust manoeuvre.

Additionally, suction may be required to clear secretions, vomit or blood.

Head positioning

Open the child's airway by performing a head tilt and chin lift (Figure 3.2) or jaw thrust manoeuvre (Chapter 4). It is extremely important to ensure that head positioning techniques are carried out properly to make certain that neither hyperextension (Figure 3.3) nor excessive flexion of the neck occurs, as both will make obstruction worse. Take care not to compress the soft tissues under the child's jaw, as this can also occlude the airway.

Suction

Standard suction devices in hospital are pipeline units. They consist of a wall terminal outlet, vacuum pressure regulator, a reservoir, tubing and a connector for an appropriate suction catheter to be attached.

In some low dependency hospital areas, during transportation and non-hospital environments such as GP surgeries, it is likely that the suction device available will be a portable device that is operated by battery or a hand/foot pump.

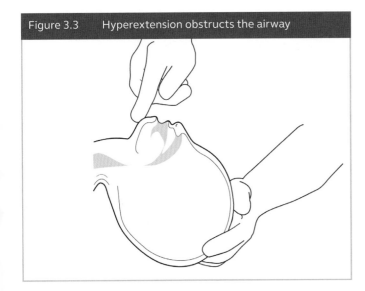

Figure 3.3   Hyperextension obstructs the airway

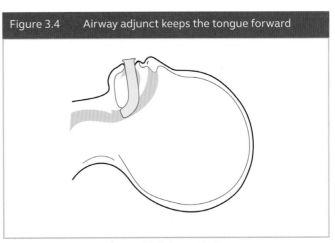

Figure 3.4   Airway adjunct keeps the tongue forward

03

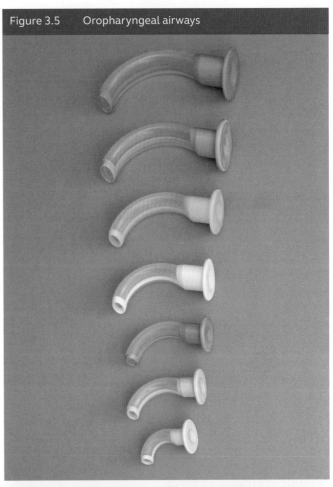

Figure 3.5   Oropharyngeal airways

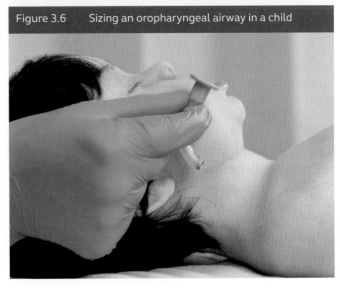

Figure 3.6   Sizing an oropharyngeal airway in a child

Large bore rigid suction catheters (e.g. Yankauer) are particularly useful for the clearance of thick or excessive secretions and vomit. Soft, flexible catheters in a range of sizes should also be available as these may be less traumatic to use and are particularly useful for nasal suction. They can also be passed through nasopharyngeal or oropharyngeal airways and tracheal tubes, but they may not allow adequate clearance of thick or copious secretions.

Whichever suction catheter types are used, they should ideally have a side hole that can be occluded by the rescuer's finger to allow greater control over the suction pressure generated. Suction pressure should not exceed 120 mmHg in infants.

Airway suction must be carried out cautiously if the child has an intact gag reflex as it may induce vomiting, which can lead to aspiration or bradycardia.

Airway opening adjuncts

Oropharyngeal airways

The oropharyngeal airway (e.g. Guedel) is a rigid curved tube designed to open a channel between the lips and the base of the tongue (Figure 3.4). They are made of plastic and are reinforced and flanged at the proximal end. Practitioners should be aware that oropharyngeal airways colour coding and size classification are being standardised. Available sizes range from ISO 3.5 (previously labelled 000) for premature infants to ISO 10.0–12.0 (previously labelled 4–5) for large adults (Figure 3.5).

The correctly sized airway is one that, when laid against the side of the face, has a length equal to the distance between the level of the patient's incisors (or where they will be) to the angle of their jaw (Figure 3.6). If an incorrect size is used, it may result in trauma, laryngospasm and/or worsening of the airway obstruction.

The oropharyngeal airway should be inserted with great care using the minimum force to avoid trauma and bleeding of the delicate palatal and pharyngeal mucosa. It is important to ensure that the tip of the oropharyngeal airway does not push the tongue back into the pharynx.

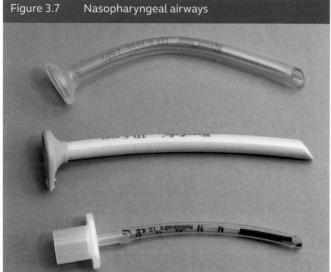

Figure 3.7   Nasopharyngeal airways

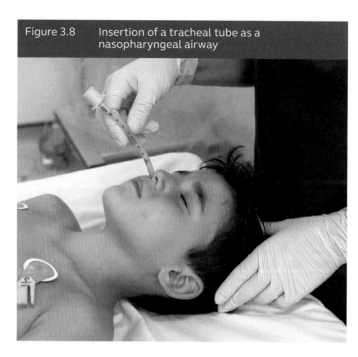

Figure 3.8   Insertion of a tracheal tube as a nasopharyngeal airway

The oropharyngeal airway can be introduced directly, sliding it carefully over the tongue or alternatively, it can be introduced upside down initially, as follows:

- place the tip with the concave side of the airway facing the roof of the mouth
- insert the airway past the teeth and gums, pushing the tongue away from the roof of the mouth with the convex side of the airway
- rotate it 180° as it passes beyond the hard palate and into the oropharynx
- ensure that the flange rests over the mouth.

Whichever technique is used, the effort required to insert the oropharyngeal airway should be minimal, do not use force.

Oropharyngeal airways are intended for use in unconscious patients. If the child is semi-conscious, they may cough, gag, vomit or develop laryngospasm. Insertion of the oropharyngeal airway should be abandoned if this occurs.

Following insertion of the oropharyngeal airway, the child's airway patency should be reassessed by the 'look, listen and feel' approach and oxygen given if indicated.

Nasopharyngeal airways

The nasopharyngeal airway is a flexible tube designed to open a channel between the nostril and the nasopharynx. They are made of soft plastic or silicone, are bevelled at the insertion end and flanged at the outer end (Figure 3.7). The flange prevents the airway from passing completely into the nasal passage. Tracheal tubes cut to the correct length may alternatively be used.

The correct insertion depth should be sized from the nostrils to the tragus of the ear. An appropriate tube size can be estimated by matching its diameter against the diameter of the child's anterior nares, and when inserted, it should not cause blanching of the nostril.

Once appropriately sized, the nasopharyngeal airway should be lubricated and introduced into the nostril. With a gentle rotating motion, the airway should be passed directly backwards and posteriorly along the floor of the nostril. The tube should not be directed upwards, as this will cause trauma and bleeding (Figure 3.8). Following insertion of the nasopharyngeal airway, the child's airway patency should be reassessed using the 'look, listen and feel' approach and oxygen given if indicated.

Nasopharyngeal airways may be better tolerated by conscious children than oropharyngeal airways and are useful as adjuncts in the management of children who may improve their level of consciousness (e.g. the fitting child who is becoming less obtunded).

Their use is contraindicated in patients where basal skull fracture is suspected or if there is a coagulopathy.

Oxygen delivery and ventilatory support

Oxygen should be given as soon as it is available. Initially, this should be at the highest available concentration for all seriously ill children; concerns about oxygen toxicity should never prevent its use during resuscitation. Oxygen should be regulated using a flowmeter capable of delivering up to 15 L min^{-1} (although this may be much higher when high-flow nasal cannulae are used via a special flowmeter). It should ideally be warmed and humidified to minimise the risks of airway irritation and hypothermia. The method used to deliver the oxygen should be selected according to the child's clinical condition. Oxygen saturation levels should be monitored by pulse oximetry (SpO$_2$). When the child's condition has stabilised, the inspired oxygen concentration should be reduced whilst monitoring SpO$_2$ to maintain adequate oxygenation. Blood gases should be taken to also monitor for adequate ventilation; aim for a PaO$_2$ of 10–13 kPa and PaCO$_2$ 4.5–6 kPa.

Oxygen concentration can be expressed as a percentage or fraction of inspired oxygen FiO$_2$ (where 100% oxygen is the equivalent to an FiO$_2$ of 1.0). Table 3.1 shows the amount of oxygen that is delivered for each oxygen delivery device.

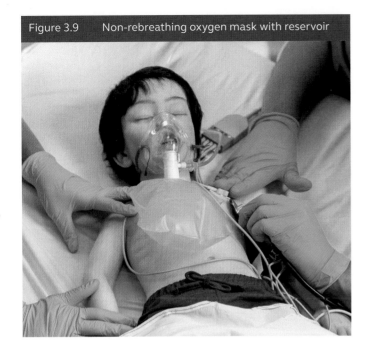

Figure 3.9 — Non-rebreathing oxygen mask with reservoir

When the side valves (or flaps) over the inspiratory holes are removed, a lower FiO_2 will be achieved, as room air will be drawn into the mask as the child inhales.

Simple oxygen mask

A simple oxygen mask without a reservoir bag can deliver oxygen concentrations of up to 60% at flow rates of 10–15 L min^{-1}. Room air is entrained around the edges of the mask and through the holes in the mask so diluting the oxygen delivery.

'Blow-by' facial oxygen

Either the end of the oxygen tubing or a face mask can be held by the child's carer at a short distance from the child's face. This is a less threatening method that can help alleviate the child's fear and maximise their cooperation. However, the inspired concentration that can be delivered is low and inconsistent, so it is only suitable for children with mild respiratory compromise who cannot tolerate other oxygen delivery methods. Oxygen flow rates need to be adjusted depending on what the child will accept.

Nasal cannulae

This method can be useful in stable children of all ages, particularly in pre-school children. The delivery of oxygen via cannulae (or 'prongs') is dependent on oxygen flow and nasal resistance, but the FiO_2 will be low and variable, so it is not suitable during resuscitation or when a high oxygen concentration is required. They are also not suitable for use in children with copious or tenacious nasal secretions, as they will easily become blocked. Flow rates should be kept below 4 L min^{-1} as higher flows are extremely irritating to the nasal passages and do not significantly increase oxygen delivery.

High-flow nasal cannula oxygen (HFNC)

Heated, humidified, high-flow nasal cannula oxygen (e.g. Optiflow, Vapotherm) is increasingly being used for critically ill patients, as it has the advantage of humidifying and warming the gases. It is also able to deliver a higher FiO_2 (up to 1.0) than standard nasal cannulae. At high oxygen flow rates, HFNC is able to increase functional residual capacity, improve mucociliary clearance of secretions, and also deliver some positive end-expiratory pressure (PEEP) which can be advantageous for hypoxic children (e.g. pneumonia, pulmonary contusion, and bronchiolitis). Flows of 2 L kg^{-1} min^{-1} are commonly used for children up to 12 kg, plus 0.5 L kg^{-1} min^{-1} for each kg thereafter to a maximum of 50 L min^{-1}.

Table 3.1 Oxygen delivery devices, flow rates and maximum inspired oxygen levels

Device	Flow rate	Maximum inspired
Nasal prongs	Maximum 4 L min^{-1}	40%
Oxygen mask without reservoir	10–15 L min^{-1}	60%
Oxygen mask with reservoir	Must be enough to avoid reservoir collapse during inspiration, e.g. 12–15 L min^{-1}	90%
Humidified High-flow nasal cannulae (HFNC)	4–50 L min^{-1}*	100%
*Will vary between manufacturers		

Oxygen mask with reservoir bag

This is the preferred method for delivering oxygen in the seriously ill child who is breathing spontaneously. The flow of oxygen must be sufficiently high to ensure the reservoir bag fills adequately (Figure 3.9). It is possible to give an oxygen concentration up to 90% with an oxygen delivery flow of 12–15 L min^{-1} depending on the child's minute volume (the product of the tidal volume of each breath and the number of breaths min^{-1}).

These devices have three 'one-way' valves; one between the reservoir bag and the mask and one on each side of the face mask over the inspiratory holes. They are designed so that when the child inhales, the valve between the mask and reservoir bag opens, allowing oxygen to flow into the mask, whilst the valves on either side of the mask close to prevent room air from drawing in. When the child exhales, the valve between the mask and reservoir bag closes whilst the ones on either side of the mask open to allow the child's expired breath to escape (i.e. there is no rebreathing of gas).

Methods of assisted ventilation

If a child stops breathing completely, or if spontaneous ventilation is inadequate, positive pressure ventilatory support is required.

When providing positive pressure ventilation for an infant/child, aim for a respiratory rate of 12–30 min^{-1} with younger children having higher rates. In a newborn, the rate should be 30 min^{-1}. The volume delivered should be sufficient to produce a normal visible chest expansion, and breath sounds on auscultation. Lower rates of ventilation are used for children and infants who have an advanced airway in place during cardiorespiratory arrest (see Chapter 8).

Continuous monitoring of the heart rate and SpO_2 should be undertaken as soon as practicable.

Mouth-to-mask devices

Rescuers should not delay giving rescue breaths until the arrival of advanced paediatric airway and ventilation equipment. Therefore, expired air breaths (e.g. mouth-to-mouth) using a barrier device such as a face shield may be more appropriate in initial resuscitation attempts. The pocket-mask is widely used in the resuscitation of apnoeic adults, and the standard size may be suitable for use in larger children and adolescents. There is a 'paediatric' pocket-mask available, but "one size" does not fit all infants and children, and an appropriate size of paediatric face mask may need to be substituted. Expired air ventilation using a pocket-mask should only be used if a manual ventilation device (e.g. self-inflating bag system) is not immediately available.

When it is deemed appropriate for use (e.g. in an adolescent), the pocket-mask is a device designed to minimise infection risks when delivering expired air ventilation. The device is made of transparent plastic with a one-way valve that directs the patient's expired breath away from the rescuer. An oxygen delivery port (which also has a one-way valve) is incorporated into some pocket-masks and allows supplemental oxygen to be administered.

Technique for mouth-to-mask ventilation

- Having assembled the pocket-mask, the rescuer positions themselves behind the supine child.
- The child's head should be placed in an appropriate position (e.g. 'sniffing' position) to achieve a patent airway.
- Apply the mask over the child's mouth and nose, pressing down with the thumbs of both hands to create a seal.
- Lift the child's jaw upwards (jaw thrust) into the mask with the other fingers, taking care not to compress the soft tissues under the mandible.

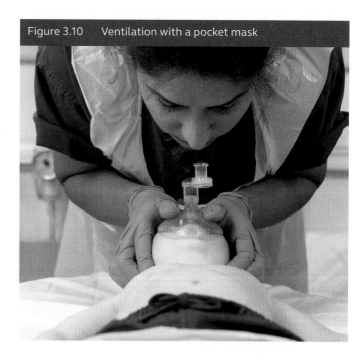

Figure 3.10   Ventilation with a pocket mask

- Blow through the mask's one-way valve until chest expansion is observed (Figure 3.10).
- Stop inflation and observe the chest falling.
- Repeat as appropriate.
- If chest expansion is not seen, assess whether this may be due to inadequate airway patency or a poor seal between the child's face and the mask, and correct as necessary.
- If the mask has an appropriate port and there is oxygen available, supplemental oxygen should be administered.

This technique can also be used with a standard face mask, but it will not protect against infection unless a breathing system filter is also used.

The self-inflating bag device (as used for bag-mask ventilation)

In a child who has inadequate/absent breathing, maintaining a patent airway is the first priority of management. Once this is achieved, adequate ventilation must be established. The self-inflating bag system with an oxygen reservoir is the first line system for providing ventilation during resuscitation. Although the self-inflating bag can be used without a supplemental oxygen source, it is usually used to deliver ventilation with high-flow oxygen in resuscitation situations. The self-inflating bag can be connected not only to a face mask but also to a tracheal tube, i-gel or laryngeal mask airway when these are in place.

A self-inflating bag system consists of a bag that the operator squeezes to deliver a breath to the patient. Exhalation occurs through a one-way valve at the patient end of the bag, whilst the device automatically refills with air (and oxygen when attached) via an inlet(s) at the opposite end.

Used without supplemental oxygen, a self-inflating bag system will ventilate with room air (21% oxygen). The oxygen concentration can be increased to approximately

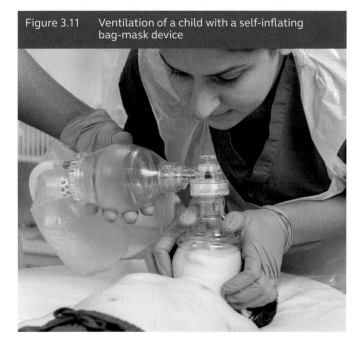

Figure 3.11   Ventilation of a child with a self-inflating bag-mask device

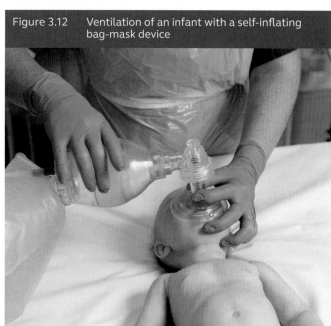

Figure 3.12   Ventilation of an infant with a self-inflating bag-mask device

50% by attaching a high-flow of oxygen via the oxygen port on the base of the bag, without a reservoir bag. The use of the reservoir bag, as described above together with high-flow of oxygen at 15 L min^{-1}, will enable the delivery of > 90% oxygen (Figure 3.11).

Self-inflating bags are available in various sizes, depending on the manufacturer (e.g. 250, 450–500, 900–1200 and 1600–2000 mL). Smaller sizes usually have a pressure-limiting valve that prevents excessive inflation pressures that otherwise may cause barotrauma. The pressure limit is pre-determined by the manufacturer (usually 30–40 cm H_2O). During resuscitation, higher than normal inflation pressures may be required, and the pressure limiting valve may need to be over-ridden. The most common reason for needing to activate the pressure-limiting valve is upper airway obstruction due to a poor airway opening technique. Thus, ensure that the child's airway is patent (e.g. check head positioning) before overriding the valve. It should be noted that such valves are now being incorporated into some of the large bag sizes.

The smallest bags (approximately 250 mL) are intended for preterm neonates < 2.5 kg only. They are not appropriate for use in full-term neonates and infants as they may be inadequate to support effective tidal volume. When selecting the bag size, rescuers should follow manufacturers' guidance for age and weight ranges. The bag volume should always be able to support sufficient tidal volume for the patient. Regardless of size, the provider should only use the force and tidal volume necessary to cause visible chest expansion (Figures 3.11, 3.12).

Self-inflating bags should not be used to deliver oxygen to spontaneously breathing patients. Depending on the valve system, this may result in the inspiration of room air (or even rebreathing of the child's own passively expired air if the mask is held tightly on the face) as the child's own respiratory efforts may not generate sufficient

pressure to open the valve. Children, who are making an adequate respiratory effort, should therefore have oxygen administered by another method.

Face mask selection

These are the interface between the ventilation device and the child. They must be capable of providing a good seal over the mouth and nose whilst ensuring minimal pressure is applied over the eyes.

Masks are available in a variety of sizes and two basic types; anatomically shaped ones for older children and adults and circular ones for infants and small children (Figure 3.13). The preferred mask is transparent (to allow rapid detection of secretions/vomit and observation of the child's central colour) and should have a low dead space.

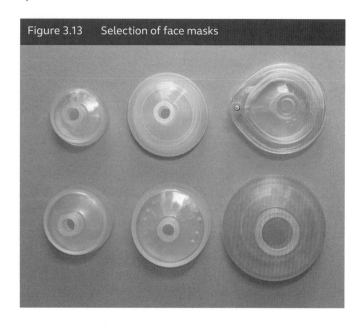

Figure 3.13   Selection of face masks

Bag-mask ventilation

Ventilatory support using assisted ventilation is indicated in the child with decompensated respiratory failure. Bag-mask ventilation (BMV) describes the use of a face mask and a self-inflating bag system with an oxygen reservoir attached that delivers positive pressure ventilation without rebreathing of expired respiratory gases, as described above.

Correctly performed BMV is a vital skill for all healthcare professionals who work with children. While the operating principle of self-inflating bags is simple, they require skill and practice to safely and effectively use them.

Hypoventilation can occur with poor technique (e.g. inadequate mask seal or incorrect head positioning) and is likely to have a negative effect on the outcome.

Excessive BMV should be avoided as it causes over insufflation of the stomach. Gastric distension will then limit the movement of the diaphragm and therefore reduce ventilation. It will also lead to an increased risk of gastro-oesophageal reflux and aspiration of gastric contents.

When self-inflating bags are used with a face mask, it can be difficult for a single rescuer to achieve an airtight seal whilst simultaneously using one hand to maintain a patent airway with a jaw thrust manoeuvre and squeezing the bag with the other. A two-person technique (one person to maintain the airway and hold the mask in position, and the second to squeeze the bag) will usually overcome these difficulties and is the recommended technique in resuscitation. The effectiveness of BMV can be seen by observing adequate chest expansion, monitoring heart rate, auscultating the chest and monitoring SpO_2.

Technique for bag-mask ventilation (two-person technique)

- Having selected the appropriate size of bag and mask, one rescuer should stand behind the supine child.
- The oxygen supply should be connected at a high-flow, and the reservoir bag should be seen to inflate.
- A second person should stand slightly to one side of the child's head.
- The child's head should be placed in an appropriate position (e.g. 'neutral' position for an infant, 'sniffing the morning air' in the older child) to achieve a patent airway. A roll placed under the infant's shoulders is often useful to assist in maintaining an appropriate airway position (unless contraindicated in trauma cases).
- The first rescuer applies the mask over the child's mouth and nose, gently pressing down with the thumb and index finger of both hands. They then lift the child's jaw upwards (jaw thrust) into the mask with the other fingers, with one finger under the angle of the jaw. Take care not to compress the soft tissues underneath the mandible.

- The second rescuer gently squeezes the bag until normal chest expansion is observed.
- Stop inflation and observe the chest falling.
- Repeat as appropriate.
- If chest expansion is not seen, assess whether this may be due to inadequate airway patency or a poor seal between the child's face and the mask, and correct as necessary.

Bag-mask ventilation frequently results in gastric distension, and therefore the placement of a gastric tube should be undertaken as early as practicable.

T-piece (flow-inflating bag) circuit

This equipment is often employed by anaesthesia and critical care staff. It requires a continuous gas source for inflation of the bag. Therefore, there must always be an appropriate self-inflating system immediately available in case there is a failure of the gas supply. This circuit does not have any valves, and the bag has an open end. To achieve ventilation, the end of the bag needs to be occluded, and the bag squeezed. To prevent rebreathing, a high gas flow is required (at least three times the patient's minute ventilation (i.e. > 30 mL kg^{-1} x respiratory rate). This circuit can deliver 100% oxygen and can be used in spontaneously breathing children. The bag of this device gives some 'feeling' of the lungs' compliance and allows some positive end-expiratory pressure (PEEP) to be applied manually. The safe and effective use of this equipment requires considerable expertise, and it should be utilised by experienced practitioners only.

Supraglottic airway devices

Laryngeal mask airway (LMA)

The LMA is a supraglottic airway device that is widely used in children undergoing routine surgical procedures as a means of providing an effective airway to ventilate and oxygenate (Figure 3.14). Like the oropharyngeal airway, it can cause gagging, coughing and laryngospasm in children who are semi-conscious, so it should only be used in unconscious patients with relaxed jaw muscles.

Trained providers should consider LMA insertion if BMV is difficult or not successful. It is an alternative to tracheal intubation when suitably skilled individuals are not available.

It consists of a tube with an inflatable cuffed mask at the distal end, which is introduced into the mouth and advanced into the pharynx until resistance is felt (Figure 3.15). The cuff is then inflated, providing a low-pressure seal over the laryngeal inlet. This leaves the distal opening of the tube just above the vocal cords. The LMA does not protect the lungs from regurgitation and aspiration of gastric contents.

Figure 3.14   Laryngeal mask airways and i-gel

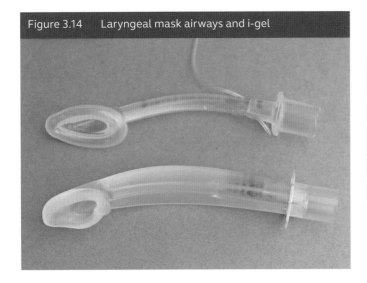

Figure 3.15   Insertion of laryngeal mask airway

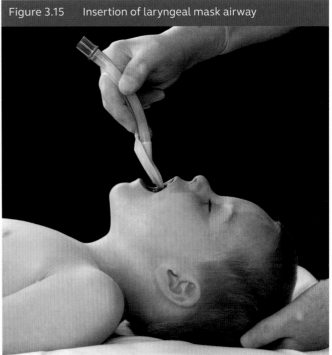

LMA insertion technique

The correct size of LMA is based on the age/weight of the child (Table 3.2). Before insertion, the device should be inspected for damage and tubing obstruction. The cuff should be checked for leaks by inflation to 50% greater than the recommended inflation volume. A water-soluble lubricant gel needs to be applied to the tip and back of the cuff just before insertion.

There have been several methods described to insert the LMA in children. In general, it is useful to consider the LMA as a slightly longer oropharyngeal airway with the distal cuff sitting over the laryngeal inlet.

The following is the standard insertion technique:

- The cuff is fully deflated, and the tubing is held by the dominant hand of the rescuer, just above the cuff (Figure 3.15).

- Whilst standing behind the child's head, the other hand holds the occiput and gently extends the head.

- The tip of the mask is inserted into the child's mouth and is pressed against the hard palate.

- The mask is advanced into the mouth until the cuff passes beyond the back of the tongue. Stop pushing the mask once resistance is felt (the cuff should not be visible in the mouth once the mask is in place).

- Once the LMA is correctly positioned, the cuff should be slowly inflated using an air filled syringe (Table 3.2).

- A small outward movement of the tube is frequently seen once the correct volume is given; this is the moment to stop inflating the cuff.

- The opening of the cuff must be facing forward once the LMA is inserted to lie above the laryngeal inlet (i.e. towards the patient's feet).

- A self-inflating bag system is connected to the LMA and gently squeezed. The chest should be seen to rise in a similar manner to that when performing BMV.

- The LMA should be secured in place using tape.

- The LMA cuff pressure should be checked with a manometer following insertion.

If resistance is felt while attempting to pass the cuff beyond the back of the tongue, various strategies can be used to aid insertion. The head can be further extended, the mask partially inflated and rotated 90° or 180° (like the rotation technique used to insert an oropharyngeal airway) and then further advanced. If the chest is not seen to rise, the LMA should be removed, and BMV should be performed.

Table 3.2   LMA size selection and cuff volume

LMA size	Child selection	Maximum cuff volume
1	Neonates < 5 kg	4 mL
1 ½	Infants 5–10 kg	7 mL
2	Infants 10–20 kg	10 mL
2 ½	Children 20–30 kg	14 mL
3	Children 30–50 kg	20 mL

i-gel

The i-gel is a supraglottic airway management device (Figure 3.14 and Table 3.3). It is used in children undergoing routine surgical procedures to provide an effective airway to achieve ventilation and oxygenation. Like the other SGAs, it can cause gagging, coughing and laryngospasm in children who are semi-conscious, so it should only be used in unconscious patients with relaxed jaw muscles.

It has advantages to its use, including ease of insertion, it has no cuff to inflate, has an integral bite block, and has a gastric channel to pass an oral gastric tube (as do some types of LMA).

Table 3.3   i-gel size selection

i-gel size	Child selection
1	Neonates < 5 kg
1 ½	Infants 5–12 kg
2	Infants 10–25 kg
2 ½	Children 25–35 kg
3	Children 30–60 kg

Other supraglottic airway devices

There are now several other SGAs that have been used successfully in children under anaesthesia. They may also be useful in resuscitation. Providers should use the equipment they are familiar with.

Tracheal intubation

Tracheal intubation should only be performed by experienced personnel who have been trained to perform the technique. It is considered the "gold standard" method to achieve and maintain a secure airway. In addition, it allows optimal control of the ventilation pressures (including PEEP), prevents gastric distension, protects the lungs from aspiration of gastric contents, and makes it easier to ventilate the lungs when chest compressions are performed. The oral route is quicker and simpler than nasal intubation, whereas the nasal route provides a more secure airway for longer term use.

Tracheal intubation should be considered in the following situations:

- ineffective BMV
- severe anatomical or functional upper airways obstruction (e.g. facial burns)
- need for protection of the airway from aspiration of gastric contents
- if high pressures are required to maintain adequate oxygenation (e.g. asthma)
- mechanical ventilation is required
- need for bronchial or tracheal suctioning
- instability or high probability of one of the above occurring before or during transport.

Intubation can be more difficult to achieve in children compared to adults. It requires extensive training, both on manikins and real patients in the operating theatre or intensive care unit. In most situations, provided there is effective ventilation using BMV, there is no need to perform tracheal intubation until experienced personnel are available. In some circumstances (e.g. head trauma and cervical spine injury), repeated attempts at intubation by the inexperienced may worsen the child's condition.

Equipment

Tracheal tubes

Traditionally uncuffed tubes have been preferred for intubation for children up to eight years (up to 6 mm internal diameter) as it was thought that the cricoid ring was the narrowest part of the airway and acted as a 'natural cuff'. However, recent studies have shown that this may not be completely accurate (see Chapter 1) and that there is no greater risk of complications for children between one month and eight years when cuffed tracheal

tubes (TT) are used. Consequently, cuffed TT can be considered for use in the resuscitation of infants and children (except neonates) provided the correct tube size is selected, the cuff inflation pressure is monitored (20–25 cm H_2O) and the tube position verified. If a cuffed TT is used, the cuff should be of a high-volume, low-pressure design and should be positioned below the cricoid ring, with the tracheal tube tip above the carina. Under certain circumstances (e.g. poor lung compliance, high airway resistance or a large glottic air leak), cuffed TT have distinct advantages over uncuffed tubes.

Regardless of whether a cuffed or uncuffed TT is used, its position should be checked to ensure that the tip of the tube lies above the carina. Tracheal tubes have markings along their length that indicate the distance the tube needs to pass along the larynx of an average child to rest in the mid-trachea.

Choice of tracheal tube

Tube sizes are based on internal diameter (ID) in millimetres:

- preterm neonates: 2.5–3.0 mm uncuffed (or gestational weeks/10)
- term neonates: 3.0–3.5 mm uncuffed
- infants six months to one year: 3.5 mm cuffed
- infants > one year: 4.0 mm cuffed
- children over one year: appropriate ID is given by the formula for uncuffed TT:
  - Age (years)/4 + 4
  - ensure a half size larger and smaller TT are available to hand
  - if a cuffed TT is used, a half size smaller diameter should be used.

Resuscitation tapes (e.g. Broselow, Sandell tapes) can also be used to estimate the TT size based on the child's length.

To estimate the length of TT for correct placement in the trachea, the following formulae can be used:

- oral TT: length (cm) = Age (years)/2 + 12
- or, up to 12 years, 3 x ID (cm)
- nasal TT: length (cm) age (years)/2 + 15.

Clinical and radiological confirmation of tube placement is essential following intubation.

Stylet

A stylet may be used to aid intubation, but its use should not be routine. It moulds the shape of TT during intubation to facilitate its direction into the glottis. It must be chosen according to TT size and should be fixed so that its tip does not protrude beyond the distal end of the tube (to avoid tracheal trauma).

Laryngoscope

This consists of a body containing batteries, a light source and a blade. It must be checked before use, and spares must always be available.

There are two types of blades; curved and straight (Figure 3.16). Their role is the same; that is to keep the tongue out of the way and displace the epiglottis allowing the vocal cords to be seen.

The choice of blade type depends on personal preference and the experience of the provider, but the following age limits can act as a guide:

*   Straight blades (numbers 0 and 1) are usually preferred for neonates and infants (< one year) and are designed to advance over the posterior border of the epiglottis so that the vocal cords can be seen. The blade may also be placed in the vallecula (between the tongue base and the epiglottis). The advantage of lifting the epiglottis is that it will then not obscure the view of the vocal cords. The disadvantage is that manipulation of the epiglottis causes vagal stimulation.

*   Curved blades are preferred in children and adolescents (numbers 0, 1 and 2 for infants and children; 3 and 4 for adolescents and adults). They are designed to have their tip resting in the vallecula and to lift the epiglottis from above.

Straight and curved blades come in several lengths. The choice of length is guided by the child's age. If in doubt, remember that it is possible to intubate with a blade that is too long but not with one that is too short.

Video laryngoscopes are becoming widely available and are especially useful in the management of the difficult airway (e.g. congenital airway problems, trauma, burns).

Procedure

Although tracheal intubation should only be performed by those with suitable training and experience, all members of the team should understand the requirements for safe and successful intubation. The ECG, heart rate, SpO_2 and end-tidal CO_2 should be monitored during intubation. There is a risk of reflex bradycardia and hypoxia during intubation. Peripheral oxygen saturation is unreliable if peripheral perfusion is inadequate (e.g. in cardiorespiratory arrest, shock or circulatory failure). An intubation checklist should be used, and the team briefed before embarking on the procedure to minimise complications. Check all necessary equipment is available before intubation:

*   medications
*   self-inflating bag system and oxygen supply
*   oropharyngeal/nasopharyngeal airway
*   laryngoscope handles and blades
*   tracheal tubes of the appropriate sizes

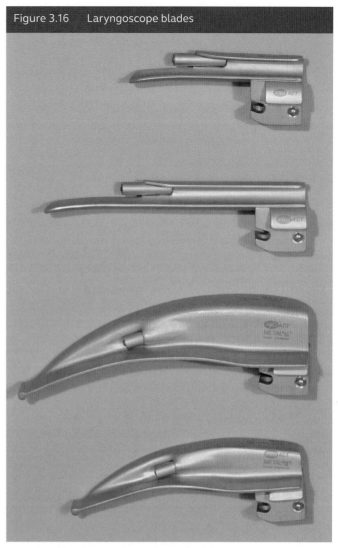

Figure 3.16   Laryngoscope blades

*   bougie
*   end-tidal CO_2 monitoring
*   stylet and Magill forceps
*   suction apparatus with the appropriate size of suckers
*   tapes or ties to secure the tube
*   nasogastric tubes.

Intubation technique

Prior to intubation, the patient should be pre-oxygenated with 100% oxygen via BMV. If, during the intubation attempt, there is a fall in peripheral oxygen saturation or bradycardia occurs, the procedure should be interrupted, and the patient ventilated again with 100% oxygen by BMV.

In infants < one year, head and neck extension may be required by placing a neck roll under the shoulders (provided there is no history of cervical spine injury).

If there is suspected cervical spine injury, in-line manual immobilisation of the neck should be maintained at all times during intubation.

Attempts to intubate should be interrupted if:

- the peripheral oxygen saturations reading begins to fall
- the heart rate begins to fall or is < 60 min^{-1}
- more than 30 s has elapsed.

BMV should be recommended until the child's condition improves before attempting intubation again.

An incorrectly placed tube or prolonged hypoxia from repeated intubation attempts can cause morbidity and even mortality.

Verification of TT placement

Displaced, misplaced or obstructed TT can occur frequently and can lead to an increased risk of death. The position of the tube should be checked after placement using end-tidal CO_2 monitoring (e.g. capnography). CO_2 should be detected if the TT is correctly placed after four to six ventilations. If no end-tidal CO_2 is present after these ventilations, the TT is likely to be in the oesophagus and not in the trachea. The tube should be immediately removed, and BMV restarted, as the patient is at risk of hypoxia. Remember: 'No trace, wrong place'.

Confirmation of correct TT placement comprises:

- clear visualisation of the tube passing through the glottis
- end-tidal CO_2 monitoring
- symmetrical chest rise and fall with each ventilation
- bilateral air entry in four zones with each ventilation – axillae and apices
- absence of bubbling noise over the stomach upon ventilation
- chest X-ray (after initial resuscitation) to confirm TT is above the carina (ideally tip between T2 and T3).

Once the correct position is confirmed, secure the TT with tape after drying and cleaning the skin with gauze.

If auscultation is asymmetrical, particularly if it is decreased on the left side of the chest and the tube is long for age, withdraw the TT cautiously by 0.5 cm increments until symmetrical breath sounds are heard. If breath sounds are now heard bilaterally, then the TT will have been in the right main bronchus before adjustment. Other causes of unilateral chest wall rise should be considered, including pneumothorax, secretions causing plugging of bronchi.

Sudden deterioration of the intubated patient

If the condition of an intubated child deteriorates, consider various possibilities, which are easily recalled by the acronym 'DOPES':

D	**D**isplacement of the tracheal tube (e.g. oesophagus, right main bronchus)
O	**O**bstruction of artificial airway (accumulated secretions (e.g. bronchiolitis), kinking of the tracheal tube)
P	**P**neumothorax (from excessive BMV pressure, rib fractures)
E	**E**quipment failure (e.g. disconnected oxygen supply)
S	**S**tomach distension (following expired air or bag-mask)

Other reasons for deterioration or inadequate ventilation include:

- TT too small with significant air leak
- tidal-volume given is too small (aim for tidal volumes of 5–7 mL kg^{-1})
- pressure-limiting valve active with non-compliant lungs (e.g. in near drowning).

Emergency anaesthesia for intubation

In cardiorespiratory arrest, as the child is unconscious, intubation does not require analgesia, anaesthesia or neuromuscular blockade (muscle relaxants). In many other emergency situations, however, combinations of these drugs may be required.

Emergency anaesthesia is delivered by a combination of drugs to facilitate and secure tracheal intubation in an emergency. It reduces the incidence of adverse events in responsive patients. These include:

- hypoxia
- pain
- cardiac arrhythmias
- rise in systemic BP and intracranial pressure
- airway trauma
- reflux and aspiration of gastric contents
- psychological trauma.

Pre-oxygenation is important to prevent hypoxia during emergency anaesthesia and intubation, with at least three minutes of oxygen delivered by BMV or an anaesthetic circuit to increase the amount of oxygen reserve. Emergency drugs, including atropine, should be immediately available. A combination of drugs in Table 3.4 should then be administered by the team.

The team delivering emergency anaesthesia must have considerable experience in intubation and BMV, as the child will not be able to breathe on their own after the drugs have been administered. An alternative plan for airway management in case of unsuccessful intubation must have been considered during the checklist and brief.

Table 3.4   Some examples of drugs for emergency anaesthesia

Analgesia	Anaesthetic agent	Neuromuscular blocking drug
alfentanil	ketamine	rocuronium
fentanyl	propofol	suxamethonium
	sevoflurane	
	thiopentone	

Care of the child with a tracheostomy

A tracheostomy is a surgical opening into the trachea, which bypasses the mouth, pharynx and larynx. Children may have a tracheostomy present because of a congenital upper airway narrowing or to facilitate long-term ventilation. They often have complex medical problems, and information about this should be gained as soon as possible. The parents/caregivers will have been taught how to care for the tracheostomy, including emergencies and paediatric basic life support.

The ABCDE approach should be used when assessing children with a tracheostomy, and resuscitation should be commenced as usual if no breathing and/or pulse are detected. The main differences to the management of the airway/breathing are discussed below.

In these children, difficulty in breathing, leading to respiratory distress, may be caused by obstruction of the tracheostomy tube leading to ineffective ventilation. The management of an obstructed tracheostomy is detailed in Figure 3.17. Try to relieve the obstruction by suctioning the tracheostomy tube. If a suction catheter cannot be passed, the tracheostomy tube should be removed immediately and replaced. If a clean tube is not available, ventilation via BMV should be given at the tracheostomy stoma site until the tube is cleaned and replaced. If the child's upper airway is patent, it may be possible to provide bag-mask ventilation via the mouth and nose using a conventional bag and mask whilst the tracheal stoma site is occluded. In an emergency situation, tracheal intubation via the tracheostomy with a classical endotracheal tube may be needed. Attention should be given to correct positioning (not endobronchial).

Cricoid pressure (Sellick manoeuvre)

Unconscious children with a full stomach are at risk of regurgitation of gastric contents and pulmonary aspiration. The application of pressure to the cricoid cartilage occludes the oesophagus and may reduce the risk of regurgitation. However, cricoid pressure is difficult to perform correctly in infants and young children and may cause airway distortion and obstruction, so routine use is not recommended. If it is thought the airway is in any way compromised, cricoid pressure should be removed immediately. On some occasions, cricoid pressure may help visualisation of the vocal cords, aiding intubation.

Cricoid pressure is performed by:

- identification of the cricoid cartilage (just below the thyroid cartilage)
- gentle application of pressure using two fingers to the cricoid cartilage
- the cricoid is displaced backwards to compress the oesophagus.

NB. This manoeuvre should not be performed if the child begins actively to vomit because it may lead to oesophageal rupture.

The difficult airway

If ventilation is not possible using BMV, call for assistance and perform simple airway manoeuvres. In the majority of situations, it should be possible to ventilate the child until expert assistance arrives.

Occasionally, despite using these simple airway manoeuvres, ventilation may not be possible due to airway abnormalities (e.g. facial trauma, epiglottitis, airway malformations).

If the obstruction is above the larynx (facial trauma, congenital facial abnormalities), supraglottic airway devices (e.g. i-gel, LMA) can be life-saving.

Nevertheless, immediate expert help should be sought as intubation may be needed using either conventional or optical laryngoscopy.

Intubation by the non-expert would only be acceptable if no such expertise were available, and it is not otherwise possible to oxygenate and ventilate a hypoxic child.

In the very rare situations when the clinician cannot ventilate the child and intubation is not possible, cricothyroidotomy should be considered.

Cricothyroidotomy

Needle cricothyroidotomy is a 'last resort' emergency technique indicated in cases of upper airway obstruction (e.g. laryngeal obstruction by oedema, foreign body or major facial trauma). It is a technique of default (i.e. only to be undertaken when ventilation by BMV or supraglottic airway device and TT intubation have failed).

Cricothyroidotomy can be performed with a large-bore over-the-needle cannula. A syringe is connected to the cannula and gently aspirated as it punctures either a prominent tracheal ring or the cricothyroid membrane percutaneously, at an angle of 45° from the head; these landmarks can be very difficult to identify in pre-school children. The trachea is situated just beneath the skin and air aspiration confirms the correct position.

Figure 3.17   Emergency Paediatric Tracheostomy Management
– resuscitation algorithm for a patient with a tracheostomy; NTSP Paediatric Working Group

Emergency Paediatric Tracheostomy Management

SAFETY - STIMULATE - SHOUT FOR HELP - OXYGEN

SAFE: Check Safe area, Stimulate, and Shout for help
AIRWAY: Open child's airway: head tilt / chin lift / pillow or towel under shoulders may help
OXYGEN: Ensure high flow oxygen to the tracheostomy AND the face as soon as oxygen available
CAPNOGRAPHY: Exhaled carbon dioxide waveform may indicate a patent airway (advanced response)

Basic Response

SUCTION TO ASSESS TRACHEOSTOMY PATENCY

Remove attachments: humidifier (HME), speaking valve
Change inner tube (if present)
Inner tubes may need re-inserting to connect to breathing circuits

The tracheostomy tube is patent
Perform tracheal suction
Consider partial obstruction

Can you pass a SUCTION catheter? — Yes → **CONTINUE ASSESSMENT (ABCDE)**

No

EMERGENCY TRACHEOSTOMY TUBE CHANGE

Deflate cuff (if present). Reassess patency after any tube change
1st change – same size tube
2nd change – one-half size smaller tube
3rd change - over suction catheter to guide

IF UNSUCCESSFUL – REMOVE THE TUBE

IS THE PATIENT BREATHING? - Look, listen and feel at the mouth and tracheostomy/stoma

No / Yes

CALL FOR HELP: 2222 in hospital, 999 in community

5 RESCUE BREATHS

Patent Upper Airway – use the nose/mouth
Obstructed Upper Airway – use the tracheostomy/stoma

NO SIGNS OF LIFE? START CPR

15 compressions : 2 rescue breaths
Ensure help or resuscitation team called

Continue oxygen
Stabilize
Reassess
Review

Plan for definitive
airway if tube
change failure

Advanced Response

Primary emergency oxygenation

Standard ORAL airway manoeuvres
Cover the stoma (swabs / hand).
Use:
Bag-valve-face mask
Oral or nasal airway adjuncts
Supraglottic Airway (SGA)
e.g. Laryngeal Mask Airway (LMA)

Tracheostomy STOMA ventilation
Paediatric face-mask applied to stoma
SGA applied to stoma

Secondary emergency oxygenation

ORAL intubation with endotracheal tube
Uncut tube, advanced beyond stoma
One half-size smaller than tracheostomy tube
'Difficult Airway' Expert and Equipment*

Attempt intubation of STOMA
3.0 ID tracheostomy or endotracheal tube
'Difficult Airway' Expert and Equipment*

*EQUIPMENT: Fibreoptic scope, bougie,
airway exchange catheter, Airway trolley

NTSP (Paediatric Working Group) www.tracheostomy.org.uk Review January 2022

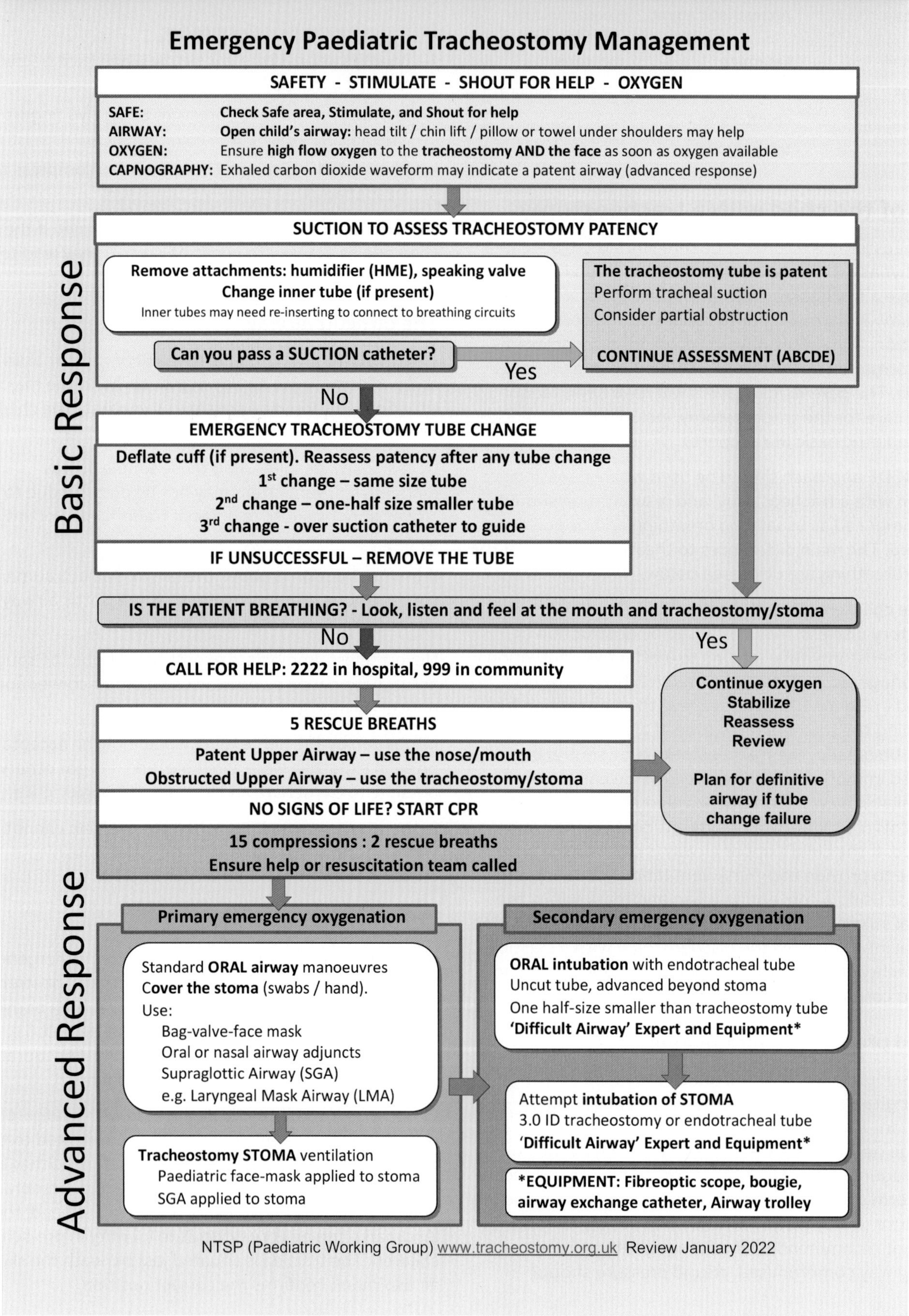

The needle is removed and the cannula connected to a 3 or 3.5 mm TT adaptor and a self-inflating bag system. An alternative is to connect directly via a 3-way tap, with all ports open to an oxygen source. Oxygen is given by obstructing the side port of the 3-way tap for 1 s and allowing 4 s for exhalation.

Oxygen flow for this technique in L min^{-1} = age of the child in years (maximum 6 L min^{-1}).

Over-the-needle cannulae have high resistances. Small tidal volumes are delivered, and there is no significant CO_2 removal. There is also a risk of barotrauma, particularly with the 3-way tap technique, if the airway is completely obstructed above the cannula. The technique only provides temporary oxygenation until a definitive airway can be provided. Expert help must be sought as soon as possible.

Surgical tracheostomy should be reserved for skilled practitioners as it is a difficult technique with major risks, including haemorrhage, laryngeal tear, pneumomediastinum and subcutaneous emphysema.

Monitoring

Pulse oximetry

The clinical recognition of cyanosis may be difficult and is not reliable. Pulse oximetry enables continuous evaluation of the peripheral oxygen saturation of haemoglobin and is a valuable non-invasive method of monitoring the child (Chapter 2). It provides an early indication of hypoxia and should be used during both stabilisation and transportation of the critically ill child (Figure 3.18). A detecting probe is placed around a finger/toe (in the child) or hand/foot (in the infant). Ideally, the pulse oximeter monitor should display a wave-form, a numerical percentage of oxygenation and produce a tone modulated sound. It is important to remember that it is a measure of oxygenation and does not indicate the adequacy of ventilation. Peripheral oxygen saturation readings should always be interpreted with reference to the inspired oxygen concentration. When peripheral perfusion is poor, recorded values will be unreliable. Furthermore, in cardiorespiratory arrest, circulatory failure or shock with severely reduced peripheral perfusion, pulse oximetry may be unrecordable.

End-tidal CO_2 monitoring (capnography)

Monitoring end-tidal CO_2 reliably confirms TT placement in a child weighing more than 2 kg with a perfusing rhythm. It should be used following intubation and during the transportation of an intubated child. It can also be used in non-intubated critically ill children (e.g. non-invasive ventilation, nasal cannulae).

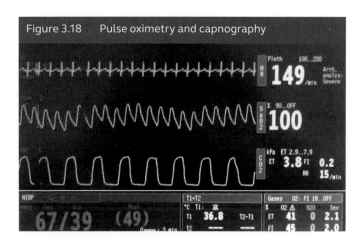

Figure 3.18   Pulse oximetry and capnography

The presence of an end-tidal CO_2 trace after 4–6 ventilated breaths indicates that the TT is in the tracheobronchial tree, both in the presence of a perfusing rhythm and during cardiorespiratory arrest. Figure 3.18 shows an example of an end-tidal CO_2 trace.

Although the CO_2 trace may be attenuated during CPR, as pulmonary blood flow is very low, the absence of CO_2 should be assumed to indicate misplacement of the TT unless its position is confirmed using other methods (e.g. direct visualisation). If the TT position is confirmed and correct, then CPR quality may be inadequate. If there is any doubt, remove the tube and return to mask ventilation. Remember, **'No trace, wrong place'**.

Types of end-tidal CO_2 sampling devices

1. Side-stream end-tidal CO_2

A connector is placed in the breathing system, usually at the end of the tracheal tube or supraglottic airway; the closer to the airway device, the better. A fine bore sampling tube then takes a continuous sample and analyses it with infrared light. The amount of infrared light absorbed is proportional to the amount of CO_2 present. This is then presented as a number (capnometry) or graphically (capnography). The latter gives more clinical information.

2. Main-stream end-tidal CO_2

The infrared source and detector are contained within a cell or cuvette which is placed directly in the breathing system, usually between the TT or SGA and the ventilation tubing. Gas is analysed as it passes through the sensor, and none is removed from the system (unlike side-stream). This usually presents the information as capnography. The disadvantage of this type of device is its size and weight; there is a potential risk of TT dislodgement, especially in small children.

Information that can be gained from end-tidal CO_2 monitoring during resuscitation

1. Tube placement: this is the most reliable method to confirm correct TT placement in the airway, although a CO_2 trace does not exclude endobronchial intubation.

2. Quality of CPR: the more effective chest compressions are, the greater the cardiac output which delivers CO_2 to the lungs where it is exhaled, thus generating a higher end-tidal concentration.

3. Return of spontaneous circulation (ROSC): there will be an immediate, sustained increase in end-tidal CO_2. This may be the first indicator of ROSC and often precedes a palpable pulse.

4. Guide to the rate of ventilation: hyperventilation is common during resuscitation and should be avoided. End-tidal CO_2 can help avoid this.

03: Summary learning

Airway management is the first priority in the care of the critically ill or injured child and is central to successful paediatric resuscitation.

The delivery of high-flow oxygen with the use of simple airway manoeuvres and BMV provides effective first-line management in the critically ill child.

Tracheal intubation is reserved for those experienced in the technique because it has many complications.

Capnography is essential for all patients with an advanced airway. If no trace is present, remember **'No trace, wrong place'**.

My key take-home messages from this chapter are:

Further reading

Blevin AE, McDouall SF, Rechner JA, Saunders TA, Barber VS, Young JD, Mason DG. A comparison of the laryngeal mask airway with the facemask and oropharyngeal airway for manual ventilation by first responders in children. Anaesthesia. 2009;64:1312-6.

Bhende MS, Thompson AE. Evaluation of an end-tidal carbon dioxide detector during pediatric cardiopulmonary resuscitation. Pediatrics 1995; 95:395-399.

P. Van de Voorde, et al., European Resuscitation Council Guidelines 2021: Paediatric Life Support, Resuscitation (2021), https://doi.org/10.1016/j.resuscitation.2021.02.015

Johnson M, Miskovic A, Ray S et al. The nasopharyngeal airway: Estimation of the nares-to-mandible and nares-to-tragus distance in young children to assess current clinical practice. Resuscitation 2019;140:50-54

Ellis DY, et al. Cricoid pressure in emergency department rapid sequence tracheal intubations: a risk-benefit analysis. Ann Emerg Med 2007;50:653-65.

Gausche M, Lewis RJ, Stratton SJ, et al. Effect of out-of-hospital pediatric endotracheal intubation on survival and neurological outcome: a controlled clinical trial. JAMA 2000;283:783-90.

Eich C, Roessler M, Nemeth M, Russo SG, Heuer JF, Timmermann A. Characteristics and outcome of prehospital paediatric tracheal intubation attended by anaesthesia-trained emergency physicians. Resuscitation 2009;80:1371-7.

Ghai B, Wig J. Comparison of different techniques of laryngeal mask placement in children. Curr opin Anesth 2009; 22:4000-404.

Grein AJ, Weiner GM. Laryngeal mask airway versus bag-mask ventilation or endotracheal intubation for neonatal resuscitation. Cochrane Database Systemic Review 2005; CD003314. http://www2.cochrane.org/reviews/en/ab003314

Kwon, JH, et al. Analysis of the functionally-narrowest portion of the pediatric upper airway in sedated children. Medicine, 2018; 97;27:, e11365. https://doi.org/10.1097/MD.0000000000011365

Warner KJ, et al. Prehospital management of the difficult airway: a prospective cohort study. J Emerg Med 2009;36:257-65.

Weiss M, Dullenkopf A, Fischer JE, Keller C, Gerber AC European Paediatric Endotracheal Intubation Study Group. Prospective randomised controlled multi-centre trial of cuffed or uncuffed endotracheal tubes in small children. Br J Anaesth. 2009;103:867-73.

Zelicof-Paul A, Smith-Lockridge A, Schnadower D et al. Controversies in rapid sequence intubation in children. Current Opinion in Pediatrics 2005;17: 355-362.

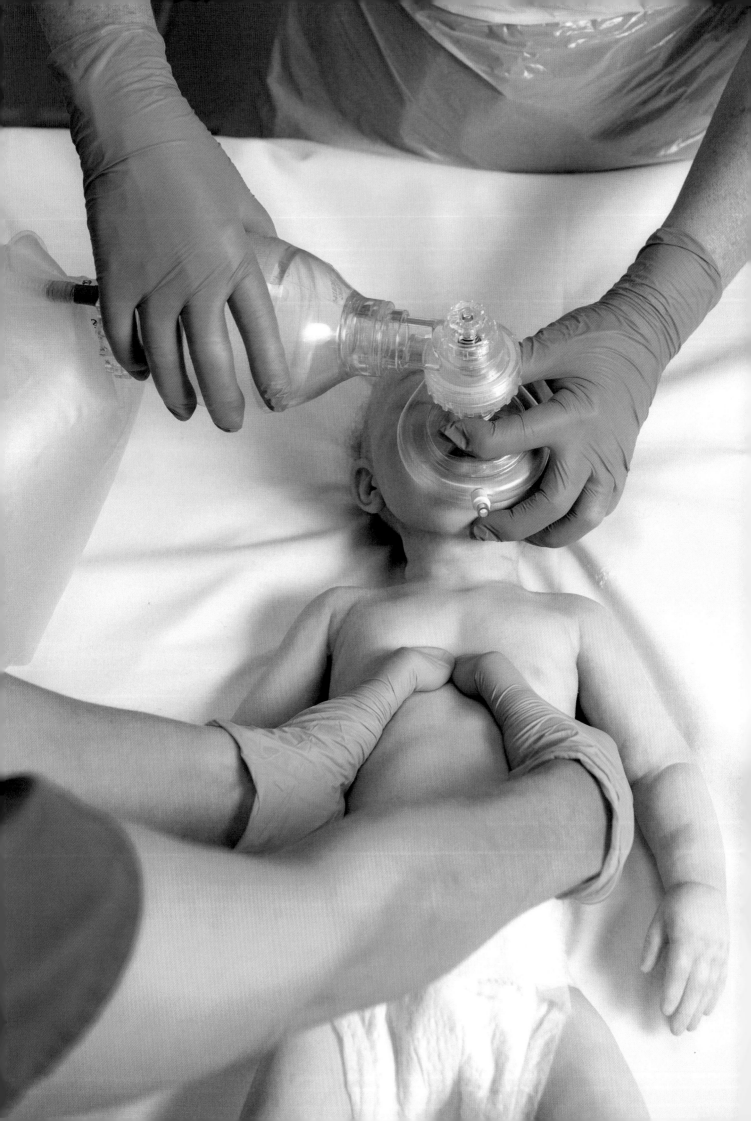

Basic life support

The learning outcomes will enable you to:

Understand the importance of early effective basic life support (BLS) for decreasing mortality and morbidity

Describe how and when to activate the Emergency Medical Service (EMS) or the in-hospital clinical emergency team

Understand the rationale for the sequence of steps in BLS both in and out of hospital

Consider the importance of early appropriate choking management

Understand the rationale for the different techniques of BLS employed in infants and children

Introduction

BLS is the combination of manoeuvres and skills that, without the use of technical adjuncts, provides recognition and management of a person in cardiac or respiratory arrest and 'buys time' until the patient can receive more advanced treatment. BLS must be started as promptly as possible. Its main objective is to achieve sufficient oxygenation and perfusion to 'protect' the brain and other vital organs. Ideally, everyone should possess BLS knowledge and skills. The sequence of actions in BLS is known as cardiopulmonary resuscitation (CPR).

Age definitions

For the purposes of basic life support (BLS), an infant is a child less than one year (excluding newborn (see Chapter 13)), and a child is aged between one year and 18 years. The differences between adult and paediatric resuscitation are largely based on different aetiology; studies have shown that the paediatric causes of arrest continue into early adulthood. If the rescuer believes the patient to be a child, then they should use the paediatric guidelines.

Background

In the management of the collapsed child, several factors are critical in maximising the chances of a good outcome. The most important is early recognition and appropriate intervention in children who exhibit signs of respiratory and/or circulatory compromise. Prevention of cardiorespiratory arrest by managing respiratory distress and/or circulatory failure will help improve the prognosis (Chapters 1 and 2).

Nevertheless, there will always be some children in whom respiratory and/or circulatory collapse cannot be prevented. For these children, early BLS, rapid activation of the Emergency Medical Service (EMS) or in-hospital clinical emergency team, and prompt, effective advanced life support are crucial in improving mortality and morbidity.

> If the rescuer believes the patient to be a child, then they should use the paediatric guidelines

Basic life support sequence

Although unusual, primary cardiac arrest of ventricular fibrillation (VF) or pulseless ventricular tachycardia (pVT) does occasionally occur in children. If this situation is likely, such as a sudden, witnessed collapse of a child with a known cardiac condition, an optimal outcome will depend on early defibrillation. It is then preferable for a lone rescuer to activate the EMS before starting BLS and to use an automated external defibrillator (AED), if available.

However, for the majority of children who suffer cardiorespiratory arrest, the recommended sequence of events is based on two facts:

1. Cardiorespiratory arrest is hypoxic in origin, and therefore the priority is prompt oxygenation provided by rescue breaths or bag-mask ventilation (BMV).

2. The most common cardiac arrhythmia is profound bradycardia deteriorating into asystole; hence effective BLS is more important than access to a defibrillator.

The sequence of actions in paediatric BLS will depend upon the level of training of the rescuer attending:

- Healthcare professionals with a duty to respond to paediatric emergencies should be fully competent in paediatric BLS as they have an obligation to deliver more comprehensive care; this specific sequence is detailed later in this chapter (Figure 4.14).

- Those trained only in 'adult' BLS (may include healthcare providers and lay rescuers) who have no specific knowledge of paediatric resuscitation should use the adult sequence they are familiar with, including paediatric modifications. (Figure 4.1).

- Bystander CPR should be started in all cases when feasible. The EMS dispatcher has a crucial role in assisting lay untrained bystanders to recognise cardiac arrest and provide CPR. When bystander CPR is already in progress at the time of the call, dispatchers may only provide instructions when asked for or when issues with knowledge or skills are identified.

It is important that rescuers follow the specific order of steps in BLS because if one manoeuvre is missed or incorrectly performed, the effectiveness of the next step is also likely to be compromised, hence the order of delivering the resuscitation sequence: Airway (A), Breathing (B) and Circulation (C).

BLS is more effective when the rescuer is proficient in its delivery, but even suboptimal CPR gives a better result than no CPR at all. Hence rescuers unable or unwilling to provide mouth-to-mouth ventilation should be encouraged to perform at least compression-only CPR. A child or infant is far more likely to be harmed if the bystander does nothing.

Out-of-hospital BLS (with paediatric modifications)

S	Safety
S	Stimulate
S	Shout for assistance
A	Airway
B	Breathing
C	Circulation

S – Safety

In all emergencies, quickly assess the situation and ensure the safety of the rescuer(s) and then the child. However, the potential hazards may be different; this is equally important whether the situation occurs within or outside the healthcare environment.

All bodily fluids should be treated as potentially infectious; put on gloves as soon as practicable and use barrier devices for ventilation (e.g. pocket mask) if possible. Whilst the efficacy of face shields is uncertain, and they may not reliably prevent transmission of infection, their use affords some protection and may make it more acceptable for the receipt or delivery of rescue breaths.

On approaching the child, and before touching them, rapidly look for any clues about what may have caused the emergency. This may influence the way the child is managed (e.g. any suspicion of head or neck injury necessitates consideration of cervical spine immobilisation (Chapter 11)).

S – Stimulate

It is important to establish the responsiveness of the unconscious child by tactile and verbal stimulation as they may not be in a critical condition. You can do this by stabilising the child's head by placing one hand on their forehead and then tugging their hair whilst calling their name or telling them to "wake up". Never shake a child vigorously.

If the child responds (e.g. moves, cries, talks):
- leave the child in the position you find them (provided they are not in further danger)
- check their condition and get help if needed
- reassess the child regularly.

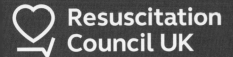
Paediatric out-of-hospital basic life support

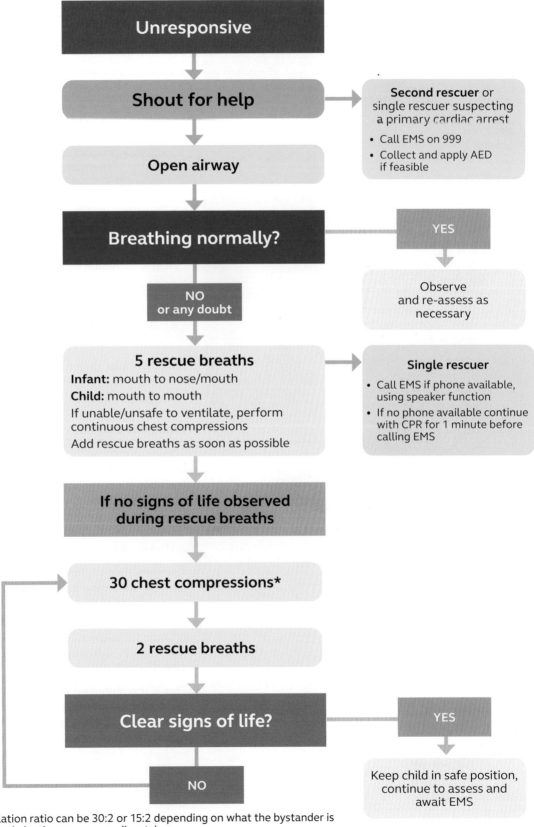

* Chest compression : Ventilation ratio can be 30:2 or 15:2 depending on what the bystander is familiar with/or is directed to do by the emergency dispatcher.

Those trained only in 'adult' BLS (may include healthcare providers and lay rescuers) who have no specific knowledge of paediatric resuscitation, should use the adult sequence they are familiar with, including paediatric modifications.

Figure 4.1   Paediatric out-of-hospital basic life support algorithm (paediatric modifiers)

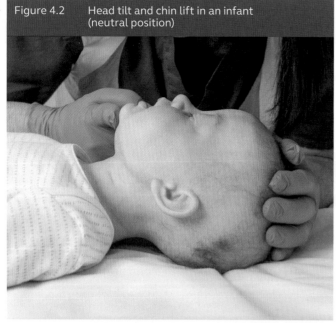

Figure 4.2   Head tilt and chin lift in an infant (neutral position)

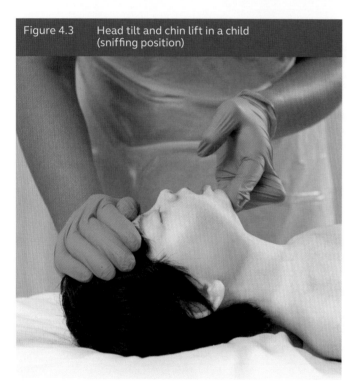

Figure 4.3   Head tilt and chin lift in a child (sniffing position)

S – Shout for assistance

If there is only one rescuer, they must not leave the child, but shout for "help" as they start BLS.

In cases where there is more than one rescuer, a second rescuer should call the EMS immediately upon recognition of unconsciousness, preferably using the speaker function of a mobile phone and collect and apply an automated external defibrillator (AED) if feasible (Table 4.1).

A lone rescuer with no phone dealing with a child who has a witnessed sudden collapse should suspect that this is a primary cardiac arrest. In this situation, a shockable rhythm is likely, and the child may need defibrillation. Seek help immediately if there is no one to go for you.

Table 4.1   **Information required when requesting EMS**

National 999 ambulance request
Is the patient breathing normally?
Precise location/address you are calling from?
What number you are calling from?
What is the reason for your call?
How many casualties?

A Airway

In the unconscious child, the tongue is likely to at least partly occlude their airway. This can usually be overcome by using a head tilt and chin lift manoeuvre or, if necessary, by performing a jaw thrust.

Head tilt and chin lift

This is a simple and effective initial manoeuvre. Turn the child on to their back. To perform the head tilt, approach the child from the side, place one hand on their forehead and gently tilt their head back. In infants, the head should be placed in a neutral position (Figure 4.2). For the child, a 'sniffing' position that causes some extension of the head on the neck will be required (Figure 4.3).

The chin lift is performed by placing the fingertips of the rescuer's other hand on the bony part of the child's lower jaw and lifting the chin upwards. Take care not to compress the soft tissues under the child's jaw as this will occlude the airway.

Jaw thrust

This is the preferred airway opening manoeuvre when cervical spine immobilisation is required. To perform a jaw thrust, approach the child from behind and place hands on either side of the child's head. Two or three fingertips of both hands should be placed under both angles of the child's lower jaw. With thumbs resting gently on the child's cheeks, lift the jaw upwards. The rescuer's elbows should rest on the surface that the child is laid on (Figure 4.4).

Have a low threshold for suspecting injury to the neck. If you suspect this, try to open the airway using jaw thrust alone. If this is unsuccessful, add head tilt gradually until the airway is open. Establishing an open airway takes priority over concerns about the cervical spine.

Whichever airway opening method is used, it is also important for rescuers to look in the child's mouth to ensure there is no obvious foreign body present. If a foreign body is seen and the rescuer is confident that they can remove it safely, this can be attempted; however, blind finger sweeps should never be performed. The management of choking is discussed later in this chapter.

B Breathing

Assessing for normal breathing

After opening the airway, the rescuer needs to assess the child for effective, normal breathing. The best way to do this is to 'look, listen and feel' whilst maintaining the airway opening manoeuvre.

LOOK for chest (and abdominal) movements.

LISTEN for airflow at the mouth and nose (+/- additional noises).

FEEL for airflow at the mouth and nose.

Keeping the airway open, look, listen, and feel for normal breathing by putting your face close to the child's face and looking along the chest whilst simultaneously looking for signs of life. (Figures 4.5 and 4.6)

Signs of life include:
- swallowing
- vocalising
- coughing
- normal (not agonal) breathing.

Look, listen and feel for breath and chest movement
- Listen at the child's nose and mouth for breath sounds.
- Feel for air movement on your cheek.
- In the first few minutes after cardiorespiratory arrest, a child may be taking infrequent, noisy gasps. Do not confuse this with normal breathing.
- Look, listen, and feel for no more than 10 s before deciding; if you have any doubts about whether the breathing is normal, act as if it is not normal.
- Simultaneously look for signs of life.

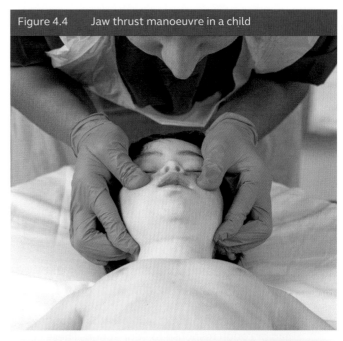
Figure 4.4   Jaw thrust manoeuvre in a child

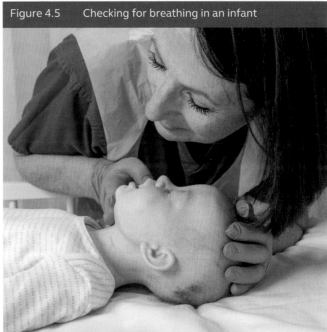
Figure 4.5   Checking for breathing in an infant

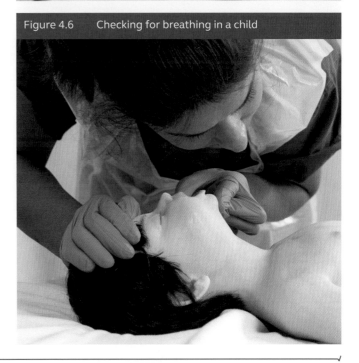
Figure 4.6   Checking for breathing in a child

If the child is breathing normally

- Consider turning the child onto their side into a recovery position (Figure 4.18) or maintain an open airway with a head tilt and chin lift or jaw thrust.
    - If not already done so, call the relevant emergency number (999) on your mobile phone using the speaker function if available. Only leave the child if no other way of obtaining help is possible.
    - Check for continued normal breathing.

If the child's breathing is NOT normal or absent

- Give 5 initial rescue breaths:
    - While performing the rescue breaths, note any gag or cough response to your action. These responses, or their absence, will form part of your ongoing assessment for signs of life.
    - BLS can be undertaken without any adjuncts; however, expired air ventilation provides only 16–17% of oxygen. Oxygen should be given as soon as possible. The trained healthcare provider must provide bag-mask ventilation (BMV) with oxygen as soon as the necessary equipment is available.

Rescue breaths for an infant (Figure 4.7)

- Ensure a neutral position of the head (as an infant's head is usually flexed when supine, this may require some gentle extension) and apply chin lift.
- Take a breath and cover the mouth and nose of the infant with your mouth, making sure you have a good seal.
- If the nose and mouth cannot both be covered in the older infant, the rescuer may attempt to seal only the infant's nose or mouth with their mouth (if the nose is used, close the lips to prevent air escape).
- Blow steadily into the infant's mouth and nose over 1 s, sufficient to make the chest rise visibly. This is the same as in adult practice.
- Maintain the head position and chin lift, take your mouth away, and watch for the chest to fall as air comes out.
- Take another breath and repeat this sequence four more times.
- Identify effectiveness by seeing the infant's chest has risen and fallen in a similar fashion to the movement produced by a normal breath.

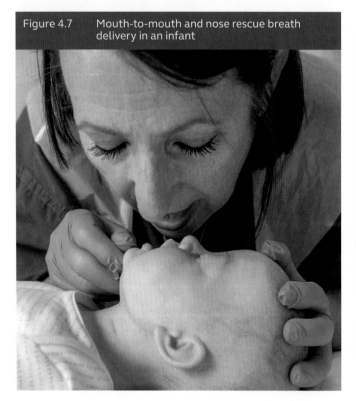

Figure 4.7   Mouth-to-mouth and nose rescue breath delivery in an infant

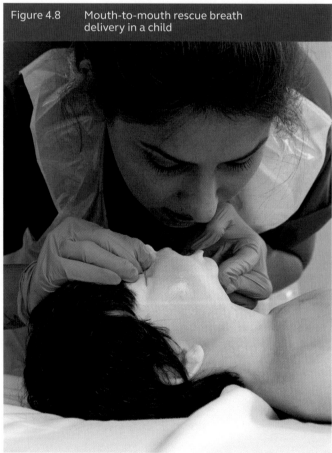

Figure 4.8   Mouth-to-mouth rescue breath delivery in a child

---

Rescue breaths for a child over 1 year (Figure 4.8)

- Ensure head tilt and chin lift, extending the head into a 'sniffing' position.
- Pinch the soft part of the nose closed with the index finger and thumb of your hand on their forehead.
- Open the mouth a little but maintain a chin lift.
- Take a breath and place your lips around the mouth, making sure you have a good seal.
- Blow steadily into their mouth over 1 s, sufficient to make the chest rise visibly.
- Maintain head tilt and chin lift, take your mouth away and watch for the chest to fall as air comes out.
- Take another breath and repeat this sequence four more times.
- Identify effectiveness by seeing the child's chest has risen and fallen in a similar fashion to the movement produced by a normal breath.

For both infants and children, if you have difficulty achieving an effective breath, the airway may be obstructed:

- Open the child's mouth and remove any visible obstruction. Do not perform a blind finger sweep.
- Ensure that there is adequate head tilt and chin lift but also that the neck is not overextended; try repositioning the head to open the airway.
- If head tilt and chin lift has not opened the airway, try the jaw thrust method.
- Take up to 5 attempts to achieve an effective breath. If still unsuccessful, move on to chest compressions.

If there is only one rescuer with a mobile phone, they should call for help (and activate the speaker function) immediately after the 5 initial rescue breaths. Proceed to the next step while waiting for an answer. If no phone is readily available, perform 1 min of CPR before leaving the child. To minimise any interruptions in CPR, it may be possible to carry an infant or small child whilst summoning help.

In cases where paediatric BLS providers are unable or unwilling to start with rescue breaths, they should proceed with chest compressions and add ventilations into the sequence as soon as this can be done.

Following the rescue breaths if you are confident that you can detect signs of life:

- Continue ventilations (12–30 breaths per min or as guided by EMS dispatcher), if necessary, until the child starts breathing effectively on their own.
- Unconscious children and infants who are not in cardiac arrest and have normal breathing can have their airway kept open by either continued head tilt and chin lift or jaw thrust. If there is a perceived risk of vomiting, positioning the unconscious child in a recovery position.
- Reassess the child frequently.

C Circulation

Following the rescue breaths, if there are no signs of life or you are unsure, immediately start high-quality chest compressions.

Principles of chest compressions

Chest compressions are serial, rhythmic compressions of the anterior chest wall, intended to cause blood to flow to vital organ tissues in an attempt to keep them viable until the return of spontaneous circulation (ROSC) is achieved.

High-quality chest compressions

- Rate: 100–120 min^{-1} for both infants and children.
- Depth: depress the lower half of the sternum by at least one-third of the anterior-posterior dimension of the chest (which is approximately 4 cm for an infant and 5 cm for a child).
- Compressions should never be deeper than the adult 6 cm limit (approximately an adult thumb's length).
  - To avoid compressing the upper abdomen, locate the xiphisternum by finding the angle where the lowest ribs join the sternum (breastbone).
  - Compress the sternum one finger's breadth above this.
- Release all pressure on the chest between compressions to allow for complete chest recoil. Avoid leaning on the chest at the end of a compression.
- Allow adequate time for chest recoil to occur (approximately 50% of the whole cycle should be the relaxation phase (i.e. from the start of one compression to the next)).
- After 30 chest compressions, tilt the head, lift the chin, and give 2 rescue breaths.
- Continue compressions and breaths in a ratio of 30:2 (healthcare professionals with a duty to respond to paediatric emergencies may use the ratio of 15:2 as described later in this chapter).
- Perform compressions on a firm surface.
- Pauses in chest compressions should be minimised so that 80% or more of the CPR cycle is comprised of chest compressions.
- The best method for compressions varies slightly between infants and children.

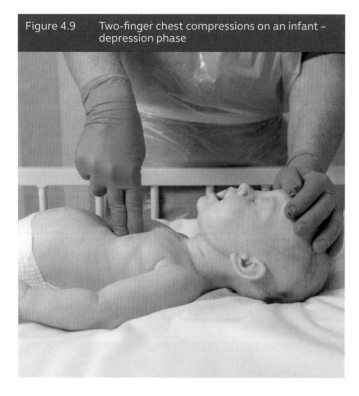

Figure 4.9   Two-finger chest compressions on an infant – depression phase

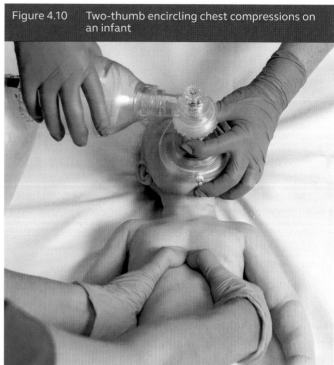

Figure 4.10   Two-thumb encircling chest compressions on an infant

Chest compressions in infants

Two-finger technique

This is the recommended method of infant chest compressions for the lone rescuer. Having landmarked as described above, place two fingers of one hand in the correct position on the sternum and depress it by at least one-third of the depth of the infant's chest, approximately 4cm (Figure 4.9).

Two-thumb encircling technique

This is the recommended method of infant chest compressions for two rescuers. There is evidence that this method delivers greater cardiac output than the two-finger technique; however, it is difficult for a single rescuer to perform and also deliver timely and effective rescue breaths. It is, therefore, usually reserved for in-hospital resuscitation, where there are two rescuers and ventilation delivery devices (Figure 4.10).

The two-thumb encircling technique:

- Place both thumbs flat, side-by-side, on the lower half of the sternum (as above), with the tips pointing towards the infant's head.

- Spread the rest of both hands, with the fingers together, to encircle the lower part of the infant's ribcage with tips of the fingers supporting the infant's back. Press down on the lower sternum with your two thumbs to depress it at least one-third of the depth of the infant's chest, approximately 4 cm.

- For small infants you may need to overlap your thumbs to provide effective compressions.

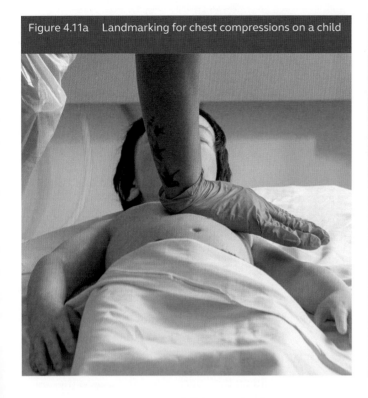

Figure 4.11a   Landmarking for chest compressions on a child

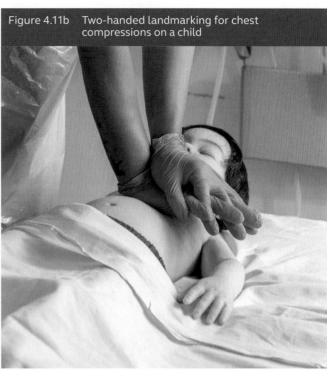

Figure 4.11b   Two-handed landmarking for chest compressions on a child

Chest compressions in children aged over 1 year

- Place the heel of one hand over the lower half of the sternum (as above).
- Lift the fingers to ensure that pressure is not applied over the child's ribs.
- Position yourself vertically above the child's chest and, with your arm straight, compress the sternum by at least one-third of the depth of the chest, approximately 5 cm.
- In larger children, or for small rescuers, this may be achieved by using both hands with fingers interlocked.

Do not interrupt CPR at any moment unless there are clear signs of life (e.g. normal breathing, coughing). Two or more rescuers should alternate who is performing chest compressions frequently; the compressing rescuer should switch hands (the hand compressing with the hand which is on top) or the technique (one to two-handed) to avoid fatigue (Figure 4.11a, 4.11b).

Continue resuscitation until:

- the child shows signs of life (e.g. normal breathing, coughing, movement)
- additional qualified help arrives
- the rescuer becomes exhausted.

Automated external defibrillators (AEDs)

- In children and infants with cardiac arrest, a lone rescuer should immediately start CPR.
- In cases where the likelihood of a primary shockable rhythm is extremely high, such as in sudden witnessed collapse, the lone rescuer should activate the EMS and apply an AED if readily available. When there is more than one rescuer, the second rescuer should immediately call for help and then collect and apply an AED (if available) while the first rescuer continues with CPR.
- Trained providers should limit the no-flow time when using an AED by performing CPR up to the point of analysis and immediately after the shock delivery or no shock decision; pads should be applied with minimal or no interruption in CPR.
- If possible, use an AED with a paediatric attenuator in infants and children younger than 8 years (e.g. energy reduced to 50–75 J). If this is not available, use a standard AED for all ages.

There have been continuing reports of safe and successful use of AEDs in children less than 8 years, demonstrating that AEDs can identify arrhythmias accurately in children and are extremely unlikely to advise a shock inappropriately.

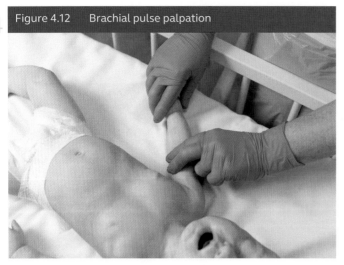
Figure 4.12   Brachial pulse palpation

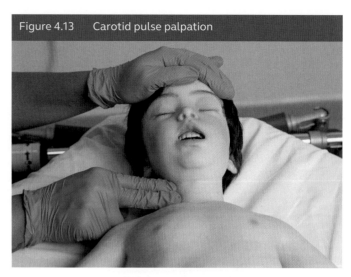
Figure 4.13   Carotid pulse palpation

In-hospital BLS

The following is the sequence to be used by health care professionals with a duty to respond to paediatric emergencies.

S	Safety
S	Stimulate
S	Shout for assistance
A	Airway
B	Breathing
C	Circulation

S – Safety

In all emergencies, quickly assess the situation and ensure the safety of the rescuer(s) and then the child. However, the potential hazards may be different; this is equally important whether the situation occurs within or outside the healthcare environment.

All bodily fluids should be treated as potentially infectious; put on the required level of personal protective equipment (PPE).

S – Stimulate

Check for a response as described earlier.

If the child responds:
- assess ABCDE (O_2, monitoring, vascular access)
- call for further assistance as appropriate.

S – Shout for assistance

If there is no response:
- call for help/emergency buzzer
- activate 2222 for clinical emergency team.

Information required when requesting in-hospital clinical emergency team - 2222
Precise location of the emergency
Specific clinical emergency team required (e.g. paediatric resuscitation, paediatric trauma)
Any other local policy requirements

A Airway

Position the child on their back, open and assess the airway as previously described.

B Breathing

Assess for normal breathing whilst simultaneously looking for signs of life. Studies have shown how unreliable feeling for a pulse is in determining the presence or absence of a circulation even for trained paediatric healthcare professionals, hence the importance of looking for signs of life. However, if a health care professional wishes to check for a pulse, this should be done simultaneously with the breathing assessment. In infants, the recommended sites for pulse palpation are the brachial or femoral artery (Figure 4.12), and in the child, it is the carotid or femoral artery (Figure 4.13).

If the child is breathing normally

- Consider turning the child onto their side into a recovery position (Figure 4.18) or maintain an open airway with a head tilt and chin lift or jaw thrust.
  - Check for continued normal breathing.
  - Check ABCDE and treat as required.

If the child's breathing is NOT normal or absent

- Give 5 initial rescue breaths.
  - Provide ventilation initially by bag-mask ventilation (BMV), using a high concentration of inspired oxygen (100%) as soon as this is available. To provide an adequate seal to the mask, a two-person technique is advocated. (Chapter 3, Figure 3.11).

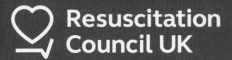

Paediatric basic life support

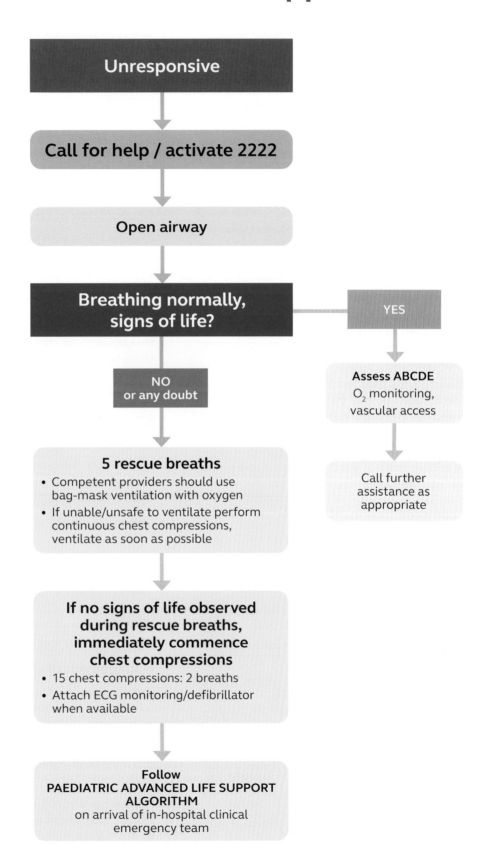

Figure 4.14   Paediatric basic life support algorithm

63

Following the rescue breaths if you are confident that you can detect signs of life

- Continue BMV if necessary until the child starts breathing effectively on their own or until the arrival of the in-hospital clinical emergency team.

c Circulation

Following the rescue breaths, if there are no signs of life or if you are unsure, immediately start high-quality chest compressions.

High-quality chest compressions

- Rate: 100–120 min^{-1} for both infants and children.
- Depth: depress the lower half of the sternum by at least one-third of the anterior-posterior dimension of the chest (which is approximately 4 cm for an infant and 5 cm for a child).
- Compressions should never be deeper than the adult 6 cm limit.
- Release all pressure on the chest between compressions to allow for complete chest recoil and avoid leaning on the chest at the end of a compression.
- Allow adequate time for chest recoil to occur (approximately 50% of the whole cycle should be the relaxation phase (i.e. from the start of one compression to the next)).
- Chest compression pauses should be minimised so that 80% or more of the CPR cycle is comprised of chest compressions.

Chest compressions in infants

Preferably use the two thumb encircling method; if this is not possible, use the two-finger technique.

Chest compressions in children over 1 year

- Use one hand; for larger children or smaller rescuers, use both hands with fingers interlocked.
- Landmarks for chest compressions are as described earlier in this chapter.
- Continue chest compressions and breaths at a ratio of 15:2.
- Attach ECG monitoring/defibrillator when available, minimising any interruptions to CPR.

Continue with this sequence until the arrival of the in-hospital clinical emergency team or until the child starts to show signs of life.

Choking

When a foreign body enters their airway, a child will react immediately by coughing in an attempt to expel it. A child who is choking on a foreign body but can still cough effectively must be actively encouraged to do so. A spontaneous cough is not only safer, but it is probably more effective than any manoeuvre a rescuer might perform.

However, if coughing is absent or becoming ineffective, the child's airway is at risk of complete obstruction, which will rapidly result in asphyxiation. Any child, who is unable to effectively cough due to foreign body aspiration, requires immediate interventions (Figure 4.15).

Recognition of choking

Choking is characterised by the sudden onset of respiratory distress associated with coughing, gagging or stridor.

The majority of choking events in infants and children occur during play or feeding and are therefore frequently witnessed by an adult, which means interventions can start immediately. However, it is important to be aware that the signs of choking (Table 4.2) can be confused with those of other causes of airway obstruction (e.g. laryngitis or epiglottitis), which require different management.

Table 4.2   Signs of choking

General signs	
Witnessed episode	
Coughing or choking	
Sudden onset	
Recent history of playing with or eating small objects	
Ineffective cough	Effective cough
Unable to vocalise	Crying or verbal response to questions
Quiet or silent cough	Loud cough
Unable to breathe	Able to take a breath before coughing
Cyanosis	Fully responsive
Decreasing level of consciousness	

Management of choking

If the child is coughing effectively, no external manoeuvre is necessary. Encourage the child to cough and observe them closely.

If the child's coughing is absent or becoming ineffective, shout for help and quickly determine the child's conscious level.

Management of obstructed airway in-hospital may include the use of suction/laryngoscopy/magills forceps by experienced personnel. Out of hospital, the use of existing anti-choking devices in the first aid of a choking infant/child is not recommended due to the lack of available evidence to date.

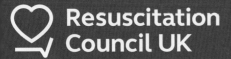

Paediatric foreign body airway obstruction

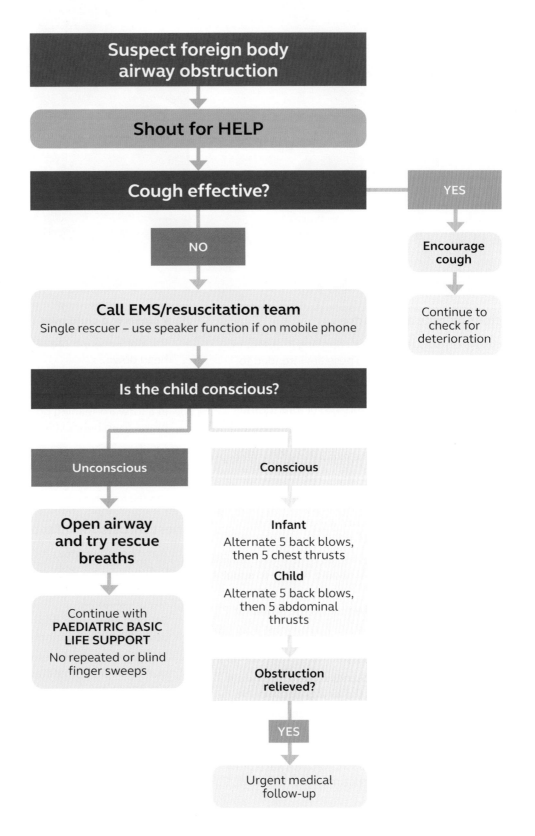

Figure 4.15   Paediatric foreign body airway obstruction algorithm

Figure 4.16	Delivery of back blows to an infant

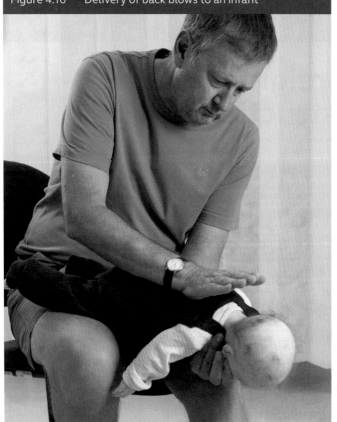

Figure 4.17	Delivery of back blows to a child

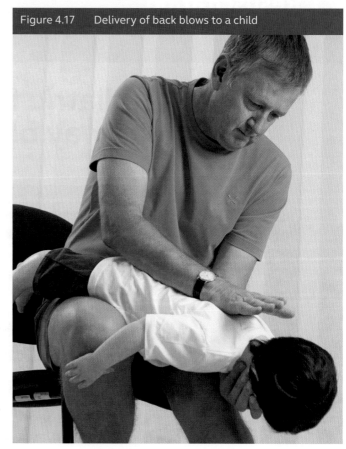

Conscious infants and children

If the child is conscious, but their coughing is absent or ineffective, deliver back blows. These are intended to loosen the object for the child to be able to then expel it. If back blows do not relieve the airway obstruction, thrusts should be given; chest thrusts for infants and abdominal thrusts for children. These thrusts are intended as an 'artificial cough'; they increase the intrathoracic pressure, which will facilitate the expulsion of the foreign body.

Back blows in an infant

- Support the infant in a head-downwards, prone position to enable gravity to assist in removing the foreign body (Figure 4.16).
- A seated or kneeling rescuer should be able to support the infant across their lap.
- Support the infant's head by placing the thumb of one hand at the angle of the lower jaw and one or two fingers from the same hand at the same point on the other side of the jaw.
- Do not compress the soft tissues under the infant's jaw, as this will exacerbate the airway obstruction.
- Deliver up to 5 sharp back blows with the heel of one hand in the middle of the back between the shoulder blades.
- The aim is to relieve the obstruction with each blow rather than to give all 5 (hence may not require all 5 if successful).

Back blows in a child over 1 year

- Back blows are more effective if the child is positioned head down.
- A small child may be placed across the rescuer's lap as with an infant. If this is not possible, support the child in a forward-leaning position and deliver the back blows from behind (Figure 4.17).

If back blows do not relieve the airway obstruction, and the child is still conscious, give chest thrusts to infants or abdominal thrusts to children. Do not use abdominal thrusts (Heimlich manoeuvre) for infants.

Chest thrusts for infants

- Turn the infant into a head-downwards supine position. This is achieved safely by placing your free arm along the infant's back and encircling the occiput with your hand.
- Support the infant down your arm, which is placed down (or across) your thigh.
- Identify the landmark for chest compression (lower sternum approximately a finger's breadth above the xiphisternum).
- Deliver up to 5 chest thrusts. These are similar to chest compressions but sharper in nature and delivered at a slower rate.
- The aim is to relieve the obstruction with each thrust rather than to give all 5 (hence, if successful all 5 may not be required).

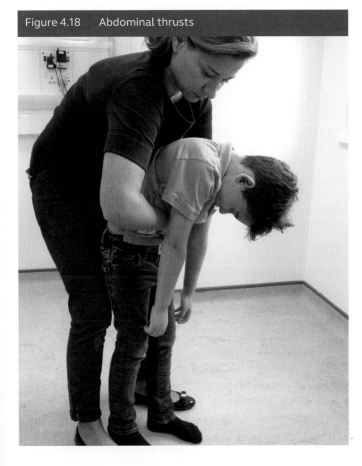

Figure 4.18   Abdominal thrusts

Abdominal thrusts for children over 1 year:

- Stand or kneel behind the child. Place your arms under the child's arms and encircle their torso (Figure 4.18).
- Clench your fist and place it between the umbilicus and xiphisternum.
- Grasp your fist with the other hand and pull sharply inwards and upwards.
- Repeat up to 4 more times.
- Ensure that pressure is not applied to the xiphoid process or the lower rib cage as this may cause abdominal trauma.
- The aim is to relieve the obstruction with each thrust rather than to give all 5 (hence, if successful all 5 may not be required).

Following chest or abdominal thrusts, reassess the infant/child

- If the object has not been expelled and the patient is still conscious, continue the sequence of back blows and chest thrusts for an infant or abdominal thrusts for children.
- Call out, or send for help if it is still not available.
- Do not leave the infant/child at this stage.
- If the object has not been expelled and the patient is still conscious, continue the sequence.

If the object is expelled successfully:

- Assess the infant or child's clinical condition.
- It is possible that part of the object may remain in the respiratory tract and cause complications.

- If there is any doubt or if the child was treated with abdominal thrusts, urgent medical follow up is mandatory.

If the infant/child with foreign body airway obstruction is, or becomes, unconscious, move to treatment with the paediatric BLS algorithm

Call for help if it is still not available.

- Airway opening:
  - When the airway is opened for attempted delivery of rescue breaths, look to see if the foreign body can be seen in the mouth.
  - If an object is seen, attempt to remove it with a single finger sweep.
  - Do not attempt blind or repeated finger sweeps; these can push the object more deeply into the pharynx and cause injury.
- Rescue breaths:
  - Open the airway and attempt 5 rescue breaths.
  - Assess the effectiveness of each breath: if a breath does not make the chest rise, reposition the head before making the next attempt.
- Chest compressions and CPR:
  - Proceed immediately to chest compressions regardless of whether the breaths are successful and perform CPR as previously described.
  - Continue with paediatric BLS using a compression and ventilation ratio of 15:2 (or the ratio you are familiar with) until help arrives or the child improves.
  - If the child regains consciousness and is breathing effectively, place them in the recovery position and monitor breathing and conscious level whilst awaiting the EMS/in-hospital clinical emergency team.

Recovery position

For children and infants with a decreased level of consciousness who do not meet the criteria for the initiation of rescue breathing or chest compressions (CPR), the recovery position may be recommended (Figure 4.19). The following describes one method of achieving a left lateral position:

- Kneel beside the child and make sure that both their legs are straight.
- Place their arm nearest to you out at a right angle to the body, elbow bent with the hand palm uppermost.
- Bring their far arm across the chest, and hold the back of their hand against the child's cheek nearest to you.
- With your other hand, grasp their far leg just above the knee and pull it up, keeping the foot on the ground.

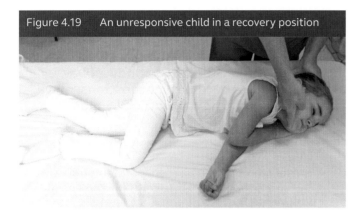

Figure 4.19   An unresponsive child in a recovery position

- Keeping their hand pressed against the cheek, pull on their far leg to roll the child towards you onto their side.
- Adjust their upper leg so that both hip and knee are bent at right angles.
- Tilt the head back to make sure the airway remains open.
- Adjust their hand under the cheek if necessary to keep the head tilted and facing downwards to allow liquid material to drain from the mouth.
- Check breathing regularly.
- Ensure the position is stable. In an infant, this may require the support of a small pillow or a rolled-up blanket placed behind their back to maintain the position.

It is important to maintain a close check on all unconscious patients until the EMS arrives to ensure that their breathing remains normal (check breathing at least once every minute).

Avoid any pressure on the child or infant's chest that may impair breathing and regularly turn the unconscious child or infant over onto their opposite side to prevent pressure injuries whilst in the recovery position (i.e. every 30 min).

In certain situations, such as when the child or infant is breathing spontaneously but requires airway management, the recovery position is not recommended. In these circumstances:

- Keep the patient flat, maintain an open airway by either continued head tilt and chin lift or jaw thrust
- For a child or infant with traumatic injuries, leave them lying flat, open and maintain their airway using a jaw thrust, taking care to avoid spinal rotation.

04: Summary learning

Rescuers must always ensure their own safety before undertaking BLS.

The preferred ratio of chest compressions to ventilations is 15:2 when BLS is being delivered by healthcare professionals but in some instances it may be appropriate to adopt the standard adult 30:2 sequence.

Management of conscious choking infants consists of back blows followed by chest thrusts.

Management of conscious choking children consists of back blows followed by abdominal thrusts.

Management of unconscious infants and children as a result of choking requires BLS to be performed.

My key take-home messages from this chapter are:

Further reading

Tsou JY, Kao CL, Chang CJ, Tu YF, Su FC, Chi CH. Biomechanics of two- thumb versus two-finger chest compression for cardiopulmonary resuscitation in an infant manikin model. Eur J Emerg Med 2020;27:132.

Nadkarni VM, Larkin GL, Peberdy MA, Carey SM, Kaye W, Mancini ME, et al. First documented rhythm and clinical outcome from in-hospital cardiac arrest among children and adults. JAMA. 2006 Jan 4;295(1):50-7.

Kitamura T, Iwami T, Kawamura T, Nagao K, Tanaka H, Nadkarni VM, et al. Conventional and chest-compression-only cardiopulmonary resuscitation by bystanders for children who have out-of-hospital cardiac arrests: a prospective, nationwide, population-based cohort study. Lancet. 2010 Apr 17;375(9723):1347-54.

Kao PC, Chiang WC, Yang CW, Chen SJ, Liu YP, Lee CC, et al. What is the correct depth of chest compression for infants and children? A radiological study. Pediatrics. 2009 Jul;124(1):49-55.

Meyer A, Nadkarni V, Pollock A, Babbs C, Nishisaki A, Braga M, et al. Evaluation of the Neonatal Resuscitation Program's recommended chest compression depth using computerised tomography imaging. Resuscitation. 2010 May;81(5):544-8.

Sutton RM, Niles D, Nysaether J, Arbogast KB, Nishisaki A, Maltese MR, et al. Pediatric CPR quality monitoring: analysis of thoracic anthropometric data. Resuscitation. 2009 Oct;80(10):1137-41.

Babbs SF, Nadkarni V. Optimizing chest compression to rescue ventilation ratios during one-rescue CPR by professionals and laypersons: children are not just little adults. Resuscitation 2004; 61:173-81.

Berg RA, Hilwig RW et al. "Simulated mouth-to-mouth ventilation and chest compressions (bystander cardiopulmonary resuscitation) improves outcome in a swine model of prehospital pediatric asphyxial cardiac arrest." Crit Care Med 1999; 27(9):1893-1899.

Berg RA, Hilwig RW et al. "Bystander" chest compressions and assisted ventilation independently improve outcome from piglet asphyxial pulseless "cardiac arrest". Circulation 2000; 101(14):1743-1748.

Tibballs J, Russell P. Reliability of pulse palpation by healthcare personnel to diagnose paediatric cardiac arrest. Resuscitation. 2009 Jan;80(1):61-4.

Couper K, Hassan A, Ohri V, Patterson E, Tang H, Bingham R, Olasveengen T, Perkins G. On behalf of the International Liaison Committee on Resuscitation Basic and Paediatric Life Support Task Force Collaborators. Removal of foreign body airway obstruction: A systematic review of interventions. Resuscitation 2020; 156:174-181

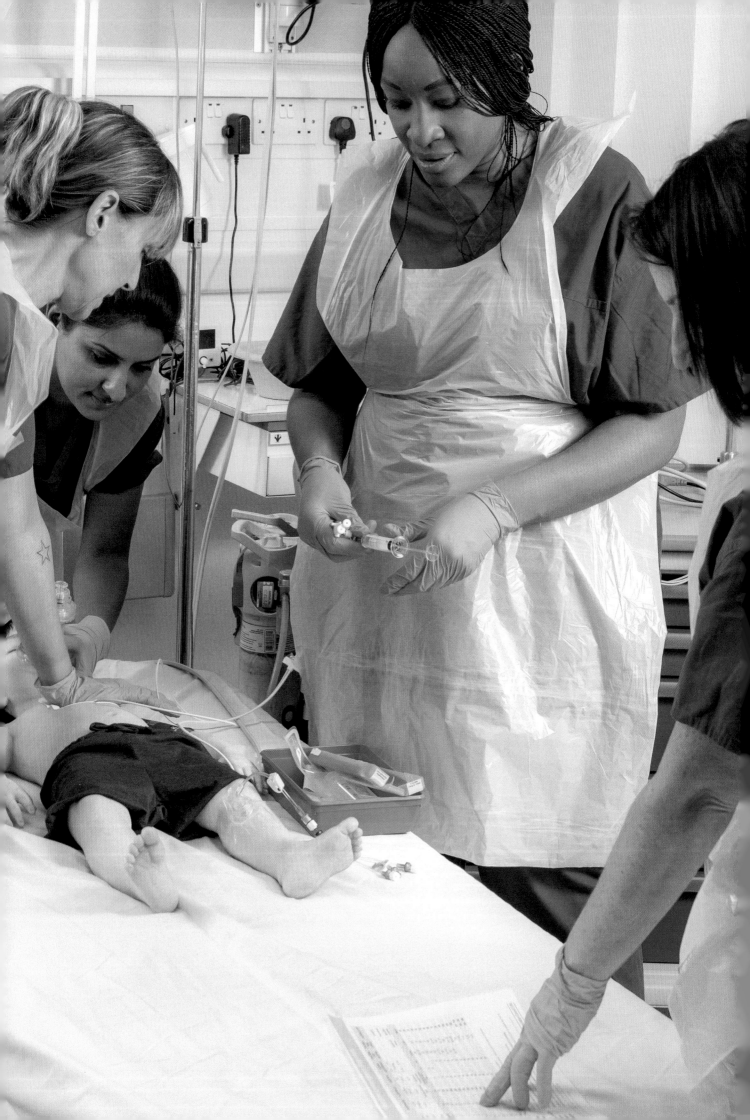

Advanced management of circulation and drugs

In this chapter

Establishment of circulatory access

Fluid administration

First-line resuscitation medications

The learning outcomes will enable you to:

Consider the requirement for circulatory access during resuscitation

Describe the different routes of emergency circulatory access and their appropriate use

Discuss the advantages and potential complications of intraosseous access

Understand the type and volume of fluids to be administered in the emergency situation

Understand the indications, dosages and actions of the first-line medications used in cardiorespiratory arrest

Circulatory access

Once the airway is patent and adequate ventilation of the child is established, attention must be focused on circulation. The exception is for the child who presents with life-threatening haemorrhage when circulation would be attended simultaneously with A and B assessment by a trauma team.

Establish circulatory access within the first few minutes of resuscitation or following the recognition of signs of shock in order that medications can be administered (e.g. adrenaline), fluids can be given, and blood samples can be obtained.

Circulatory access may be achieved via the intravenous (IV) or intraosseous (IO) routes. The tracheal route is no longer recommended because of the variability in alveolar drug absorption.

Circulatory access may be achieved via the intravenous (IV) or intraosseous (IO) routes

For children who are unwell but remain responsive to pain, IV access is preferred over IO if possible, as infusions of fluids and drugs via the IO route can be painful. Children and infants have small calibre, mobile veins and are uncooperative and stressed during intravenous access attempts. The use of transillumination, near-infrared light and ultrasound may improve visualisation of superficial veins if available. Other methods to aid successful insertion include techniques to reduce anxiety such as breastfeeding or oral sucrose in infants, tourniquets, tapping the veins, local warming of the area and topical anaesthetic creams in children. If there is an IV cannula already in situ, check its patency before use; otherwise, insert the largest possible IV cannula in a peripheral vein e.g. the antecubital fossa (Figure 5.1a), the long saphenous vein (Figure 5.1b) or the back of the hand (or feet in smaller children). The length of time employed attempting intravenous access will be guided by the clinical state of the child. In cardiorespiratory arrest and/or severe shock states, when peripheral circulation is severely compromised, the IO route is the preferred method of gaining vascular access. If intravenous access attempts are made, they should be limited to 2 attempts in 5 mins before gaining intraosseous access.

The use of scalp veins during resuscitation is not advisable due to the risk of extravasation, leading to potential tissue necrosis. Their use may also interfere with the management of the airway and ventilation. If the child requires chest compressions, these should not be interrupted by access attempts or other procedures apart from defibrillation.

Some drugs and fluids cannot be given via peripheral IV access; these include calcium solutions, hyperosmolar fluids and those with a pH < 5 or > 9. Catecholamines (e.g. adrenaline, noradrenaline, dopamine) may be given peripherally initially (in dilute solutions), and should ideally be infused through a dedicated line. If continuous catecholamine therapy is required as part of the ongoing resuscitation of the child, then IO or central IV access is preferred as tissue necrosis may occur if extravasated.

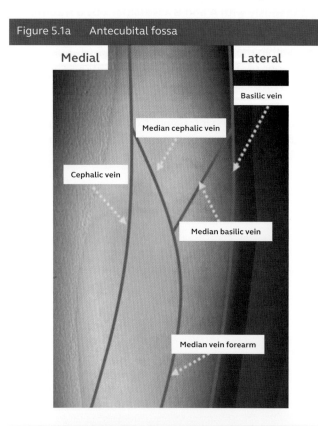

Figure 5.1a   Antecubital fossa

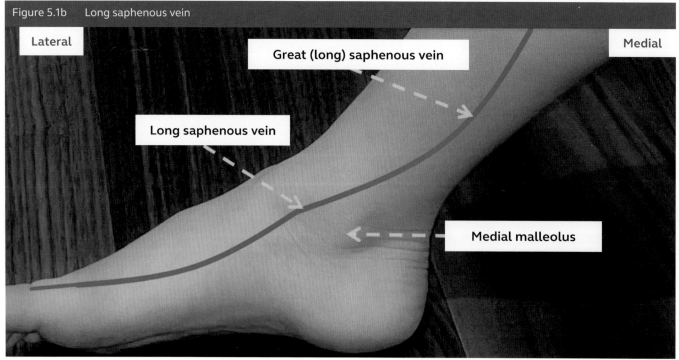

Figure 5.1b   Long saphenous vein

Intraosseous access

IO access is indicated in children, infants, or newborns in any clinical situation where vascular access is urgently required but not immediately available via a peripheral vein. This may include cardiorespiratory arrest, shock, life-threatening status epilepticus and burns.

In these situations, gaining vascular access via the IO route rather than the peripheral, umbilical or central routes may be safer, faster to achieve and associated with fewer complications. It requires less skill and practice on the part of practitioners who may use the techniques only rarely and has a high success rate.

Additionally, further IV access is easier to obtain once a fluid bolus and medications have been administered via the IO needle. Usually, IO needles are removed as soon as another means of vascular access (either peripheral or central) is available and ideally within 24 h.

IO needles are usually placed in the proximal or distal ends of long bones. The IO needle is inserted through the skin, periosteum, then cortex of the bone so that the needle lies in the medullary (or marrow) cavity. The medullary cavity provides access to a non-collapsible venous plexus which drains into the central venous circulation via emissary veins. When accessed with an IO needle, medications and fluid will pass from the medullary space through the vascular system into the central circulation (Figure 5.2).

The main advantages of IO access are:

- The relative ease and speed of insertion.
- It can be used to deliver all resuscitation fluids, medications and blood-derived products.
- It allows rapid adequate plasma concentration of medications similar to that of central venous administration (more rapid and reliable than that achieved through a peripheral IV).
- It allows bone marrow aspiration, which can be used for analysis. In this situation, the laboratory should be informed as the fat in a marrow sample may cause damage to auto-analysers. There are currently no point of care tests able to analyse a bone marrow sample.

Insertion of an intraosseous cannula

Before undertaking this procedure, the appropriate equipment must be available, and there should be no contraindications to IO insertion.

Insertion site – anatomical landmarks

The site used for IO access will vary as appropriate for the age of the patient. The insertion site of choice in infants and children is the proximal tibia with the distal tibia and distal femur as alternative access sites. With increasing age, the cortical thickness of long bones, particularly the tibia increases, making penetration more difficult and requiring greater force. Therefore, in older children and adults, the distal tibia or proximal humerus may be preferable.

Figure 5.2   Intraosseous space and relationship with circulation

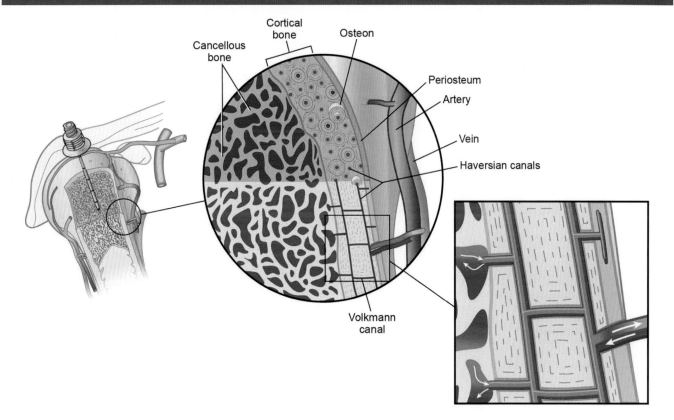

Proximal tibia

This is the most common insertion site for IO in infants and children because there is a flat wide surface of bone with a thin layer of overlying tissue (this allows easy identification of landmarks). Additionally, the tibia is away from the airway and chest so that resuscitation efforts are not impeded by access attempts (Figure 5.3).

Landmarks – newborns, infants and small children

The insertion site is located approximately 1 cm (1 fingerbreadth) below and 1 cm (1 fingerbreadth) medial to the tibial tuberosity on the anteromedial surface of the tibia. In some, the tuberosity cannot be palpated as it may not have developed sufficiently; in this situation, the insertion point is 2–3 cm distal to and 1 cm medial to the lower end of the patella.

Landmarks – older children and adolescents

2–3 cm below and medial to tibial tuberosity on the anteromedial surface of the tibia.

Distal tibia

Landmarks – newborns, infants and small children

1–2 cm proximal to the most prominent aspect of the medial malleolus.

Landmarks – older children and adolescents

3 cm proximal to the most prominent aspect of the medial malleolus on the flat centre aspect of the bone (Figure 5.4). This site is preferred in older children as there is less cortical thickening.

Distal femur

Landmarks – newborns, infants and small children (< 6 years) only

Hold the leg straight with the knee held straight and immobilised; insert the IO needle into the centro-medial aspect of the distal femur (medial to avoid the central tendon), 1–2 cm above the patella and 1–2 cm medial to the midline (Figure 5.5). The knee must remain immobilised until the IO is removed.

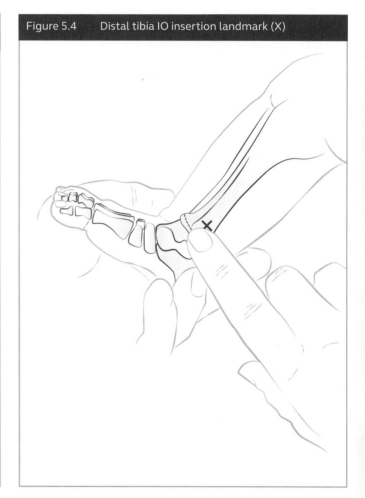

| Figure 5.3 | Proximal tibia IO insertion landmark (X) circulation |
| Figure 5.4 | Distal tibia IO insertion landmark (X) |

Proximal humerus

Landmark

The most prominent aspect of the greater tubercle of the humeral head. Only use in young children if landmarks can be reliably identified and if there is pelvic and/or lower limb trauma preventing the use of the tibia. Generally, successful insertion in the humeral head requires more training and experience.

To identify this landmark:

1. Place the patient's hand on their abdomen (to adduct the elbow and internally rotate the humerus).

2. Place the palm of your hand over the humeral head anteriorly (it should feel like a ball and is the general area where the IO will be inserted (Figure 5.6).

3. Place the ulnar aspect of your hand vertically over the axilla, then the ulnar aspect of your other hand along the midline of the upper arm laterally, then join your thumbs together – this point will identify the vertical line of insertion on the proximal humerus.

4. Feel proximally along the insertion line identifying the surgical neck of the humerus (this is where the humeral bone shaft meets the ball-like head of the humerus). The insertion site is 1–2 cm above the surgical neck on the most prominent aspect of the greater tubercle.

5. Insert the needle using a downward angle.

Contraindications
Contraindications to the insertion of an IO include osteogenesis imperfecta ('brittle bone' disease) and haemophilia or other known coagulopathies.
IO cannulation should not be sited through an area of infected skin or wounds.
Fractured bones must not be used, nor should the cannula be inserted into a bone immediately distal to a fracture site, as this may predispose to the development of compartment syndrome; similarly, if the bone has had a previous IO inserted in it within the last 48 h it should not be used.

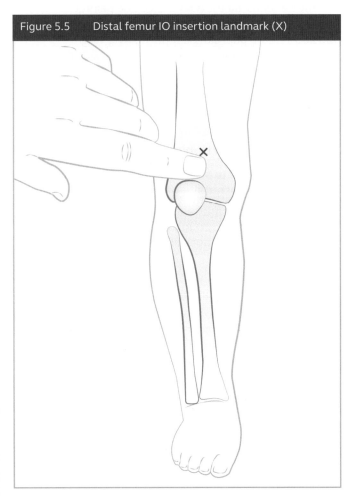

Figure 5.5   Distal femur IO insertion landmark (X)

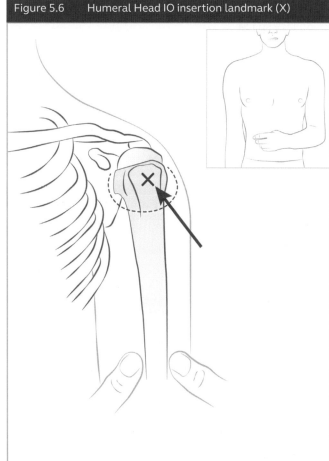

Figure 5.6   Humeral Head IO insertion landmark (X)

Equipment required

1. IO cannulae

Several IO needles are available commercially, such as the Cook and Jamshidi needles (Figure 5.7), but powered needle devices such as the EZ-IO drill (Figure 5.8) are becoming more popular. There appears to be little difference in the success rate of obtaining IO access between powered and manual devices, but studies have shown that powered devices are more readily used by staff.

IO cannulae have a trocar, and manual varieties come in a variety of sizes. Generally, it is recommended that size 18 gauge is used for a newborn to 6 months of age, 16 gauge for a child between 6–18 months, and 14 gauge for children > 18 months.

The powered EZ-IO device needles are all 15 gauge but come in a variety of lengths for different weights (15, 25, 45 mm). There is a black 5 mm depth marking on the side of the needle, which should remain visible after pushing the needle through the soft tissue to rest on the periosteum (prior to utilising the drill mechanism); otherwise, the needle will not be long enough to reach the medullary space.

Additional IO cannulae should be available in case of insertion difficulties or the need to secure further vascular access (e.g. infusion of vasoactive medications; in cases of trauma where large volumes of fluid need to be rapidly infused). If there is no dedicated IO cannula available, bone marrow aspiration or spinal (lumbar puncture) needles can be used.

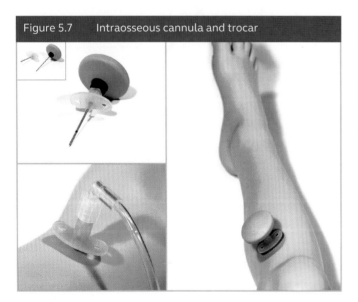

Figure 5.7   Intraosseous cannula and trocar

2. Alcohol-based skin preparation solution

This minimises the risk of infection.

3. Three-way tap with integrated IV extension tubing

This is primed with 0.9% sodium chloride and attached to a syringe also filled with 0.9% sodium chloride to minimise air emboli risk, confirm correct placement, and allow for flushing of medications.

4. Syringe

This is to aspirate bone marrow once the IO is inserted (e.g. to obtain a sample and/or confirm correct position).

5. Emergency medications and/or fluids

Have these to hand to ensure prompt delivery when access is achieved.

6. Local anaesthetic agent

If the child is still conscious, this should be considered to minimise pain along the intended track of the IO cannula; use 1 or 2% preservative and adrenaline free lidocaine.

Additionally, in the conscious child, infusion of drugs and medications via the IO route can be painful. If there is time, before administering drugs and fluids, infusion-related pain can be reduced by giving (preservative and adrenaline free) 1% lidocaine 0.5 mg kg^{-1} (0.05 mL kg^{-1} of 1%), maximum dose 40 mg, over 2 min. Allow a dwell time of 60 s, then flush with 0.9% sodium chloride 5 mL; then give a further dose of the 1% lidocaine at half the dose (i.e. 0.25 mg kg^{-1}) over another 60 s.

Technique for insertion of an IO cannula

1. Identify the site to be accessed and clean the skin around the selected site with an alcohol-based antiseptic solution.

2. Infiltrate the skin through to the periosteum with a local anaesthetic agent (i.e. 1% lidocaine) if appropriate.

3. Immobilise the limb with your non-dominant hand ensuring no hands are placed under the limb.

4. Using your dominant hand, grasp the needle or drill with the needle attached and position it at a 90° angle to the skin at the prepared site. If using the EZ-IO drill, push the needle through the skin until the needle reaches the periosteum, making sure the depth marker (described above) is still visible once this has been done.

5. Using a firm rotating action for the manual needle or using the drill, the needle should be advanced (approximately 1–2 cm) until loss of resistance is felt; this 'give' indicates penetration of the cortex. The needle should now feel as if 'gripped' by the bone.

6. Unscrew and withdraw the trocar.

7. The 3-way tap with integrated IV extension tubing should be attached and marrow aspirated and/or fluid flushed into the cannula to confirm position. If it is vital to obtain a marrow sample, this can be attempted at this point. However, this must not delay the administration of adrenaline in cardiorespiratory arrest.

8. Rapidly flush the IO needle with at least 5–10 mL of 0.9% sodium chloride to ensure patency and check the soft tissues around the insertion site for any swelling.

9. Administer resuscitation medications and/or fluid boluses as indicated (Figure 5.9). It should be noted that, with the smaller size cannulae, a fluid bolus may be easier to deliver with a 20 mL rather than a 50 mL syringe. Pressure will be required to deliver fluids and medications as the pressure in the medullary cavity is high. A simple drip or other low-pressure devices (< 300 mmHg) will not be useful. If the child is conscious, give lidocaine as above.

10. Although the cannula will be stable once correctly sited, it is advisable to secure it further to prevent accidental dislodgement, particularly during the child's transfer to a definitive care facility.

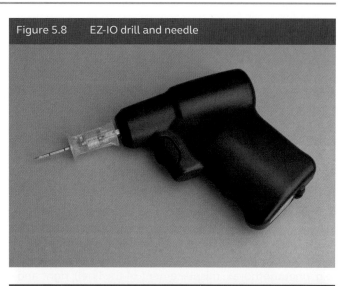

Figure 5.8   EZ-IO drill and needle

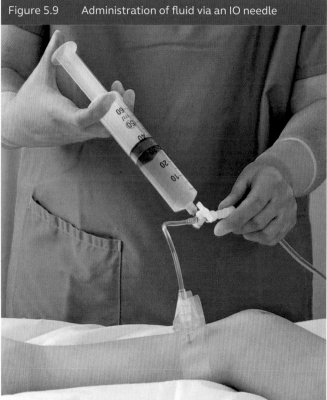

Figure 5.9   Administration of fluid via an IO needle

Complications	
Although these are uncommon, complications can occur. The potential for most of these complications can be minimised by removing the cannula as soon as alternative secure intravenous access has been obtained. These include:	
Extravasation	True extravasation ('tissuing') of an IO cannula may occur, but more frequent is the transient trivial swelling of subcutaneous tissue commonly seen as fluid leaks from the marrow cavity into surrounding tissues. If the swelling does not rapidly subside or there is concern that the cannula is misplaced, the rescuer should withdraw a small amount of fluid; this aspirate should be blood-stained if the cannula is in the correct place.
Embolism	There is a potential risk of fat or bone marrow embolism, but in practice, no cases have been reported.
Infection (e.g. osteomyelitis or cellulitis)	A serious but rare complication. The risk is very low if the IO needle is removed as soon as possible.
Compartment syndrome	May result from a large extravasation into a fascial compartment or misplacement of the IO needle. This can compromise the blood supply distally, causing limb ischaemia. This is a more common complication and requires ongoing surveillance and urgent plastic surgery referral if it occurs.
Skin necrosis	
Fracture	
Damage to the growth plate of epiphyses	Although this is a theoretical risk, no cases causing harm have been reported.

This is more difficult to achieve in children, is time-consuming and has a higher complication rate than in adults, so it should only be attempted by an experienced provider. Continuous infusions of inotropes, corrosive agents (e.g. potassium) and the monitoring of central venous pressure are best performed by the central venous route. Central venous access permits rapid infusion of large volumes of fluid, quicker onset of action and an earlier peak level of resuscitation drugs if they are given via this route. Vasospasm and extravasation are less likely to occur with central venous than with peripheral access.

Central venous access sites include: the right and left internal jugular veins (the right side is preferred as the vein's route is less tortuous and the dome of the lung is lower on the right, and hence there are fewer complications (e.g. pneumothorax, misplacement of the line)), right and left subclavian veins, left and right femoral veins.

Urgent insertion of central venous line

The Seldinger technique is the safest method of central line placement, and this should always be done under aseptic conditions with ultrasound guided control.

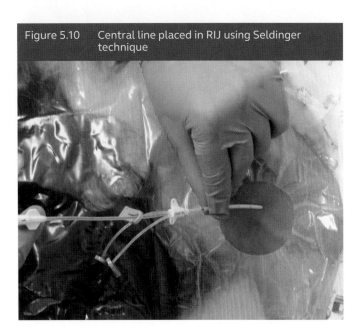

Figure 5.10   Central line placed in RIJ using Seldinger technique

Equipment required

- Alcohol-based antiseptic solution
- Lidocaine 1% for local anaesthesia with a 2 mL syringe and G23 needle (in the conscious child, consider a general anaesthetic)
- Syringe containing 0.9% sodium chloride
- Suture material
- Infusion set
- Adhesive tape
- Drapes to create a sterile field
- Over-the-needle cannula
- Double or triple lumen central lines (pre-flushed with 0.9% sodium chloride) 4–5 French gauge of different lengths depending on the age of the child
- Ultrasound machine with sterile cover for probe.

Complications
General complications include haematoma, venous obstruction, thrombosis, thrombophlebitis, air embolism and sepsis.
Specific complications of superior vena caval access (i.e. via the subclavian or internal jugular vein) include haemothorax, pneumothorax, cardiac tamponade, arrhythmias, diaphragmatic paralysis, Horner's syndrome and puncture of the internal carotid artery.
Complications seen in obtaining inferior vena cava access (i.e. via the femoral vein) include intestinal perforation, haematoma of the inguinal or retroperitoneal areas, septic arthritis of the hip and renal vein thrombosis.

Femoral vein access

The inguinal site is most commonly used during cardiopulmonary resuscitation as its distance from the head and chest allows cannulation without interrupting the management of the airway and breathing. This is a technique best carried out by the experienced clinician.

Technique

1. Remember the aseptic technique.

2. Place the leg in slight external rotation and clean the skin at the site of insertion and create a sterile field with drapes.

3. Identify the puncture site using an ultrasound probe covered with a sterile cover. The vein is directly medial to the femoral artery, which should be palpable. If the artery is not palpable, its location corresponds to the point midway between the anterior superior iliac spine and the pubic symphysis. During chest compressions, pulsations should be felt in the femoral artery.

4. If the child is aware of pain, lidocaine 1% should be used to infiltrate the puncture site. General anaesthesia should be considered in the conscious child.

5. Attach a short cannula with a needle to a sodium chloride-filled syringe, introduce it at a 45° angle (less in infants), using the ultrasound to guide entry (the bevel of the needle should be pointing towards the child's head), into the vein and keep the syringe in line with the child's thigh.

6. Advance the needle, pulling back on the plunger once the needle is below the surface of the skin. The needle will be seen entering the vein and as soon as blood flows back into the syringe, stop advancing it.

7. Gently remove the needle with the syringe, leaving the cannula in the vein whilst occluding the end of the cannula to prevent blood loss.

8. Thread the guidewire through the cannula to ensure it passes easily into the femoral vein. Remove the short cannula leaving the wire in situ (never lose hold of the end of the guidewire).

9. Thread a dilator over the guidewire to dilate the tract sufficiently for the central line to pass easily; remove the dilator, still keeping hold of the guidewire, then thread the double or triple lumen 4/5 French catheter (flushed with 0.9% sodium chloride pre-procedure) over the guidewire then remove the guidewire.

10. Confirm the location of the cannula by aspirating blood from each lumen; then flush with 0.9% sodium chloride and attach each port to a pre-flushed 3-way tap. Additional checks for correct placement may include transducing the line to ensure a venous rather than arterial waveform.

11. Suture the catheter in place and cover it with a transparent sterile fixing; some centres place an antibiotic patch around the catheter entry site through the skin before securing to reduce infection rates.

Fluid administration for volume resuscitation

Intravascular fluids are primarily administered to restore circulatory volume and ensure adequate perfusion of vital organs.

During cardiorespiratory arrest, hypovolaemia is often a primary contributory factor, and fluid resuscitation may play a critical part in achieving a return of spontaneous circulation (ROSC).

The administration of fluids is indicated for any child exhibiting signs of circulatory failure (e.g. decreased skin perfusion, prolonged capillary refill time, hypotension). However, although adequate fluid resuscitation is essential, fluid overload confers considerable morbidity. Hence fluid administration MUST always be followed by careful re-assessment to ensure that only the minimum fluid volume required to maintain volume homeostasis is given. Caution is advised in children and infants with suspected cardiogenic shock where the heart is unable to deal with the volume load or those with diabetic ketoacidosis when large fluid shifts are undesirable (Chapter 10).

Fluid volumes

There has been much debate about the appropriate size of fluid bolus volume for resuscitation in children following a large study in a number of African countries which suggested that aggressive fluid administration may worsen outcomes. The application of this study to children treated in more advanced health care systems is not known but should prompt all healthcare providers to carefully assess the effect of each fluid bolus on the child's clinical condition. Children and infants with a febrile illness, and no signs of shock do not require fluid bolus therapy. During the resuscitation of a child with compromised circulation due to hypovolaemia (including sepsis and anaphylaxis), initial resuscitation fluid is administered as a bolus of 10 mL kg^{-1} of isotonic fluid (balanced crystalloid solutions are preferred but 0.9% sodium chloride is an acceptable alternative). The child's circulatory status should then be reassessed, and if signs of circulatory failure persist, this should be repeated. Re-assessment after each fluid bolus is important to prevent over-transfusion of fluid; signs of overload include moist sounds ('crackles') at the lung bases, jugular venous distension in children and/or liver distension in infants.

If there is no improvement in circulatory status following 40–60 mL kg^{-1}, ongoing losses must be suspected (e.g. diarrhoeal fluid, bleeding). The aim in the management of hypovolaemic shock is to prevent the onset of decompensated circulatory failure, as this may lead to irreversible cardiorespiratory failure and death.

Septic shock

In septic shock, fluid resuscitation is specifically required as vasodilatation may be considerable, and there may be a relatively hypovolaemic state.

Up to 60–80 mL kg^{-1} of volume expansion is often required in the first hour of resuscitation; larger volumes (> 100 mL kg^{-1}) can be required within the first few hours. Inotropes (and intubation) may also be required in children with septic shock and should be considered at an early stage (e.g. after 40-60 mL kg^{-1}) (see Chapter 10). Call for senior help early as intubation is safer when cardiovascular stability has been achieved. The use of balanced isotonic crystalloid solutions is recommended (or 0.9% sodium chloride is an acceptable alternative).

Fluids must be infused during cardiorespiratory arrest if hypovolaemic shock is a likely cause of the arrest. However, as in other clinical states, excessive amounts of fluid may be harmful in cardiac arrest from other causes and in post-resuscitation states, so fluid administration should be done with care. Measurement of blood pressure (BP) alone is not the critical determinant in deciding circulatory status. BP can remain normal in compensated circulatory failure and only starts to drop as decompensation develops.

Circulatory failure without hypovolaemia

If circulatory failure is due to other causes, such as cardiac failure, a smaller initial volume (5–10 mL kg^{-1}) should be used. The effect of each smaller bolus should be carefully assessed to ensure that fluid administration is not causing worsening of the circulation (e.g. appearance of crackles at the lung bases and increasing size of liver edge). In some patients with cardiac failure, diuretics such as furosemide may be indicated for fluid overload.

Fluid bolus in trauma

Initial fluid bolus size should be 10 mL kg^{-1} isotonic balanced crystalloid or 0.9% sodium chloride with careful re-assessment after each bolus; this is to prevent large fluid boluses destabilising any early clots that have formed, resulting in further bleeding. If the child is haemorrhaging, consider blood and blood products for subsequent boluses guided by bedside, point of care, haemoglobin (Hb) measurement. An exception would be for children with massive haemorrhage on presentation when blood would immediately be given and the massive transfusion protocol activated. Over-transfusion is not desirable and may add to morbidity, so careful re-assessment and haemoglobin measurements are required. Most children with traumatic injuries have head injuries (70–80%), and it is extremely important to maintain a good blood pressure to support cerebral perfusion. Surgical referral should be made for full patient evaluation as haemostasis may only be achieved by surgery. The principles of management adhere to the < C > AcBCDE (potential catastrophic haemorrhage, airway including c-spine, breathing, circulation, disability, exposure) approach with fluid administration forming part of the 'C' phases of resuscitation.

Types of fluid

In the initial phase of resuscitation, isotonic crystalloid solutions should be used. Isotonic in this setting means that the solution has approximately the same concentration of sodium and thus osmotic pressure as found in extracellular fluids (ECF) and blood. There are no clear advantages to using colloid solutions over crystalloids. Glucose containing solutions (such as dextrose-saline) should never be used for volume replacement as they can cause hyponatraemia (which can cause seizures) and hyperglycaemia, which in turn, can lead to further fluid loss.

Crystalloids

Examples of appropriate resuscitation crystalloids include:

- 0.9% sodium chloride
- Ringer's lactate (lactate buffered solution)
- Hartmann's solution (lactate buffered solution)
- Plasma-Lyte (acetate and gluconate buffered solution).

Crystalloids are cheap, readily available and do not cause allergic reactions. Previously they have been considered less effective than colloids at expanding the circulating volume (due to rapid dispersal to the interstitial space), but in practice, this effect is minimal.

The most commonly used isotonic crystalloid is 0.9% sodium chloride, but when given in large amounts, 0.9% sodium chloride can cause hyperchloraemic acidosis. This is because although the sodium content of 0.9% sodium chloride is similar to that in serum plasma, the chloride content is much higher. Some studies have indicated that hyperchloraemic acidosis may be harmful to patients and promote inflammation and acute kidney injury (although most evidence is in adults, there is also some evidence in children). Balanced crystalloids have a sodium, potassium and chloride content close to ECF and plasma. They also contain molecules that are metabolised to bicarbonate (e.g. lactate) in order to maintain a normal plasma pH.

Bolus infusion of fluids containing a high concentration of potassium must be avoided during resuscitation. This is particularly important in children with anuria or oliguria, as hyperkalaemia could arise.

Crystalloids may also be indicated to replace fluid loss from the interstitial space and to correct electrolyte deficiencies, as seen in patients with burns or those who are dehydrated.

Glucose solutions should never be used for volume expansion as they can cause hyperglycaemia, resulting in osmotic diuresis. This increases urine production and so increases circulatory volume loss. Additionally, the glucose is quickly metabolised to water, so the net effect is that of a hypotonic infusion which can cause a drop in serum sodium concentration and undesirable fluid shifts.

Glucose solutions should only be used to correct hypoglycaemia following measurement of blood sugar levels. 2 mL kg^{-1} of 10% glucose is given, and the patient's blood sugar should be re-measured shortly afterwards (2–5 min) to ensure it is within the normal range; this must be followed up with a maintenance infusion containing glucose to prevent recurrence of the hypoglycaemia. In the newborn 2.5 mL kg^{-1} of 10% glucose may be given during resuscitation at birth to correct hypoglycaemia.

Blood products

The administration of blood products is reserved for situations where there is a specific indication for their use (i.e. blood loss or coagulopathy). If the infusion of 20 mL kg^{-1} (i.e. 10 mL kg^{-1} bolus x 2) of a balanced salt solution does not improve the circulatory status of a child who has suffered trauma, transfusion of blood must be considered, as well as urgent surgical referral. In an emergency, Group O Rhesus-negative 'flying squad' blood or type-specific uncross-matched blood may be used for transfusion until fully cross-matched blood is available. If a trauma patient has required > 40 mL kg^{-1} of blood, the massive transfusion protocol should be activated (if it has not already been) so that there is a replacement of other blood products in addition to red cells (Chapter 11).

Fresh frozen plasma should only be used in resuscitation situations for the treatment of coagulation abnormalities or as part of a massive transfusion protocol. Other blood products (e.g. cryoprecipitate and platelets) are usually given based on the findings of laboratory or near-patient testing.

Although blood products are now very safe, the risks of blood product administration must always be considered.

First-line resuscitation medications

Only a few medications are indicated during the initial resuscitation phase of a child in cardiorespiratory arrest. Administration of medications should be considered only after adequate ventilation and chest compressions have been established, and in the case of a shockable arrhythmia (VF or pVT), following delivery of the first three defibrillation shocks.

For safety reasons, as well as speed and ease of use, the use of pre-filled medication syringes is advocated.

All medications administered should be followed by a flush of 2–5 mL 0.9% sodium chloride to ensure they reach the circulation and minimise the risks of interactions with any other medications or fluids given via the same cannula. All medications and fluids should be recorded as they are administered and then documented at the end of the resuscitation attempt.

Adrenaline

Indications for use
- cardiorespiratory arrest of any aetiology
- bradycardia < 60 min^{-1} with signs of inadequate perfusion after the initial steps to restore satisfactory oxygenation and ventilation have been taken
- first line inotrope as an infusion centrally or peripherally in fluid resistant septic shock.
- anaphylaxis.

In cardiac arrest with non-shockable rhythms, adrenaline should be given as soon as circulatory access has been achieved, as early administration is associated with better outcomes. In shockable rhythms, adrenaline should be given after the third defibrillation and then following alternate shocks after that (e.g. following the third shock, then following the fifth shock etc.).

Dosage
For all children (excluding newborns) in cardiorespiratory arrest (shockable/non-shockable rhythms, or bradycardia) with signs of inadequate perfusion, the dose of adrenaline is 10 mcg kg^{-1} (or 0.1 ml kg^{-1} of 1:10 000 solution) IV or IO. This is repeated every 3–5 min as necessary. (For the dose of adrenaline in anaphylaxis see Chapter 10).

Actions
Adrenaline is an endogenous, directly acting sympathomimetic amine with both alpha and beta-adrenergic activity.

Alpha-adrenergic effects cause splanchnic and mucocutaneous vasoconstriction and increase systolic and diastolic blood pressure. Beta 1 and 2 adrenergic effects increase the force and rate of myocardial contractions and cause vascular smooth muscle vasodilatation and bronchiolar smooth muscle relaxation. Adrenaline's pharmacological effects are dose-related.

In cardiorespiratory arrest, alpha adrenergic-mediated vasoconstriction is the most important pharmacological action of adrenaline as this increases the diastolic pressure, so enhancing coronary and cerebral perfusion and oxygen delivery to the heart and brain. This is a critical determinant for successful resuscitation.

Other beneficial effects include
- elevation of systolic BP
- increased tendency for a normal cardiac perfusing rhythm to develop during cardiorespiratory resuscitation
- enhanced contractile state of the heart and stimulates spontaneous cardiac contractions
- increased intensity of ventricular fibrillation, therefore, increasing the likelihood of successful response to defibrillation (i.e. return to a perfusing rhythm).

The most commonly observed rhythms in paediatric patients with cardiorespiratory arrest are asystole and bradyarrhythmia; adrenaline may generate a perfusing rhythm in these children. As the action of catecholamines may be depressed by acidosis, paying careful attention to oxygenation, ventilation and circulation is essential (i.e. ABCDE).

The ideal time interval for giving adrenaline is unknown, but higher or more frequent doses of adrenaline administered by any route are not recommended as they do not improve survival or neurological outcome after cardiorespiratory arrest and can, in fact, worsen them. Higher doses may, however, be required in exceptional circumstances such as adrenoceptor blocker overdose.

Catecholamines are inactivated by alkaline solutions and should never be given simultaneously with sodium bicarbonate via the same vascular access cannula. If only one cannula is available and both these medications are to be used, their administration must be separated by a bolus of 0.9% sodium chloride (2–5 mL).

In newborns, the dose is 20 mcg kg^{-1} (or 0.2 mL kg^{-1} of a 1:10 000 solution) by IV or IO route. The tracheal route is not recommended. Large doses of adrenaline may increase the risk of intracranial haemorrhage in newborns, especially in preterm infants.

The half-life of adrenaline is short (2 min), and doses are repeated until the desired effect is achieved; hence, a continuous infusion of adrenaline may occasionally be necessary once spontaneous circulation is restored.

The haemodynamic effects are dose-related:
- Low-dose infusions (< 0.1 mcg kg^{-1} min^{-1}) produce beta-adrenergic effects.
- High-dose infusions (> 0.1 mcg kg^{-1} min^{-1}) produce alpha-adrenergic mediated vasoconstriction.

Precaution
Boluses of adrenaline should be administered via a secure vascular (IV or IO) cannula. If ongoing post-resuscitation care requires an adrenaline infusion, this should be through a central venous cannula when possible.

Adrenaline frequently causes tachycardia and may produce or exacerbate ventricular ectopics.

Amiodarone

Indication for use
Refractory VF or pVT.

If VF or pVT persists after the third defibrillation, a dose of amiodarone should be given as well as adrenaline. This can be repeated after the fifth shock if defibrillation is still unsuccessful.

Dosage
5 mg kg^{-1}.

Actions
Amiodarone is a membrane-stabilising anti-arrhythmic medication that increases the duration of the action potential and refractory period in both the atrial and ventricular myocardium.

Other effects include
Atrioventricular conduction is also slowed, and a similar effect is seen in accessory pathways.

Amiodarone has a mild negative inotropic action and causes peripheral vasodilatation through non-competitive alpha-blocking effects. The hypotension that occurs with IV amiodarone is related to the rate of delivery and is due more to the solvent (Polysorbate 80 and benzyl alcohol), which causes histamine release than the drug itself. The oral form is not well absorbed, but the intravenous form has been successfully used for tachyarrhythmia management.

Precaution
Amiodarone should be given as a pre-filled syringe preparation or diluted in 5% glucose. Ideally, it should be administered via a central vascular (IV or IO) route as it can cause thrombophlebitis. If it has to be given peripherally, it should be liberally flushed with 0.9% sodium chloride or 5% glucose.

In the treatment of shockable rhythms, give an initial IV bolus dose of amiodarone 5 mg kg^{-1} after the third shock. Repeat the dose after the fifth shock if still in VF/pVT.

If defibrillation was successful, but VF/pVT recurs, amiodarone can be repeated (unless two doses have already been injected), in which case a continuous infusion should be started. One recent observational study in children showed that ECG resolution and survival to discharge was similar in a group treated with lidocaine instead of amiodarone, but the evidence was not sufficiently robust to recommend a change in practice.

The delivery rate of the amiodarone is important in patients who have a perfusing rhythm, and it should be infused slowly (no less than 20 min) when given in the setting of ventricular tachycardia with a pulse or supraventricular tachycardia (preferably with expert paediatric cardiology advice) to avoid bradycardia and cardiac arrest. Another rare but significant side effect is polymorphic VT. Systemic BP and ECG should be continuously monitored.

Second line resuscitation medications

Adenosine

Adenosine is an endogenous purine nucleoside causing atrioventricular block of a very short duration. It impairs accessory bundle re-entry at the atrioventricular node (AVN). An accessory bundle is responsible for most supraventricular tachycardia (SVT) in children.

Adenosine is rapidly metabolised by red blood cells, and its half-life is only 10 s. Therefore, it should be injected rapidly and as close to the heart as possible (via a central or upper limb peripheral intravenous route) and immediately followed by a rapid bolus of 0.9% sodium chloride. Unfortunately, it is often seen to be ineffective when given via IO access in the tibia.

Side effects (flushing, headache, hypotension, bronchospasm, anxiety and a sense of impending doom) are short-lived, owing to its short half-life.

Indication for use

Adenosine is used in the management of SVT as it impairs accessory bundle re-entry at the AV node.

Dosage (BNFc)

Neonates

Initially 150 mcg kg^{-1} then increased in steps of 50–100 mcg kg^{-1} every 1–2 min if required; dose to be repeated until tachycardia terminated or maximum single dose of 300 mcg kg^{-1} given.

Child 1–11 months

Initially 150 mcg kg^{-1}, then increased in steps of 50–100 mcg kg^{-1} every 1-2 min if required; dose to be repeated until tachycardia terminated or maximum single dose of 500 mcg kg^{-1} given.

Child 1–11 years

Initially 100 mcg kg^{-1} then increased in steps of 50–100 mcg kg every 1–2 min if required; dose to be repeated until tachycardia terminated or maximum single dose of 500 mcg kg^{-1} given (max 12 mg).

Child 12–17 years

Initially 3 mg, followed by 6 mg after 1–2 min if required, followed by 12 mg after 1–2 min if required.

Continuous cardiac monitoring with printout is required so that a cardiologist can interpret the initial rhythm later and to monitor the effect of adenosine, which may be diagnostic.

Precautions

Children treated with theophylline are less sensitive to the effects of adenosine. Adenosine should be used with caution in asthmatics (as it can invoke severe bronchospasm) and children who have undergone a heart transplant.

Atropine

Indication for use

Bradycardia resulting from vagal stimulation. There is no evidence that atropine has any benefit in asphyxial bradycardia or asystole, and its routine use has been removed from the advanced life support algorithms.

Dosage

Up to 11 years

20 mcg kg^{-1}.

Child 12–17 years

300–600 mcg (larger doses may be used in emergencies).

These dosages may be repeated but, once the vagus nerve has been fully blocked, there is no further beneficial effect.

Until recently, a minimum dose of 100 mcg was recommended as there was thought to be a paradoxical bradycardia with lower doses. However, recent data does not support this, so 20 mcg kg^{-1} doses are acceptable in babies weighing less than 5 kg.

Actions

Atropine blocks the effect of the vagus nerve on the sinoatrial (SA) and atrioventricular (AV) nodes, increasing sinus automaticity, facilitating AV node conduction and increasing heart rate. The functions of the vagus nerve include pupillary constriction, contraction of the gut and production of salivary and gastrointestinal secretions. During resuscitation, atropine may be of benefit in treating bradycardia which accompanies actions that result in vagal stimulation such as laryngoscopy.

Sodium bicarbonate

Cardiorespiratory arrest results in combined respiratory and metabolic acidosis, caused by the cessation of pulmonary gas exchange and the development of anaerobic cellular metabolism respectively. The best treatment for acidaemia in cardiorespiratory arrest is a combination of effective chest compressions and ventilation (high-quality CPR). Administration of sodium bicarbonate generates carbon dioxide, which diffuses rapidly into the cells, exacerbating intracellular acidosis if it is not rapidly cleared via the lungs. It also has the following detrimental effects.

- It produces a negative inotropic effect on an ischaemic myocardium.
- It presents a large, osmotically active sodium load to an already compromised circulation and brain.
- It produces a shift to the left in the oxygen dissociation curve, further inhibiting the release of oxygen to the tissues.
- It causes an intracellular shift of potassium, lowered VF threshold, and decreased plasma calcium.

The routine use of sodium bicarbonate in CPR is not recommended. It may be considered in prolonged arrests, and it has a specific role in hyperkalaemia and the arrhythmias associated with tricyclic antidepressant overdose (and other specific toxicities). The potential negative effects of sodium bicarbonate outweigh any benefits unless the metabolic acidosis is severe, and even then, it should be used with caution.

Dosage

The initial dose is 1 mmol kg^{-1}. This equates to 1 mL kg^{-1} of 8.4% solution, although in newborns and infants < 3 months the weaker concentration (i.e. 4.2%) solution should be used to limit the osmotic load. The decision to give further doses should be based on blood gas analysis.

Precautions

Care should also be taken to ensure that an adequate flush of 0.9% sodium chloride is given between delivery of sodium bicarbonate and any other medications via the same cannula, as incompatibilities may occur.

Calcium

Calcium is essential to myocardial contraction. However, its routine administration does not improve the outcome of cardiorespiratory arrest. High plasma concentrations achieved after injection may be harmful to the ischaemic myocardium and may also impair cerebral recovery. After ischaemia and during reperfusion of ischaemic organs, cytoplasmic calcium would appear to contribute to cellular necrosis. The administration of calcium during cardiorespiratory arrest has been associated with increased mortality.

Indication for use

Routine administration of calcium in advanced life support is not recommended. It is only indicated for the treatment of documented hypocalcaemia, hyperkalaemia, hypermagnesaemia and overdose of calcium channel blockers. Hypocalcaemia is frequently seen in septic patients who need repeated fluid boluses or trauma patients needing multiple blood transfusions.

Dosage

0.2 mL kg^{-1} (max 10 mL) of 10% calcium chloride.

0.5 mL kg^{-1} (max 20 mL) of 10% calcium gluconate.

Precautions

Rapid calcium injection may induce bradyarrhythmia and asystole in patients treated with digoxin. The dose should be infused by slow injection via central intravenous access, as calcium may produce chemical burns if it leaks into surrounding tissues.

Glucose

Indication for use

Documented hypoglycaemia. Neonatal, child and adult data show that both hyper- and hypo-glycaemia are associated with worse outcomes after cardiorespiratory arrest. Plasma glucose concentrations should be monitored closely in any ill or injured child, including after cardiorespiratory arrest.

Do not give glucose-containing fluids during CPR except for the treatment of hypoglycaemia. Hyper and hypo-glycaemia should be avoided following ROSC. However, tight glucose control has not shown survival benefits when compared with moderate glucose control in adults or children (and it increases the risk of inadvertent hypoglycaemia). Infants have high glucose requirements and low glycogen storage. They can readily become hypoglycaemic during coma, circulatory and respiratory failure. It is, therefore, necessary to closely monitor their blood glucose concentrations.

The clinical signs of hypoglycaemia and shock may have similarities, (i.e. hypotension, tachycardia, decreased peripheral perfusion and sweating). Always check the blood glucose in any child with these symptoms or any child with coma or seizures (which may also be symptoms of hypoglycaemia).

Dosage

200 mg kg^{-1} (2 mL kg^{-1} of 10% glucose solution. Newborn 2.5 mL kg^{-1} of 10% glucose solution). Re-checking the blood glucose value should be performed shortly afterwards (e.g. 2–5 min following administration) to determine if further dosages are required.

Actions

Glucose is a principal energy substrate of all body tissues, including the brain and myocardial cells. Low blood levels mean that myocardial contractility and, therefore, cardiac output may be reduced. The association between hypoglycaemia and seizures is well documented. Prevention of seizures is essential to minimise the risk of neurological insult. Additionally, studies have shown a correlation between poor neurological outcome and hyperglycaemia. Therefore, it is important that blood glucose measurements be repeated regularly to maintain the normal range.

Once resuscitation has been completed, a continuous infusion of a glucose-containing solution is preferable to serial bolus therapy with hypertonic glucose. Repeated hyperglycaemia may increase serum osmolarity with the risk of osmotic diuresis. There is also a risk of intraventricular haemorrhage in the premature neonate if boluses of hypertonic solutions are used. A risk of cutaneous necrosis exists if hypertonic glucose leaks into surrounding tissues.

Naloxone

Naloxone is a fast-acting (2 min after injection) opiate antagonist with a duration of action up to 45 min. In cases of overdose with drugs such as methadone, which has a slow-release form, continuous naloxone infusion may be required to counteract further effects of the opiate.

Indication for use

Symptomatic opiate poisoning. Clinical signs of poisoning include respiratory depression, coma, pupillary constriction (miosis), hypotension and decreased perfusion.

Dosage

The recommended initial dose for full reversal of opiate effects is 100 mcg kg^{-1} in children under five years (maximum 2 mg) and 2 mg in those over five years, administered via IV, IO or intramuscular route. If necessary, naloxone can be repeated every 3 min. Titrated smaller doses can be used to partially reverse an opiate effect, where full reversal may result in extreme pain, for example, in a drowsy post-operative patient with a low respiratory rate.

A continuous naloxone infusion may be used if it is suspected that the patient has received a large amount of opiates. The infusion can range between 10–160 mcg kg^{-1} h^{-1} and is titrated until a satisfactory sustained response is obtained.

Precautions

Serious complications after naloxone treatment are uncommon (< 2%). However, if used for abrupt withdrawal from opiates, severe complications have been described (e.g. seizures, pulmonary oedema, ventricular arrhythmia and hypertension).

Dopamine

Dopamine is a catecholamine that may be used as an inotrope (a drug increasing the force of cardiac contraction) in paediatric sepsis; however, it is no longer a first line choice recommendation for inotrope in international sepsis guidelines. Some studies indicate that it may be less effective than adrenaline at reversing fluid refractory shock in children in the early stages. It can be given centrally or peripherally as as an intravenous infusion.

Dosage

In the dose range 5–10 mcg kg^{-1} min^{-1}, beta-adrenergic agonist effects predominate with increased cardiac index (CI) and increased heart rate.

At doses > 10 mcg kg^{-1} min^{-1} alpha-adrenergic agonist effects occur with vasoconstriction and subsequent increased systemic vascular resistance (SVR) and further increases in heart rate.

Furosemide

Furosemide is a loop diuretic that binds to a sodium transporter in the ascending loop of Henle in the kidney. This results in an increase of sodium and hence water lost in the urine. Furosemide is useful in reducing the intravascular fluid volume in fluid overload states and in cardiac failure. It causes increased losses of both calcium and potassium in the urine, and patients should be monitored, particularly for hypokalaemia.

Ketamine

Ketamine is a potent sedative, amnesic, analgesic and anaesthetic agent. It inhibits the activation of NMDA receptors by glutamate. It can provide anaesthesia and sedation with relatively little effect on the respiratory drive. Protective airway reflexes are largely maintained. Ketamine also has a relatively stable haemodynamic profile as it blocks the re-uptake of catecholamines, so it may be beneficial in intubation in septic shock.

Dosage

Doses are dependent on indication for use, but typically, 1–2 mg kg^{-1} IV is used for procedures. Ketamine can also be given by the intramuscular route when there is no circulatory access (typical dose 4 mg kg^{-1}); always check local protocols and the BNFc.

Side effects

These include hallucinations (which can be ameliorated by benzodiazepine administration) and hypersalivation.

Lidocaine

Lidocaine (or lignocaine) is a commonly used anaesthetic agent and a class 1B anti-arrhythmic drug which blocks sodium channels, shortening the cardiac action potential and decreasing the rate of contractions of the heart. Evidence indicates that either amiodarone or lidocaine may be used to treat paediatric shock-resistant VF or pVT. loading dose 1 mg kg^{-1} (maximum 100 mg) followed by an infusion of 20–50 mcg kg^{-1} min^{-1}. Toxicity can occur if there is underlying renal or hepatic disease.

Lorazepam

Lorazepam is a benzodiazepine with anti-seizure, sedation and amnesic properties. Benzodiazepines are first-line agents when seizures are prolonged (> 5 min). Lorazepam is longer-acting and a more potent anti-convulsant than diazepam.

Dosage

It is given intravenously, at a dose of 0.1 mg kg^{-1} (max dose 4 mg); this can be repeated if no effect after 5–10 min.

Caution: respiratory depression.

Levetiracetam

Levetiracetam is an anti-epileptic drug that inhibits neurotransmitter release from nerve end terminals. It is used as a second-line agent in the management of prolonged seizures (> 5 min). It is equally as effective as phenytoin at terminating seizures. It can be given more rapidly than phenytoin and has a good safety profile which has led to its increasing use.

Dosage
40 mg kg^{-1} (max 3 g; given over 5 min).

Milrinone

Milrinone Is a type 3 phosphodiesterase inhibitor that potentiates the effects of beta-receptor stimulation in cardiac and vascular tissue resulting in increased inotrope effect (increased force of cardiac contraction) and peripheral vasodilatation (which can cause hypotension). It also lowers preload by increasing diastolic myocardial relaxation (lusitropy), which improves coronary perfusion. Milrinone is used in low cardiac output states, shock and congestive heart failure.

Noradrenaline

Noradrenaline is a catecholamine with predominantly alpha-1 adrenergic agonist effects resulting in increased SVR and BP with less effect on heart rate. It is useful in the management of septic shock, particularly warm shock.

Phenobarbital

Phenobarbital is a barbiturate that increases GABA activity in the brain and depresses glutamate activity; the overall effect is to decrease CNS electrical activity hence its effectiveness in seizures. It can also cause sedation, respiratory depression and hypotension, particularly in combination with benzodiazepines.

Phenytoin

Phenytoin is a membrane stabilising drug which inhibits the spread of seizure activity in the motor cortex. It is one of the second line medications used in the status epilepticus algorithm if benzodiazepines have failed to terminate seizures.

Dosage
Dose is 20 mg kg^{-1}, and it must be given slowly intravenously over 20 min, as it can cause profound bradycardia, hypotension, cardiac arrhythmia and even asystole.

Magnesium

This is a major intracellular cation and serves as a co-factor in many enzymatic reactions. Magnesium treatment is indicated in children with documented hypomagnesaemia or with polymorphic VT (torsade de pointes), regardless of cause.

Dosage
For polymorphic VT 25–50 mg kg^{-1} magnesium sulphate 10% (0.25–0.5 mL kg^{-1} of 10% solution); max dose 2 g. Administer over 10–15 min and can repeat if needed.

Magnesium may also be a useful drug in the treatment of acute asthma as it causes airway smooth muscle relaxation, and for infants with pulmonary hypertensive crises as it causes pulmonary arterial smooth muscle relaxation.

Salbutamol

Salbutamol has a beta-2 agonist effect relaxing the smooth muscle in the airways of patients with asthma. It is also used in the treatment of hyperkalaemia. Side effects include tachycardia, hypertension, hypokalaemia, arrhythmias.

For asthma

IV injection

Indication for use
Acute asthma

Dosage (BNFc)

Child 1–23 months: 5 micrograms kg^{-1} over 5 min (for those in whom inhaled therapy cannot be used reliably or there is no current effect).

Child 2–17 years: 15 micrograms kg^{-1} (max. per dose 250 micrograms) for 1 dose, dose to be administered over 5 min (for those in whom inhaled therapy cannot be used reliably or there is no current effect).

IV infusion

Indication for use
Acute asthma

Dosage (BNFc)

Child: 1–2 micrograms kg^{-1} min^{-1} adjusted according to response and heart rate. It can be increased in an intensive care setting. This should be reserved for those in whom inhaled therapy cannot be used reliably, or there is no current effect.

Inhalation nebuliser solution

Indication for use
Moderate, severe or life-threatening asthma

Dosage (BNFc)

Child 1 month-4 years: 2.5 mg, repeat every 20–30 min or when required, give via oxygen driven nebuliser.

Child 5–11 years: 2.5-5 mg, repeat every 20–30 min or when required, give via oxygen driven nebuliser.

Child 12–17 years: 5 mg, repeat every 20–30 min or when required, give via oxygen driven nebuliser.

Inhalation of aerosol

Indication for use
Moderate and severe acute asthma

Dosage (BNFc)

Child: 2–10 puffs, repeat every 10–20 min or when required, give via a large volume spacer (and a close-fitting face mask in children under 3 years); each puff is equivalent to 100 micrograms.

For severe hyperkalaemia

IV injection

Dosage (BNFc)

Neonate: 4 micrograms kg^{-1}, repeated if necessary, administered over 5 min.

Child: 4 micrograms kg^{-1}, repeated if necessary, to be administered over 5 min.

Inhalation of nebulised solution

Neonate: 2.5–5 mg, repeated if necessary, IV injection route preferred over inhalation of nebulised solution.

Child: 2.5–5 mg, repeated if necessary, IV injection route preferred over inhalation of nebulised solution.

05: **Summary learning**

Intraosseous access is the circulatory access of choice in cardiorespiratory arrest and decompensated circulatory failure if IV access is not immediately available.

Fluid resuscitation for hypovolaemia starts with 10 mL kg^{-1} boluses.

After each fluid bolus, the child's condition must be reassessed.

The role of medications is secondary to effective ventilation and chest compressions (and defibrillation where indicated) in the management of cardiorespiratory arrest.

The main medication used in cardiorespiratory arrest is IV or IO adrenaline, which can be repeated as necessary every 3–5 min but no more frequently.

Amiodarone is used in refractory VF or pVT after the third and fifth shock.

Hypoglycaemia and hyperglycaemia should be avoided.

My key take-home messages from this chapter are:

Further reading

Sarisoy O, Balaogh K, Tugay S, Barn E, Gokalp AS. Efficacy of magnesium sulphate for treatment of ventricular tachycardia in Amitriptyline overdose. Paediatric Emergency care 2007; 23: 9, 646-648.

Dauchot P, Gravenstein JS. Effects of atropine on the electrocardiogram in different age groups. Clin Pharmacol Ther 1971;12:274-80.

Griesdale DE, de Souza RJ, van Dam RM, et al. Intensive insulin therapy and mortality among critically ill patients: a meta-analysis including NICE- SUGAR study data. CMAJ 2009;180:821-7.

Wiener RS, Wiener DC, Larson RJ. Benefits and risks of tight glucose control in critically ill adults: a meta-analysis. JAMA 2008;300:933-44.

Krinsley JS, Grover A. Severe hypoglycemia in critically ill patients: risk factors and outcomes. Crit Care Med 2007;35:2262-7.

Padkin A. Glucose control after cardiac arrest. Resuscitation 2009;80:611-2.

Brenner T, Bernhard M,Helm M et al. Comparison of two Intraosseous systemsfor adult emergency use. Resuscitation 2008; 78: 3, 314-319.

Nadkarni VM, Larkin GL, Peberdy MA, Carey SM, Kaye W, Mancini ME, et al. First documented rhythm and clinical outcome from in-hospital cardiac arrest among children and adults. JAMA. 2006 Jan 4;295(1):50-7.

Finfer S, Bellomo R, Boyce N, French J, Myburgh J, Norton R. A comparison of albumin and saline for fluid resuscitation in the intensive care unit. N Engl J Med. 2004 May 27;350(22):2247-56.

Dumas F, Dumas F, Bougouin W, Geri G, et al. Is Epinephrine During Cardiac Arrest Associated With Worse Outcomes in Resuscitated Patients? J Am Coll Cardiol. 2014;64(22):2360-2367.

Hagihara A, Hasegawa M, Abe T, Nagata T, Wakata Y, Miyazaki S. Prehospital Epinephrine Use and Survival Among Patients With Out-of-Hospital Cardiac Arrest; JAMA 21 March 2012, Vol 307, No. 11, pp 1161-1168;

Santhanam I, Sangareddi S, Venkataraman S, Kissoon N, Thiruvengadamudayan V, Kasthuri RK. A prospective randomised controlled study of two fluid regimens in the initial management of septic shock in the emergency department. Pediatr Emerg Care. 2008 Oct; 24 (10):647-55.

Maitland K, Kiguli S, Opoka RO, Engoru C, Olupot-Olupot P, Akech SO, Nyeko R, Mtove G, Reyburn H, Lang T, Brent B, Evans JA, Tibenderana JK, Crawley J,Russell EC, Levin M, Babiker AG, Gibb DM; FEAST Trial Group. Mortality after fluid bolus in African children with severe infection. NEJM. 2011, Jun 30;364(26):2483-95.

Valdes SO, Donoghue AJ, Hoyme DB, Hammond R, Berg MD, Berg RA, Samson RA; American Heart Association Get With The Guidelines- Resuscitation Investigators.. Outcomes associated with amiodarone and lidocaine in the treatment of in-hospital paediatric cardiac arrest with pulseless ventricular tachycardia or ventricular fibrillation. Resuscitation 2014, Mar;85(3):381-6.

Eisa L et al. Do small doses of atropine (< 0.1 mg) cause bradycardia in young children? Arch Dis Child 2015;100:684-8.

Andersen LW, Berg KM, Saindon BZ et al. Time to Epinephrine and Survival After Pediatric In-Hospital Cardiac Arrest. JAMA 2015;314(8):802-810.

Ramaswamy KN, Singhi S, Jayashree M, Bansal A, Nallasamy Double-Blind Randomised Clinical Trial Comparing Dopamine and Epinephrine in Pediatric Fluid-Refractory Hypotensive Septic Shock. Pediatr Crit Care Med. 20216;17(11):e502-e512.

Scott-Warren VL, Morley RB. Paediatric vascular access. BJA Education. 2015;15(4):199-206.

Ohshimo S, Wang CH, Couto TB, Bingham R, Mok YH, Kleinman M, Aickin R, Ziegler C, DeCaen A, Atkins DL, Maconochie I, Rabi Y, Morrison L; International Liaison Committee on Resuscitation (ILCOR) Pediatric Task Force. Pediatric timing of epinephrine doses: A systematic review. Resuscitation 2021;160:106-117.

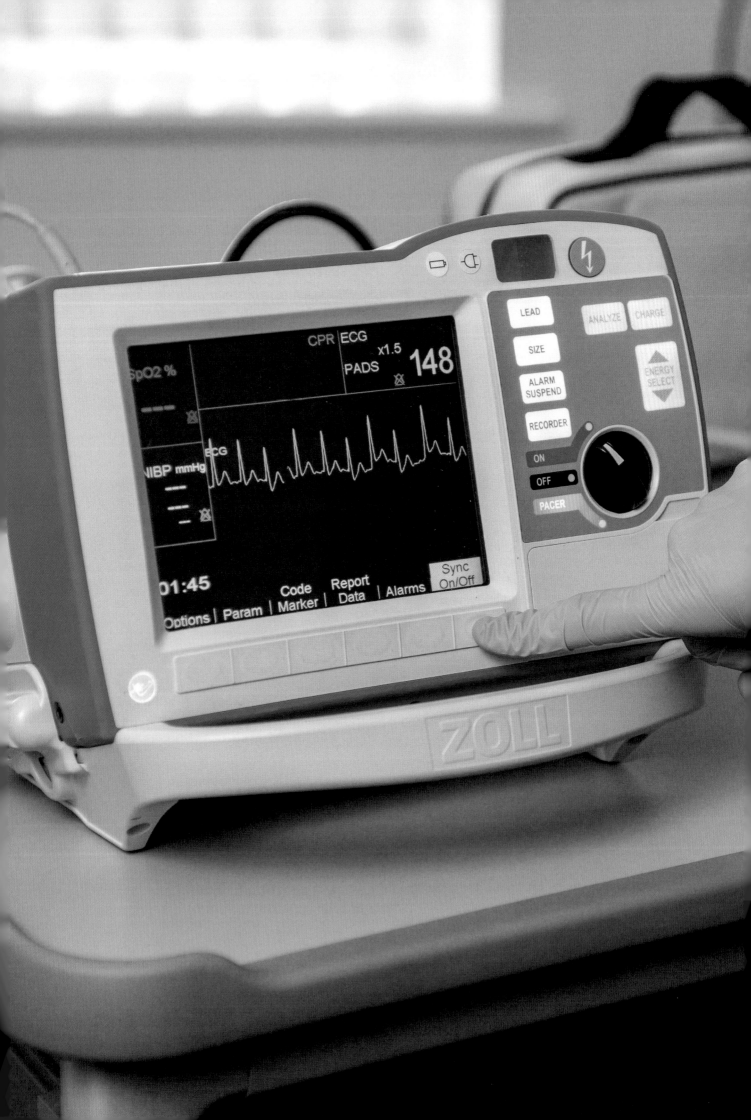

Rhythm recognition

ECG monitoring

Once optimal ventilation and oxygenation have been established, all seriously ill children should have their ECG monitored continuously via lead II, and at least one 12-lead ECG should be performed.

This facilitates the observation of heart rate and rhythm changes, which are important indicators of the response to treatments or the evolution of the disease process. Normal heart rates vary for physiological reasons (e.g. pain, pyrexia and wakefulness) and with age (Table 6.1).

Acute illness in children can result in cardiac arrhythmias. Less frequently, the cardiac arrhythmia may be the precipitant for the episode of acute illness. In these cases, there is commonly an underlying cardiac anatomic anomaly or reason for electrolyte disturbance causing abnormal cardiac electrical conductivity.

Examples include:

- acquired cardiac disease (e.g. cardiomyopathy, myocarditis)
- congenital heart disease or following cardiac surgery
- electrolyte disturbances (e.g. renal disease).

Additionally, some medications in therapeutic or toxic amounts may also cause arrhythmias (e.g. digoxin, beta-blockers, tricyclic antidepressants).

By monitoring the ECG, it is possible to detect those arrhythmias that are (or have the potential to become) life-threatening.

Table 6.1   Heart rate ranges (beats min^{-1})

Age	Mean	Awake	Deep sleep
Newborn – 3 months	140	85–205	80–140
3 months – 2 years	130	100–180	75–160
2–10 years	80	60–140	60–90
> 10 years	75	60–100	50–90

By monitoring the ECG, it is possible to detect those arrhythmias that are (or have the potential to become) life-threatening

Basic electrocardiography

The ECG trace represents electrical activity within the heart, not the effectiveness of myocardial contraction or tissue perfusion. The child's clinical status needs to be considered alongside the ECG trace: treat the patient, not the monitor.

When evaluating the ECG, possible artefacts may occur; detachment of ECG electrodes or leads can simulate asystole, whilst vibrations transmitted to the leads (e.g. during patient transportation) can mimic ventricular fibrillation (VF).

A normal ECG complex consists of a P wave, a QRS complex and a T wave (Figure 6.1).

Looking at an ECG rhythm strip

Standard ECG paper is composed of small squares; when the paper speed is 25 mm sec^{-1}, each square represents 0.04 s. The larger squares are 5 mm in length on the ECG paper and represent 0.2 s. The heart rate can be calculated by counting the number of QRS complexes in 6 s (30 large squares) and multiply this by 10.

The ECG

The electrical impulse normally starts from the sinoatrial (SA) node in the right atrium and stimulates atrial contraction. As the impulse moves through the atrium to the Atrioventricular node (AVN), a positive deflection is seen on the ECG rhythm strip known as the P wave. P waves are normally 2 small squares lasting 0.08–0.1 s on the ECG paper and represent electrical depolarisation of the atria. The time it takes for depolarisation to pass through the atria, AV node and His-Purkinje system to the ventricles (Figure 6.2) is represented by the P–R interval (lasting 0.08–0.15 s (2–4 small squares on the ECG paper)). A prolonged P-R interval suggests a degree of heart block.

The QRS complex represents depolarisation of the ventricles, which stimulates the right and left ventricles to contract. This is seen on the ECG as the large QRS complex (lasting around 0.08–0.12 s (2–3 small squares on the ECG paper)). Abnormalities in conduction pathways through the ventricles can cause abnormalities in ventricular conduction. This may be seen as the widening of the QRS complex. The ST segment and the T wave represent ventricular repolarisation in preparation for the next impulse. A prolonged QT interval (a delay between the beginning of ventricular depolarisation and repolarisation) is a risk factor for arrhythmias and sudden death.

It is important to remember that the ECG complex relates to the electrical activity of the heart, not muscular contraction. Therefore, always assess and treat the patient, not the monitor.

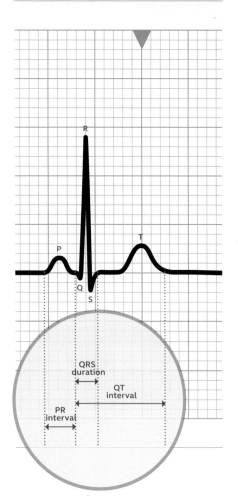

Figure 6.1	The normal ECG complex

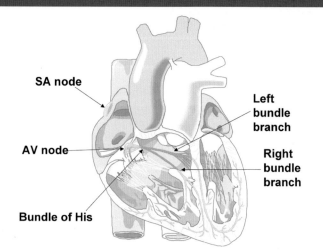

Figure 6.2	Electrical conduction through the heart

Paediatric cardiac arrhythmias

Assess with ABCDE approach – recognise and treat reversible causes
Oxygen if SpO$_2$ < 94%, respiratory rate, heart rate, CRT, cardiac monitoring, blood pressure, vascular access, AVPU

Signs of circulation?

NO → Follow **ADVANCED LIFE SUPPORT ALGORITHM**

YES

Compensated

Normal LOC, +/- respiratory distress and signs of circulatory compromise, BP > 5th centile*

Monitor for clinical deterioration and seek expert help

Treat the cause:
If bradycardia, consider oxygenation and vagal tone
If SVT, consider vagal manoeuvres
Reassess
Consider adenosine

Decompensated – seek expert help

Signs of vital organ perfusion compromise:
Reduced LOC, tachypnoea, bradycardia /tachycardia, BP < 5th centile*, CRT > 2 secs, weak or impalpable peripheral pulses

Bradycardia

< 1 year < 80 min^{-1}
> 1 year < 60 min^{-1}

Optimal oxygenation with positive pressure ventilation if required

If unconscious and HR < 60 min^{-1} despite oxygenation, start chest compressions

No response to oxygenation:
If vagal stimulation possible cause – atropine
If no response to oxygenation or atropine consider adrenaline

Pacing – very rarely required and guided by aetiology.

Tachycardia

Narrow complex

Sinus tachycardia
Infant typically 180–220 min^{-1}
Child typically 160–180 min^{-1}
Gradual onset

Treat the cause:
Physiological response:
– Crying
– Exercise
– Anxiety/fear
– Pain

Identify precipitant
Compensatory mechanism:
– Respiratory/circulatory failure
– Hypovolaemia
– Sepsis
– Anaemia

SVT
Infant > 220 min^{-1}
Child > 180 min^{-1}
Abrupt onset

Synchronised cardioversion with appropriate sedation + analgesia (e.g. IM/intranasal ketamine if delay in IV access)

Chemical cardioversion may be 1st choice if suitable IV access is in place and delay in synchronised cardioversion.

Adenosine
Consider amiodarone before 3rd shock

Broad complex

VT
Could be VT or SVT, if unsure treat as VT

If conscious:
Synchronised cardiove·sion with appropriate sedation + analgesia (e.g. IM/int anasal ketamine if delay in IV access, do not delay cardioversion).

If unconscious:
Immediate synchronised cardioversion
Consider amiodarone before 3rd shock

Drug	Atropine	Adrenaline	Adenosine	Amiodarone	Synchronised cardioversion	Magnesium
Treatment	**Up to 11 years:** 20 mcg kg^{-1}. **12–17 years:** 300–600 mcg, larger doses may be used in emergency.	For **bradycardia:** 10 mcg kg^{-1} repeat if necessary.	**Up to 1 year:** 150 mcg kg^{-1}, increase 50–100 mcg kg^{-1} every 1–2 min. Maximum single dose: Neonates 300 mcg kg^{-1}, Infants 500 mcg kg^{-1}) **1–11 years:** 100 mcg kg^{-1} increase 50–100 mcg kg^{-1} every 1–2 min. Maximum single dose: 500 mcg kg^{-1} (max. 12 mg) **12–17 years:** 3 mg IV, if required increase to 6 mg after 1–2 min, then 12 mg after 1–2 min	5 mg kg^{-1} – by SLOW IV infusion (> 20 min) before 3rd cardioversion in discussion with paediatric cardiologist/expert	With appropriate sedation + analgesia (e.g. IM/intra nasal Ketamine if delay in IV access + airway management) – IV access attempts must not delay cardioversion **1st shock:** 1 J kg^{-1} **2nd shock:** 2 J kg^{-1}, consider up to 4 J kg^{-1}	25–50 mg kg^{-1} Maximum per dose 2 g to be given over 10–15 min, may be repeated once if necessary, in Torsades de pointes VT

Age	*Systolic BP 5th centile mmHg
1 month	50
1 year	70
5 years	75
10 years	80

Figure 6.3 Managing the child with a cardiac arrhythmia   95

Cardiac rhythm disturbances

The approach to managing a child with a cardiac rhythm disturbance is summarised in Figure 6.3. This approach is based on determining the following four factors:

1. presence or absence of circulation (i.e. a central pulse and other signs of life)
2. clinical status – compensated (haemodynamically stable) or decompensated (haemodynamically unstable)
3. heart rate (bradycardia or tachycardia)
4. width of QRS complexes on ECG (i.e. narrow or broad).

1. Presence or absence of circulation

Adopt the ABCDE approach and quickly establish the absence or presence of cardiac output (i.e. signs of life and a palpable central pulse).

Absent pulse

The absence of signs of life and no palpable central pulse indicates cardiorespiratory arrest. BLS should be started immediately. The rhythms associated with cardiorespiratory arrest are:

- asystole (or severe bradycardia, < 60 min^{-1} with signs of inadequate perfusion
- pulseless electrical activity (PEA)
- ventricular fibrillation (VF)
- pulseless ventricular tachycardia (pVT).

The commonest cardiorespiratory arrest arrhythmia in paediatrics is asystole (generally preceded by progressive bradycardia). The term PEA describes the situation where there is organised electrical activity displayed on the ECG monitor but no cardiac output. The principles of managing both asystole and PEA are the provision of effective CPR, early administration of adrenaline and the treatment of any reversible causes.

Both VF and pVT are less common in children but are more likely in those with underlying cardiac disease (congenital or acquired). The priority of management in these arrhythmias is effective CPR and rapid defibrillation. VF and pVT may also occur as a secondary rhythm during reperfusion of the myocardium during a cardiorespiratory arrest.

Any possible causes (or aggravating factors) that have specific treatments, including reversible causes, must be considered during all cardiorespiratory arrests. The management of cardiorespiratory arrest arrhythmias is outlined in Chapter 8.

Pulse present

If there is a central pulse present, determine whether the child is compensated (haemodynamically stable) or decompensated (haemodynamically unstable).

2. Clinical status

Compensated circulatory failure

The child with compensated circulatory failure, who is conscious and haemodynamically stable, must be monitored, including an ECG. If the ECG displays an arrhythmia, the child may need treatment, but it is reasonable to await expert help such as from a paediatric cardiologist. Preparations should be made to intervene (along the principles described below) should the child deteriorate and become decompensated. (See Chapter 2.)

Decompensated circulatory failure

The child who is decompensated (haemodynamically unstable) should be monitored and, if the ECG displays a life-threatening arrhythmia, the immediate interventions that may be required are outlined below. Urgent expert help must also be sought. This should include an anaesthetist as sedation or anaesthesia may be required to manage a conscious child requiring cardioversion.

3. Heart rate

Both bradycardia and tachycardia are relatively common in paediatrics. Their typical defining heart rates are listed in Table 6.2.

Table 6.2   Typical bradycardia and tachycardia heart rates

Age	Bradycardia	Tachycardia
< 1 year	< 80* beats min^{-1}	> 180 beats min^{-1}
> 1 year	< 60 beats min^{-1}	> 160 beats min^{-1}
*although 80 min^{-1} is defining rate for bradycardia in an infant, chest compressions are not indicated until the heart rate is < 60 min^{-1} (with signs of inadequate perfusion).		

Bradycardia

Bradycardia may be due to hypoxia, acidosis and respiratory or circulatory failure. It may be a pre-terminal event prior to cardiorespiratory arrest (Figure 6.4).

A bradycardic child with signs of decompensation or a child with a rapidly dropping heart rate associated with poor systemic perfusion requires immediate oxygenation (i.e. airway opening, 100% oxygen administration

Figure 6.4   Bradycardia

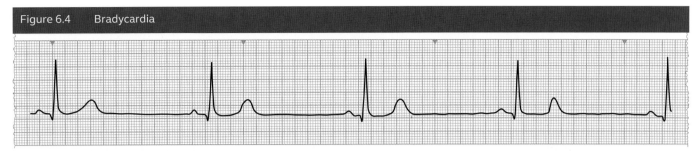

Figure 6.5   Sinus tachycardia rhythm strip

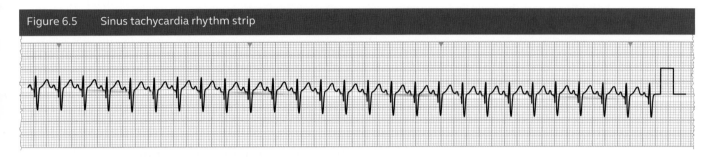

Figure 6.6   Supraventricular tachycardia rhythm strip

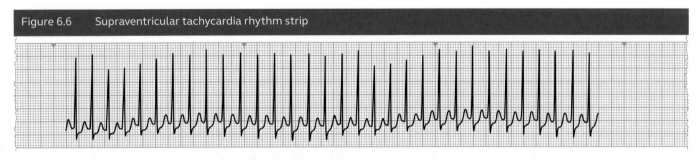

Figure 6.7   Ventricular tachycardia rhythm strip

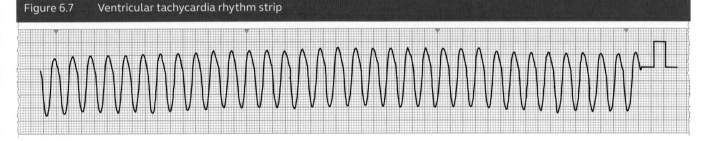

and positive pressure ventilation as necessary). If the heart rate remains < 60 min^{-1} (all ages) and the child is unconscious with decompensated circulatory failure, chest compressions must also be started. The cause of the bradycardia must be sought and treatment directed at the underlying cause.

By far, the most common causes of bradycardia in infants and children are hypoxia and vagal stimulation. Less commonly, hypothermia and hypoglycaemia can slow conduction through cardiac tissues and result in bradycardia. Infants and children with a history of heart surgery are at increased risk of damage to the AV node or other parts of the conduction system.

Atropine is indicated when increased vagal tone is the cause of bradycardia (e.g. induced by tracheal intubation, suctioning). Otherwise, adrenaline is the medication of choice but only once oxygenation has been restored, and the HR remains < 60 min^{-1} with circulatory failure. Very occasionally, in a child with congenital heart disease, the bradycardia is due to complete heart block, and emergency cardiac pacing is required. Pacing is not indicated and is ineffective in children with bradycardia secondary to hypoxic/ischaemic myocardial insult or respiratory failure.

Tachycardia

An elevated heart rate is frequently the normal physiological response to anxiety, pain or pyrexia. This is sinus tachycardia (ST) and is managed by treating the primary cause.

Other causes of ST include:

- respiratory conditions: early hypoxia, hypercapnia, obstructed airway and pneumothorax
- circulatory conditions: hypovolaemia, cardiac failure, anaphylaxis, sepsis and pulmonary hypertension
- miscellaneous causes: drugs, seizures.

The other cause of tachycardia is an arrhythmia, either supraventricular tachycardia (SVT) or ventricular tachycardia (VT).

Of these, SVT is far more common in children. The priority of management is to establish whether the child is stable or if they are displaying signs of circulatory decompensation. If the child is in a compensated state, expert help should be sought for definitive management.

The child who has decompensated circulatory failure requires chemical or electrical cardioversion whilst their ABCDE is continually assessed and appropriately supported.

4. Width of QRS complexes

In children with a tachycardia, the most important thing to establish is whether this is ST or an abnormal rhythm (tachyarrhythmia). The history and clinical examination are key in determining this. The ECG features and width of the QRS complexes can also be helpful, but it is always the child's clinical status that determines the urgency of management, regardless of the type of arrhythmia.

Narrow QRS complex tachycardia

Both ST (Figure 6.5) and SVT (Figure 6.6) have narrow QRS complexes making it potentially difficult to differentiate between them. The clinical and ECG differences that help to make this distinction are listed in Table 6.3.

Table 6.3   Distinguishing features between ST and SVT

	ST	SVT
Onset and termination	Gradual	Abrupt
History	Clues (e.g. pyrexia, fluid or blood loss)	Non-specific Previous arrhythmia
Heart rate (beats min⁻¹)	Infant < 220 min⁻¹ Child < 180 min⁻¹	Infant > 220 min⁻¹ Child > 180 min⁻¹
P wave	Present and normal (NB not clearly seen at heart rates > 200 min⁻¹)	Absent or abnormal
Beat-to-beat variability (R–R)	Yes – can be altered with stimulation	None

Broad QRS complex tachycardia

In children, broad complex tachycardia is uncommon and is usually due to an SVT. However, if uncertain, carefully consider VT (Figure 6.7) as this has more immediately serious consequences if inadequately treated (i.e. it can deteriorate to VF or pVT).

VT is usually found in a child with an underlying cardiac disease (congenital or acquired) or after certain drug ingestions.

VT is a broad complex, regular rhythm. The P waves are either absent or unrelated to the QRS complexes. It can present with or without a pulse; pulseless VT (pVT) is managed in the same manner as VF (i.e. with CPR and urgent defibrillation).

Management of pulsed VT

The management of VT with a pulse involves urgent expert consultation, as it has the potential to rapidly deteriorate to pVT or VF. The ongoing management of these children may involve electrical cardioversion or chemical cardioversion (usually with amiodarone). An anaesthetist or paediatric intensivist should be contacted in addition to a cardiologist, as amiodarone can cause hypotension and may result in rapid circulatory decompensation. If electrical cardioversion is required, anaesthesia may be necessary.

Supraventricular tachycardia

SVT is the most common primary cardiac arrhythmia observed in children. It is a paroxysmal, regular rhythm with narrow QRS complexes caused by a re-entry mechanism through an accessory pathway or the atrioventricular conduction system. A heart rate of > 220 min^{-1} in infants or > 180 min^{-1} in children (older than one year) is highly suggestive of SVT. The other features that differentiate SVT from ST are listed in Table 6.3.

Management of SVT

Once a diagnosis of SVT is made, the child's clinical status will determine the management. As described previously, a child with compensated circulatory status should be referred for expert help. Treatment may include vagal manoeuvres, adenosine or cardioversion.

Vagal manoeuvres

In infants and small children, this can be performed by soaking a flannel in ice-cold water and then placing it briefly over their face. In cooperative children, a Valsalva manoeuvre can be induced by asking the child to blow through a drinking straw. A variation on this is to blow through the outlet of a syringe in an effort to expel the plunger.

Cardioversion

The procedure for undertaking synchronised electrical cardioversion is described in Chapter 7. It is the procedure of choice for decompensated children with tachyarrhythmias, particularly if they are unconscious. Analgesia and sedation with airway management, by an experienced provider, preferably an anaesthetist will be required if the child is conscious (e.g. intramuscular or intranasal ketamine can be considered if the child has no intravenous access). Most importantly, cardioversion should not be unnecessarily delayed by intravenous access attempts. The first shock should be delivered at the energy level of 1 J kg^{-1}, and the second (if required) at 2 J kg^{-1}. Clinicians can consider increasing to 4 J kg^{-1} under expert guidance. Additionally, if the tachyarrythmia fails to convert after the second shock, an amiodarone infusion over > 20 min may be recommended before further shocks are delivered; again, this should ideally be under the guidance of a paediatric cardiologist or paediatric intensivist.

Adenosine

If intravascular access is already established in a conscious, compensated child with SVT, chemical cardioversion with adenosine may be possible. Adenosine should be given rapidly via a vein as close to the heart as possible, as it is metabolised by red blood cells as soon as it enters the bloodstream. It is very helpful to have an ECG rhythm strip running during administration as this may help in diagnosis when reviewed by a paediatric cardiologist.

Give adenosine as a rapid bolus followed with a rapid flush of 2–5 mL 0.9% sodium chloride. If the initial dose is ineffective, it can be increased.

Dosage (BNFc)

Neonates

Initially 150 mcg kg^{-1} then increased in steps of 50–100 mcg kg^{-1} every 1–2 min if required; dose to be repeated until tachycardia terminated or maximum single dose of 300 mcg kg^{-1} given.

Child 1–11 months

Initially 150 mcg kg^{-1}, then increased in steps of 50–100 mcg kg^{-1} every 1-2 min if required; dose to be repeated until tachycardia terminated or maximum single dose of 500 mcg kg^{-1} given.

Child 1–11 years

Initially 100 mcg kg^{-1} then increased in steps of 50–100 mcg kg every 1–2 min if required; dose to be repeated until tachycardia terminated or maximum single dose of 500 mcg kg^{-1} given (max 12 mg).

Child 12–17 years

Initially 3 mg, followed by 6 mg after 1–2 min if required, followed by 12 mg after 1–2 min if required.

Caution

Adenosine can precipitate severe bronchospasm. It causes unpleasant feelings of impending doom in the child and should ideally only be given under the guidance of a paediatric cardiologist.

Adenosine should be used with caution in heart transplant recipients and asthmatics.

06: **Summary learning**

Life-threatening cardiac arrhythmias are more frequently the result, rather than the cause, of acute illness.

The child's clinical status dictates management priorities – treat the patient, not the monitor.

The cause of the arrhythmia should be sought and treated.

My key take-home messages from this chapter are:

Further reading

Paediatric Formulary Committee. BNF for Children (online) London: BMJ Group, Pharmaceutical Press, and RCPCH Publications http://www.medicinescomplete.com [Accessed on 29 January 2021]

Maconochie IK, Aickin R, Hazinski MF, et al. Pediatric life support: 2020 international consensus on cardiopulmonary resuscitation and emergency cardiovascular care science with treatment recommendations. Resuscitation 2020;156:A120 55.

Lewis J, Arora G, Tudorascu DL, Hickey RW, Saladino RA, Manole MD. Acute management of refractory and unstable pediatric supraventricular tachycardia. J Pediatr 2017 181 e2.

Kim JH, Jung JY, Lee SU, Park JW, Choi JY. Delayed adenosine therapy is associated with the refractory supraventricular tachycardia in children. Am J Emerg Med 2020;38:2291 6.

Brugada J, Katritsis DG, Arbelo E, et al. 2019 ESC Guidelines for the management of patients with supraventricular tachycardia the task force for the management of patients with supraventricular tachycardia of the European Society of Cardiology (ESC). Eur Heart J 2020;41:655 720, doi:http://dx.doi.org/10.1093/eurheartj/ ehz467.

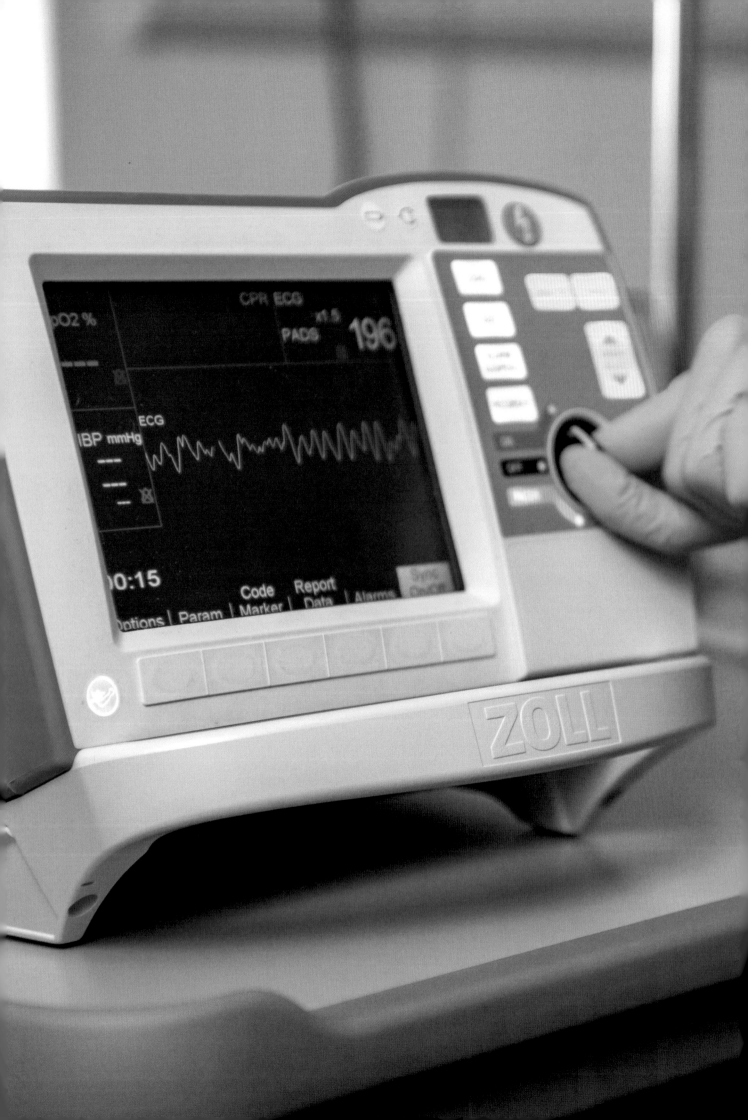

Defibrillation and cardioversion

Incidence of shockable arrhythmias

Although the initial rhythm in a paediatric cardiorespiratory arrest is far more likely to be asystole or pulseless electrical activity (PEA) than ventricular fibrillation (VF) or pulseless ventricular tachycardia (pVT), a shockable rhythm is present in up to 27% of paediatric in-hospital arrests at some point during the resuscitation. When a shockable rhythm is present, the likelihood of a successful outcome is critically dependent on rapid, safe defibrillation.

A defibrillator can also be used in the management of a child with circulatory compromise due to VT with a pulse or supraventricular tachycardia (SVT). In these situations, the machine is used to perform synchronised DC (direct current) cardioversion, which is also described in this chapter.

A shockable rhythm is present in up to 27% of paediatric in-hospital arrests at some point during the resuscitation

When a shockable rhythm is present, the likelihood of a successful outcome is critically dependent on rapid, safe defibrillation

Defibrillation

Defibrillation is the generic term used to describe the procedure of passing an electrical current across the myocardium with the intention of inducing global myocardial depolarisation and restoring organised spontaneous electrical activity. This electrical current may be delivered asynchronously when there is no cardiac output (in VF or pVT), or it may be synchronised with the R wave when there is an output (in SVT or VT with a pulse), the latter being called cardioversion.

The energy dosage should cause minimal myocardial injury. The electrical current delivered to the heart depends on the selected energy (in Joules) and the resistance to current flow (thoracic impedance). If the impedance is high, the energy requirement will be increased.

Factors determining thoracic impedance

The factors that potentially affect thoracic impedance and therefore, the energy required, include:

- defibrillator pads/paddles size
- interface between pads/paddles and the child's skin
- positioning of the pads/paddles on the chest wall
- chest wall thickness and obesity.

Types of defibrillators

Defibrillators are either automatic (i.e. automated external defibrillators (AEDs)) or manually operated. They may be capable of delivering either monophasic or biphasic shocks. AEDs are pre-set for all parameters, including the energy dose.

Manual defibrillators capable of delivering the full range of energy requirements for newborns through to adults must be available within all healthcare facilities caring for children at risk of cardiorespiratory arrest. In children requiring cardioversion (e.g. a child with circulatory failure from SVT), a manual defibrillator should be used as AEDs do not have synchronisation technology.

Biphasic defibrillators

There are various types of biphasic waveform, but there is no data to support one being superior to another. However, there is good evidence that biphasic defibrillators are more effective than monophasic. A biphasic defibrillator delivers a current that flows in a positive direction and then in reverse for a specified duration. The first shock efficacy for long-lasting VF/pVT is better with biphasic than monophasic waveforms. Biphasic waves also appear to cause less post-shock cardiac dysfunction.

Paddles or pads?

Manual defibrillation is now more commonly performed using self-adhesive pads (i.e. 'hands-free') rather than manual defibrillator paddles. Self-adhesive pads are safe, effective and generally preferable to defibrillator paddles. A major advantage of using self-adhesive pads is that they allow the rescuer to defibrillate from a safe distance, rather than having to lean across the patient; this is particularly important when access to the patient is restricted in a confined space. They deliver the shock more rapidly and with less interruption to CPR as the machine can be charged whilst chest compressions are in progress. Some self-adhesive pads have a sensor attached which measures the rate, depth and recoil of chest compressions so that the rescuer can monitor the quality of CPR delivered.

Rarely manual paddles are used; if they are, separate defibrillation gel pads need to be applied to the child's chest wall to ensure good contact and reduce transthoracic impedance. These contact gel pads tend to fall off during chest compressions, often requiring repositioning or replacing during the resuscitation attempt. Additionally, they can lead to spurious asystole on ECG analysis as the gel becomes dry and less effective as a conducting agent on repeated defibrillation attempts. This phenomenon is not encountered with self-adhesive pads.

If using the defibrillator paddles, the aim is to ensure the maximal contact with the chest wall. The largest available paddles should be selected, but they must not come in to contact with each other. Generally, the standard (adult) size paddles are appropriate for use in children over 10 kg body weight. If the child is smaller than this, the infant paddles (approximately 4.5 cm diameter) should be used. If infant paddles are unavailable for use on a small child, then the standard paddles can be placed in an anteroposterior (front and back) position instead. When delivering the shock, firm pressure needs to be exerted onto the paddles by the rescuer.

Position of self-adhesive pads

Self-adhesive pads should be placed on the child's chest in a position that 'brackets' the heart to facilitate the flow of electrical current across it.

The anterior-posterior (A-P) pad position (Figure 7.1): place the anterior pad on the lower half of the chest slightly to the left of the sternum and the posterior pad between the scapulae. The A-P position may be preferred in infants because of the size of the chest. In older children, where the chest may be larger, and it is believed CPR will be interrupted, and defibrillation delayed placing the posterior pad, the antero-lateral pad position may be preferred.

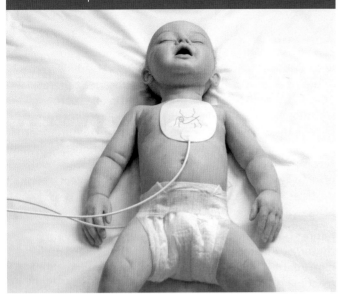

Figure 7.1   Self-adhesive pads in the anterior-posterior position on an infant

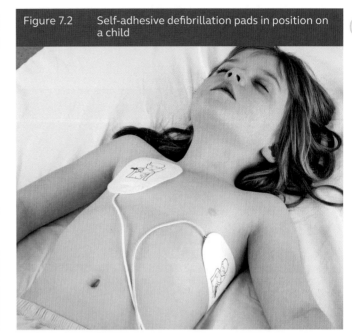

Figure 7.2   Self-adhesive defibrillation pads in position on a child

The antero-lateral (A-L) pad position (Figure 7.2): one pad is placed just below the right clavicle to the right of the sternum and the other in the mid-axillary line on the left of the chest in the V5-V6 position of a 12-lead ECG.

There is no evidence to suggest one position is superior to the other; however, it is important that the defibrillator pads must not touch. If the defibrillation pads touch, the energy arcs across the chest from pad to pad and not through the chest.

A selection of appropriate pads relating to the child's size/age may also be necessary, 8–12 cm is recommended for children and 4.5 cm for infants, although this varies between manufacturers. The pads should be smoothed onto the child's chest, ensuring that no air is trapped underneath, as this will increase impedance and reduce the efficiency of the defibrillation shock. Although the pads are generally labelled right and left or have a diagram of their correct positioning on the chest, it does not matter if they have been reversed. Therefore, if they have accidentally been placed the wrong way round, they should be left in place and not repositioned. Repositioning results in time-wasting, and the self-adhesive pads may stick less effectively.

Care must be taken when placing defibrillator pads/paddles on children who have an implantable cardioverter-defibrillator (ICD) or cardiac pacemaker, since the current delivered by an external defibrillator may travel along the wire/lead, resulting in burns where they are in contact with the myocardium. This may increase the resistance at the contact point and the 'threshold' for pacing over a period of time. If resuscitation of these children is successful, the pacemaker threshold must be regularly checked for some months after the event. Manual defibrillation pads/paddles must be placed at least 12 cm from the pacemaker/ICD site; this may necessitate anterior-posterior positioning in some children.

Energy levels

Manual defibrillators

Manual defibrillators (Figure 7.3) have several advantages over AEDs. Therefore, they must be readily available in all healthcare settings where children at risk of cardiorespiratory arrest may be cared for, even when AEDs are located nearby. The advantages include:

- ability to alter energy levels
- trained operators can diagnose arrhythmias and, when appropriate, deliver shocks more rapidly (with AEDs, this diagnosis must await the results of the machine's rhythm analysis)
- additional facilities permit other treatments (e.g. synchronised cardioversion or external pacing).

When using a manual defibrillator, an energy dose of 4 J per kg body weight (4 J kg^{-1}) should be used for all shocks, regardless of whether they are monophasic or biphasic waveforms. Consider escalating energy doses after seeking expert help for the 6th shock in refractory VF/pVT; doses up to 8 J kg^{-1} may be used. It seems reasonable not to use doses above those suggested for adults.

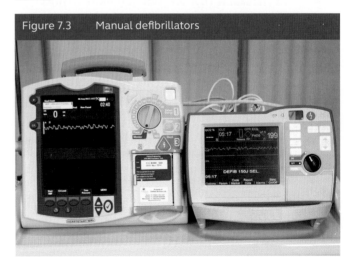

Figure 7.3   Manual defibrillators

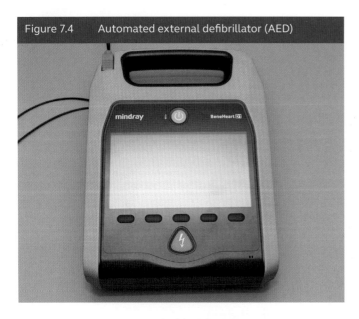

Figure 7.4   Automated external defibrillator (AED)

Automated external defibrillators

These machines are now widely available, including through Public Access Defibrillation (PAD) schemes as fully or semi-automated devices (Figure 7.4). They are safe, reliable and sophisticated and are increasingly used by health professionals and lay rescuers.

If there is any likelihood of use in infants and small children, check with the manufacturer that the machine is suitable. Machines with paediatric attenuation devices are preferable.

The AED will analyse the patient's ECG rhythm, determine whether a defibrillation shock is indicated and facilitate the delivery of a shock. In the semi-automated models, follow the AED prompts and press the relevant button.

Some of the models available to healthcare professionals have the facility for the operator to override the AED and deliver a shock independently of any prompting by the machine.

The main advantages of AEDs are that they recognise VF and pVT shockable rhythms, and therefore a shock can be delivered by a lay-person. They are also relatively cheap and lightweight and have therefore replaced many manual defibrillators. Available AEDs have been tested extensively against libraries of adult ECG rhythms and in trials in adults and children. They are extremely accurate in rhythm recognition in both adults and children. The voice prompts from the AED must be followed to ensure safe, effective practice.

In a child > 8 years requiring defibrillation, standard adult AED energy levels can be used.

If a child < 8 years requires emergency defibrillation, and there is no manual defibrillator available, an AED can be used. The AED should ideally be equipped with a dose attenuator, which decreases the delivered energy to a lower, more appropriate dosage (generally 50–75 J). If such an AED is unavailable in an emergency situation, then a standard AED with adult energy levels may be used. The upper dose limit for safe defibrillation is unknown, but higher doses than the previously recommended 4 J kg^{-1} have defibrillated children effectively and without significant adverse effects. Higher doses are acceptable because defibrillation is the only effective treatment for VF/pVT.

Infants have a much lower incidence of shockable rhythms, and good quality CPR is the treatment priority. If an infant is in a shockable rhythm and a manual machine is not available, using an AED (preferably with an attenuator) may be considered.

Minimal interruption to chest compressions

Every time chest compressions are interrupted, even for a brief period, a low flow state is created, where coronary artery and cerebral perfusion pressures fall dramatically. Several chest compressions are required to return these pressures to optimum levels. Interruptions can be minimised during defibrillation by good team communication and coordination:

- Charging the defibrillator whilst chest compressions are ongoing during the shockable arm of the ALS algorithm.

- Minimising the delay between stopping chest compressions and the delivery of shocks or checking for signs of life at the end of 2 min cycles (< 5 s is ideal).

- Resuming chest compressions immediately after the delivery of a shock with no check of either the monitor or patient.

Safety issues when undertaking defibrillation

The safety of the rescuers, as well as that of the child, is paramount. The following factors must be considered.

Oxygen

All free-flowing oxygen delivery devices (O_2 masks or nasal cannulae) must be removed from the immediate area and placed at least one metre from the child. If the child is being ventilated via a sealed advanced airway (TT/SGA), the ventilation bag or ventilator tubing can be left connected if it forms part of a closed circuit. If the circuit is disconnected for whatever reason, the devices must be placed at least one metre away from the child.

Dry surfaces

Any wet clothing should be removed from the immediate area. The surface the child is laid on, and the child's chest should be wiped dry if necessary before shock delivery.

Contact with patient

The person delivering the shock must ensure that neither they nor any other rescuers/relatives are in direct or indirect contact with the child during shock delivery.

There should be no contact between the pads and any metal objects (e.g. jewellery) or items such as transdermal medication or diathermy pads.

Operator instructions

Familiarity with the defibrillator being used increases safety for all the team and operator efficiency. Operators must also ensure that they issue clear instructions to the rest of the team/bystanders to facilitate safe practice throughout the procedure.

Sequence of actions for defibrillation

If the ALS rescuer is first on scene the entire BLS sequence needs to be followed. If, however, the rescuer is part of a response team arriving to find BLS already ongoing, they should reconfirm cardiac arrest, taking no more than 5 s to do so.

Having confirmed cardiorespiratory arrest, CPR should be started (or restarted) while the team member operating the defibrillator prepares as follows:

1. Confirms presence of shockable rhythm (VF/pVT) via self-adhesive/ monitoring pads or ECG monitor during a brief pause in chest compressions.

2. Instructs the team to resume chest compressions, preferably using a sensor allowing CPR feedback and metronomic support if available.

3. Selects the appropriate energy (4 J kg^{-1}).

4. Warns all team members (other than the individual performing the chest compressions) to "stand clear" and remove any oxygen delivery device as appropriate.

5. Charge the defibrillator to the required energy level whilst chest compressions are ongoing.

6. Once the defibrillator is charged, tell the team member doing the chest compressions to "stand clear"; when clear and after confirming continued VF/pVT, deliver a safe shock.

7. Without reassessing the rhythm or feeling for a pulse, instructs the team to restart CPR starting with chest compressions. The team should then continue CPR for two minutes; the team leader resumes coordination of the team and prepares for the next pause in CPR. If VF/pVT persists after 2 minutes of CPR, deliver a second/subsequent shock.

Further management of shockable cardiac arrest rhythms, including the reversible causes of cardiopulmonary arrest, are described in Chapter 8.

Considerations when using an AED

The AED pads are placed in the same position as manual defibrillators.

Sequence of actions for using an AED

The following guidance should be used for all AEDs, with or without a paediatric dose attenuating device:

1. Ensure the safety of the rescuers/bystanders and child.

2. Start BLS (see chapter 4).

3. Switch on the AED and attach self-adhesive pads. If more than one rescuer is present, BLS should be continued whilst the AED is attached.

4. Follow the AED prompts.

5. Ensure no one touches the child while the rhythm is being analysed. This is extremely important as artefact from chest compressions given during the analysis phase may be interpreted by the AED as VF and the machine may charge and advise a shock.

6. If defibrillation is indicated:
   - ensure no-one touches the child
   - press the shock delivery button as directed
   - continue as directed by the AED prompts.

7. If no shock is indicated:
   - resume BLS immediately
   - continue as directed by the AED prompts.

8. Continue resuscitation until:
   - help arrives and takes over management
   - the child starts to show signs of life
   - the rescuer becomes too exhausted to continue.

Note: do not switch off the AED whilst CPR is continued.

Testing the defibrillator

Defibrillators should be regularly tested as per manufacturer and local policies. All potential operators should familiarise themselves with the specific operating procedures of their available machines.

Considerations when undertaking synchronised DC cardioversion

Cardioversion is the first line of treatment for children and infants presenting with decompensated circulatory failure due to supraventricular tachycardia (SVT) or ventricular tachycardia with a pulse (VT). Cardioversion is the timed delivery of an electrical shock at a dose of 1 J kg⁻¹ body weight from the defibrillator with an increase to 2 J kg⁻¹ if the initial shock is unsuccessful. The delivery of the shock is synchronised with the R wave of the ECG to minimise the risk of inducing VF. In some instances, consideration may be given to increase the energy to 4 J kg⁻¹, but this decision should be guided by expert help.

Expert help must be sought if cardioversion is required.

The application of the pads and the safety precautions are the same as for defibrillation, but there are some additional patient safety considerations. These include:

- For children and infants who are conscious, use adequate analgesia and sedation (e.g. intranasal or intramuscular ketamine if no intravenous line in-situ) with airway management, preferably with the help of an anaesthetist or other expert provider. If an intravenous (IV) line can be rapidly sited, IV analgesia and sedation (e.g. ketamine) can be used, but IV access attempts MUST NOT delay cardioversion.

- Synchronisation mode on the defibrillator must be activated. On some machines, it may need to be re-selected if repeat shocks are required or if the machine is accidentally turned off between shocks.

- When the synchronised function is activated, a marker will appear above or on the R wave, indicating where the shock will be delivered in the cardiac cycle.

- If lead II does not display a synchronised mark for every R wave, select another lead such as lead I or III, this may help the defibrillator recognise the R wave. Not all defibrillators are the same; it is important to know how the synchronised mark is displayed on your device.

- Confirm energy values.

- Delays in shock delivery can occur between the operator depressing the delivery button and the actual shock being delivered. This is because the machine will only deliver the shock when it identifies an R wave. In practice, it means that the operator must keep the shock delivery button depressed until this occurs.

07: Summary learning

For the patient in VF/pVT, early defibrillation is the only effective means of restoring a spontaneous circulation.

When using a defibrillator, minimise interruptions in chest compressions to reduce no-flow times.

Good communication and teamwork are essential to optimise outcome and overall safety.

Use an AED if you are not confident in rhythm recognition or manual defibrillation.

My key take-home messages from this chapter are:

Further reading

Atkinson E, Mikysa B et al. Specificity and sensitivity of automated external defibrillator rhythm analysis in infants and children. Ann Emerg Med 2003;42: 185-96

Hunt EA, Duval- Arnould JM, Bembea MM, et al. Association between time to defibrillation and survival in pediatric in-hospital cardiac arrest with a first documented shockable rhythm. JAMA Netw Open 2018;1: e182643, doi:http://dx.doi.org/10.1001/jamanetworkopen.2018.2643.

Tsuda T, Geary EM, Temple J. Significance of automated external defibrillator in identifying lethal ventricular arrhythmias. Eur J Pediatr 2019,178.1333.

Berg RA, Chapman FW et al. Attenuated adult biphasic shocks compared with weight-based monophasic shocks in a swine model of prolonged pediatric ventricular fibrillation. Resuscitation 2004; 61: 189-197.

Berg RA, Samson RA et al. Better outcome after pediatric defibrillation dosage than adult dosage in a swine model of pediatric ventricular fibrillation. J Am Coll Cardiol 2005;45: 786-9.

Clark CB, Zhang Y et al. Pediatric transthoracic defibrillation: biphasic versus monophasic waveforms in an experimental model. Resuscitation 2001;51: 159-63.

Edelson DP, Abella BS, Kramer-Johansen J, et al. Effects of compression depth and pre-shock pauses predict defibrillation failure during cardiac arrest. Resuscitation 2006;71:137-45.

Eftestol T, Sunde K, Steen PA. Effects of interrupting precordial compressions on the calculated probability of defibrillation success during out-of-hospital cardiac arrest. Circulation 2002;105:2270-3.

Faddy SC, Powell J et al. Biphasic and monophasic shocks for transthoracic defibrillation: A meta analysis of randomised controlled trials. Resuscitation 2003;8: 9-16.

Jorgenson D, Morgan C, Snyder D et al. Energy attenuator for pediatric application of an automated external defibrillator. Crit Care Med 2002;30:S145-7.

Meaney P, Nadkarni V et al. Effect of defibrillation dose during in-hospital pediatric cardiac arrest. Pediatrics 2011;127(1):e16-23.

Rodriguez-Nunez A, Lopez-Herce J. Shockable rhythms and defibrillation during in-hospital pediatric cardiac arrest. Resuscitation 2014;85:387-91.

Tibbals J, Carter B et al. External and internal biphasic direct current shock doses for pediatric VF and pulseless VT. Pediatric Crit Care Med 2011;12:14-20.

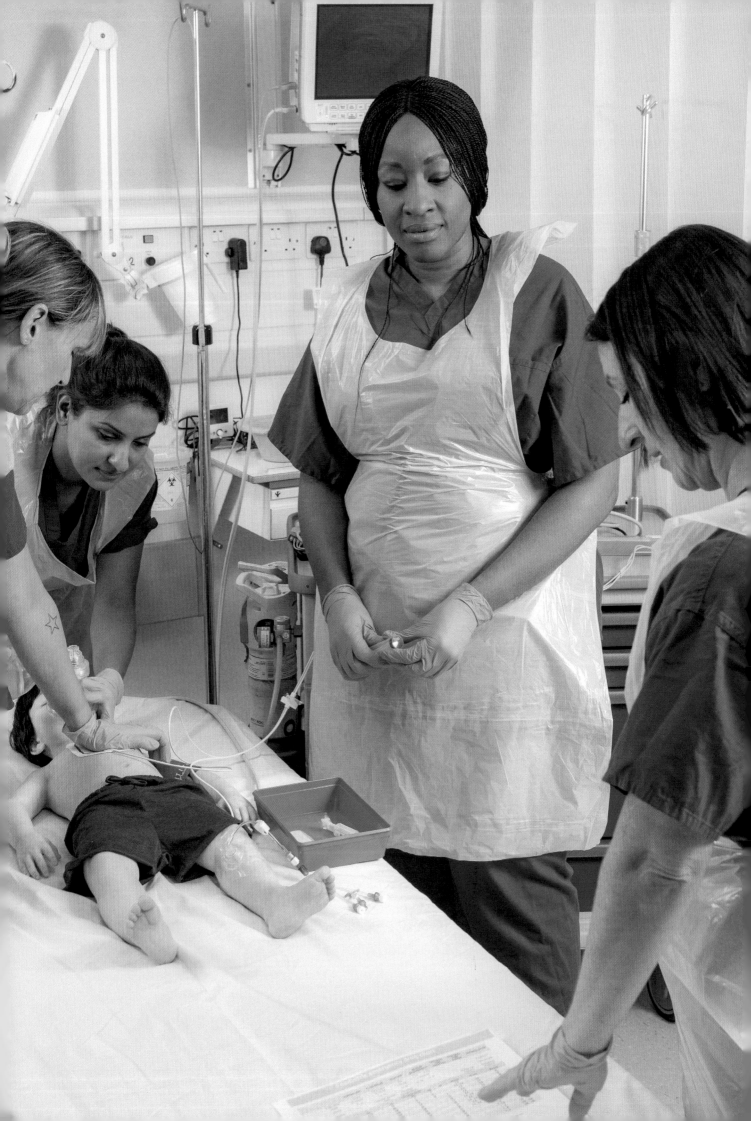

Management of cardiorespiratory arrest

Resuscitation process

Resuscitation is a continuous process from basic life support (BLS) to advanced life support (ALS). High-quality BLS provides the most important foundation for successful resuscitation.

The elements of BLS must be continued until a return of spontaneous circulation (ROSC), even when experienced help arrives (i.e. the EMS or clinical emergency team), and appropriate equipment can be used to facilitate the delivery of advanced techniques. It is important that the on-call resuscitation team prepare for this event at the changeover of staff and team huddles (Chapter 15).

All clinical staff within a healthcare facility should be able to:

- immediately recognise cardiorespiratory arrest
- start appropriate resuscitation (BLS with available adjuncts)
- summon the clinical emergency team using the standard telephone number (2222 in-hospital) and/or EMS (via national 999 system).

The exact sequence of actions will be dependent on several factors, including:

- location of the event (clinical or non-clinical area)
- number of first responders
- skills of first responders
- availability of resuscitation equipment
- local policies.

High-quality BLS provides the most important foundation for successful resuscitation

Preventing cardiorespiratory arrest

If a child is seriously ill on a ward, it is likely that they will have been deteriorating over a period of time. Measures must be put in place to ensure any critically ill child is identified and transferred to a safe area with early admission to ICU/HDU where appropriate, the aim being to ensure the child is in the right bed at the right time. Many wards now employ early warning scores (EWS) systems based on physiological parameters to help identify seriously ill children. Evidence from a large randomised trial indicated that whilst the implementation of an EWS system does not affect mortality it does improve recognition of the physiologically unstable child, reducing the number of critical incidents associated with deterioration on the wards. Whilst EWS are useful as part of the overall clinical response system; there must also be a focus on improving health carers' ability to recognise and intervene for patients with a deteriorating illness. Monitored physiological parameters are particularly useful in looking at trends that can provide more useful information than a single elevated EWS score, and it is always important to take note of any parental or nursing concern. All findings need to be escalated early, and appropriate management strategies are initiated to prevent cardiorespiratory arrest from occurring. The chain of prevention (Smith 2010) helps structure the processes required to detect and prevent patient deterioration and cardiopulmonary arrest (Figure 8.1).

Summoning senior clinical support such as a rapid response team may reduce the risk of respiratory and/or cardiac arrest in hospitalised children and infants. Most cardiorespiratory arrests in children and infants arise from decompensated respiratory or circulatory failure causing hypoxia. Secondary cardiorespiratory arrests have a poor outcome, and hence the identification of the seriously ill or injured child is an absolute priority. Any unwell child should be assessed using the ABCDE assessment process and findings communicated to ensure the child is in a safe setting. The right bed at the right time. When preventative measures and systems for early escalation for expert support are in place, a paediatric cardiopulmonary arrest outside of HDU, ITU or ED is thankfully a rare event.

Cardiorespiratory arrest in a clinical area

When a child does suffer a cardiorespiratory arrest in a clinical area, staff should be able to promptly initiate BLS and place a 2222 call to summon the clinical emergency/cardiac arrest team. Appropriate resuscitation equipment and trained staff should be readily available.

Cardiorespiratory arrest in a non-clinical area

There may be occasions when a child suffers a cardiorespiratory arrest in a non-clinical area (e.g. corridors, car park, play area). In these areas, equipment or trained staff may not be readily available, and these children may have a more prolonged period of BLS before expert help arrives.

In hospital cardiac arrest (IHCA)

The guidance in the first section of this chapter is primarily aimed at healthcare professionals who may be initial responders in a clinical emergency and have rapid access to resuscitation equipment. The guidance in the second section of this chapter is primarily aimed at the team, providing experienced help, including guidance for the team leader.

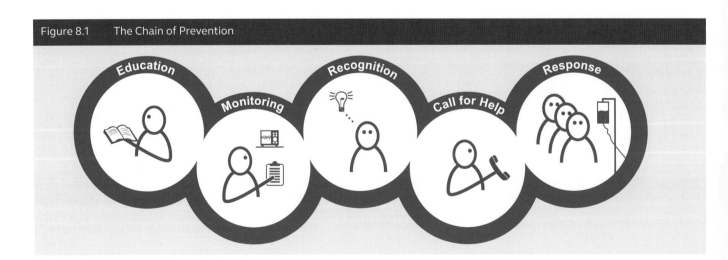

Figure 8.1   The Chain of Prevention

Number of first responders

A single rescuer must not leave the collapsed child but should start appropriate resuscitation (e.g. BLS or BLS with BMV) and ensure that further help is summoned.

Within a clinical area, there are usually more staff nearby who can be alerted, either by the first responder shouting for help and/or using an emergency call button system. As soon as a second rescuer arrives, they should be sent to summon further assistance in line with local policy (i.e. activate the clinical emergency team; in hospitals, this will be via a 2222 call). On their return (or on the arrival of other staff), simultaneous interventions can be undertaken, according to the skills of the available staff.

Skills of first responders

Healthcare providers should be able to recognise cardiorespiratory arrest, shout for help and start resuscitation to the level to which they have been trained. After training, the decay in resuscitation skills is well documented, with skills retention probably lasting about 3 months. Recent studies indicate that short, targeted refresher training for staff looking after the sicker patients at their bedside may be beneficial, so-called 'just in time' training.

Staff will have been trained to different levels according to local policies; some may only undertake BLS, whilst others would be expected to undertake additional techniques to manage airway, breathing and circulation. The initial priority for first responders in paediatric cardiorespiratory arrest, should be to ensure effective ventilation and oxygenation with good quality BLS. As more experienced help arrives, other interventions can be undertaken.

Availability of resuscitation equipment

All clinical areas where children are likely to be cared for should be equipped with resuscitation equipment to help manage a clinical emergency. The staff in each area should have responsibility for maintenance and regular checking of this clinical emergency equipment, as this will facilitate their familiarity with it. Standardised resuscitation equipment hospital-wide enables the clinical emergency team to know what equipment is readily available to them when called to deal with a child in any area. Equipment capable of delivering CPR feedback for rescuers will improve the quality of CPR given and is strongly recommended.

Quality standards

Healthcare organisations have an obligation to provide a high-quality resuscitation service and to ensure that staff are trained and updated regularly and with appropriate frequency to a level of proficiency appropriate to each individual's expected role. The Resuscitation Council UK's 'Quality Standards for Cardiopulmonary Resuscitation Practice and Training' provides further detailed information.

All 2222 calls should be audited as recommended by the RCUK Quality Standards. In-house clinical audits of all 2222 calls is vital to identify any patient safety issues or breakdown in the chain of prevention. This will also enable staff to be supported following adverse events and improve the debriefing process that may be required. Lessons for learning that arise from each 2222 event are invaluable and will help improve the hospital systems for identifying and managing critically unwell children and infants.

The National Cardiac Arrest audit (NCAA) is a UK national study incorporating both adult and paediatric in-hospital arrests in the UK attended by a 2222 team. Data collected provides feedback to each participating hospital with benchmarking against similar hospitals allowing quality improvement initiatives (see Chapter 15).

Hospitals should have policies regarding the calling criteria for their clinical emergency teams. In some centres, there might be more than one emergency team (dictated by the geographical layout or the clinical specialities of the hospital), or there may be different types of team (e.g. a cardiac arrest team and a medical emergency team). Staff must be aware of their local systems and trained to act accordingly. Operational issues should be audited. Continuous measurement of compliance with processes and patient outcomes at a national and local level provides information on the impact of changes in practice, identifies areas for improvement, and also enables comparison in outcomes between different organisations.

As resuscitation team members will differ daily, it is invaluable that cardiac arrest teams huddle/meet at the beginning of each shift. These 'huddles' enable the team members to introduce themselves to each other, discuss each team member's skills, assign roles and identify those patients at high risk of deterioration across the hospital. These 'huddles' can improve teamwork, particularly communication in a subsequent emergency scenario. Cardiac arrest teams will operate more efficiently if skills

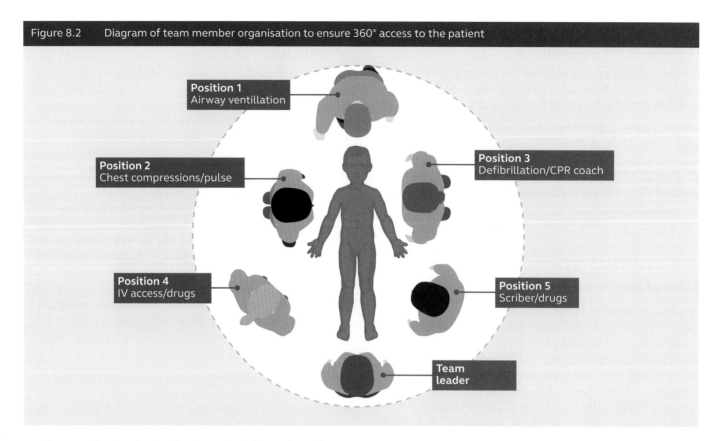

Figure 8.2 Diagram of team member organisation to ensure 360° access to the patient

Position 1
Airway ventilation

Position 3
Defibrillation/CPR coach

Position 2
Chest compressions/pulse

Position 4
IV access/drugs

Position 5
Scriber/drugs

Team
leader

can be practiced and refreshed regularly by undertaking 'mock' emergency calls; these will enable team members to refresh ALS knowledge and practice team 'choreography' which will improve performance (Figure 8.2).

The sequence of actions in cardiopulmonary resuscitation (CPR)

The initial management of a collapsed child is summarised in Figure 8.3.

Safety

The approach described in Chapter 4 should be followed to ensure firstly the safety of the rescuers and then that of the child. Whilst the risk of contracting an infection is low, personal protective measures should be used as soon as practicable (e.g. gloves, aprons, eye protection, face masks). In situations where the child may have a severe infection (e.g. open TB, COVID-19, Swine flu or SARS), rescuers must be equipped with full protective measures. In areas where such children may be treated, this equipment should be immediately available.

Stimulate

The approach described in Chapter 4 should be followed to establish the responsiveness of an unconscious child.

Responsive child

If the child responds (i.e. they demonstrate signs of life), the child should be assessed using the ABCDE approach. Appropriate interventions should be initiated and further relevant assistance summoned.

Unresponsive child

If the child is unresponsive (i.e. they do not demonstrate signs of life), start BLS immediately whilst simultaneously shouting for more assistance.

Shout for help

The single-rescuer must not leave the child but shout loudly for help and start BLS, using basic airway adjuncts and BMV if they are immediately available and activating the bedside emergency call button system if this is available.

If there is a second rescuer available, they should be sent to summon more assistance and return to help with the resuscitation attempt.

If resuscitation equipment is nearby, they should bring this to the bedside, but this must not delay calling the clinical emergency team.

Airway

The airway should be opened, as described in Chapter 4. If suction is available, it may be necessary to use this to clear any secretions in the upper airway before proceeding to ventilation.

Breathing

The rescuer should perform a breathing check, as described in Chapter 4, for 10 s whilst looking for signs of life (responsiveness, coughing, spontaneous movements, and normal breathing).

Paediatric basic life support

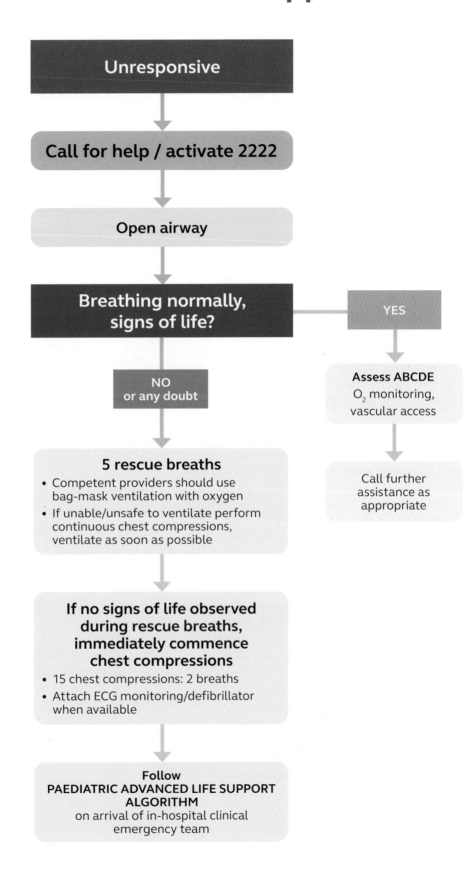

Unresponsive

↓

Call for help / activate 2222

↓

Open airway

↓

Breathing normally, signs of life? ——— **YES**

NO or any doubt

Assess ABCDE
O_2 monitoring, vascular access

↓

Call further assistance as appropriate

↓ (NO branch)

5 rescue breaths
- Competent providers should use bag-mask ventilation with oxygen
- If unable/unsafe to ventilate perform continuous chest compressions, ventilate as soon as possible

↓

If no signs of life observed during rescue breaths, immediately commence chest compressions
- 15 chest compressions: 2 breaths
- Attach ECG monitoring/defibrillator when available

↓

Follow
PAEDIATRIC ADVANCED LIFE SUPPORT ALGORITHM
on arrival of in-hospital clinical emergency team

Figure 8.3   Initial resuscitation management

If the child is not breathing or only gasping ineffectively, initial rescue breaths should be delivered by the most appropriate method available. In the hospital setting, this will usually be with a BMV device with supplemental oxygen (if not available, expired air rescue breaths with a barrier device may be used until a BMV device can be retrieved).

If there are two rescuers available and at least one is trained in the use of BMV, the rescuer managing the airway and delivering the rescue breaths should be positioned behind the child's head. A second rescuer should be positioned at the side of the child to perform chest compressions if indicated. As soon as resuscitation equipment is available, the emphasis is on ensuring that effective CPR is enhanced by BMV with supplemental oxygen. When using BMV, a two-person technique is advocated to provide an adequate seal of the mask.

Circulation

Assessment

The presence or absence of signs of life, such as response to stimuli, normal breathing (rather than abnormal gasps) or spontaneous movement, must be looked for during the breathing assessment and during rescue breaths to determine the need for chest compressions. If there is still doubt at the end of the rescue breaths, start chest compressions.

Feeling for a pulse is not a reliable way to determine if there is an effective or inadequate circulation, and palpation of the pulse is not the determinant of the need for chest compressions. Rescuers are no longer taught to feel for a pulse as part of the assessment of the need for chest compressions in BLS. If a healthcare provider still wishes to do a pulse check in an unresponsive child, they must be certain that one is present for them NOT to start CPR. In this situation, there are often other signs of life present.

High-quality chest compressions are extremely important to maximise the chances of successful CPR. The components are:

- correct compression rate, 100–120 min^{-1} for both infants and children

- correct depth: release all pressure on the chest between compressions to allow for complete chest recoil and avoid leaning on the chest at the end of a compression

- chest compression pauses should be minimised so that 80% or more of the CPR cycle is comprised of chest compressions (this is also known as chest compression fraction)

- ventilations and compressions are then delivered in 15:2 ratio until monitoring is attached.

Rhythm recognition

Establish the child's cardiac rhythm by attaching ECG monitoring (available on manual defibrillators). The priority is deciding whether the cardiac rhythm is shockable or non-shockable in order to determine the ongoing management of the cardiorespiratory arrest. Briefly pause chest compressions to allow for rhythm recognition on the monitor. If an AED is used, it will guide the rescuers through the sequence of actions.

Shockable or non-shockable cardiac rhythms

In children, the most common initial cardiorespiratory arrest rhythms are non-shockable (i.e. profound bradycardia, asystole or pulseless electrical activity (PEA). CPR should be started in children who become bradycardic (heart rate < 60 min^{-1}) with signs of inadequate perfusion despite adequate respiratory support and oxygenation.

The shockable cardiorespiratory arrest rhythms (i.e. ventricular fibrillation (VF) and pulseless ventricular tachycardia (pVT)) are less common. When these occur, it is often in a child with underlying cardiac disease (congenital or acquired).

The management of shockable and non-shockable cardiorespiratory arrest is outlined below.

Non-shockable rhythms (asystole and PEA)

Asystole

This rhythm is characterised by the total absence of effective electrical and mechanical activity in the heart (Figure 8.4). It can be simulated by artefact (e.g. detached ECG leads or electrodes); it is important to quickly check the equipment. In asystole, there is no ventricular function, but occasionally there is some atrial activity, which may be seen on the ECG as P waves (Figure 8.5). It is often preceded by severe bradycardia. The most common cause of bradycardia in a child is hypoxia, but hypotension, hypothermia or hypoglycaemia can depress normal cardiac activity and slow conduction through cardiac tissues.

Pulseless electrical activity (PEA)

This rhythm is defined as organised cardiac electrical activity in the absence of a palpable central pulse or signs of life. Some of these children may have some myocardial contraction, but it is too weak and ineffective to produce a detectable pulse, blood pressure or signs of life. The ECG rhythm displayed is often a slow, broad complex one, although any variation of regular QRS complexes may be seen.

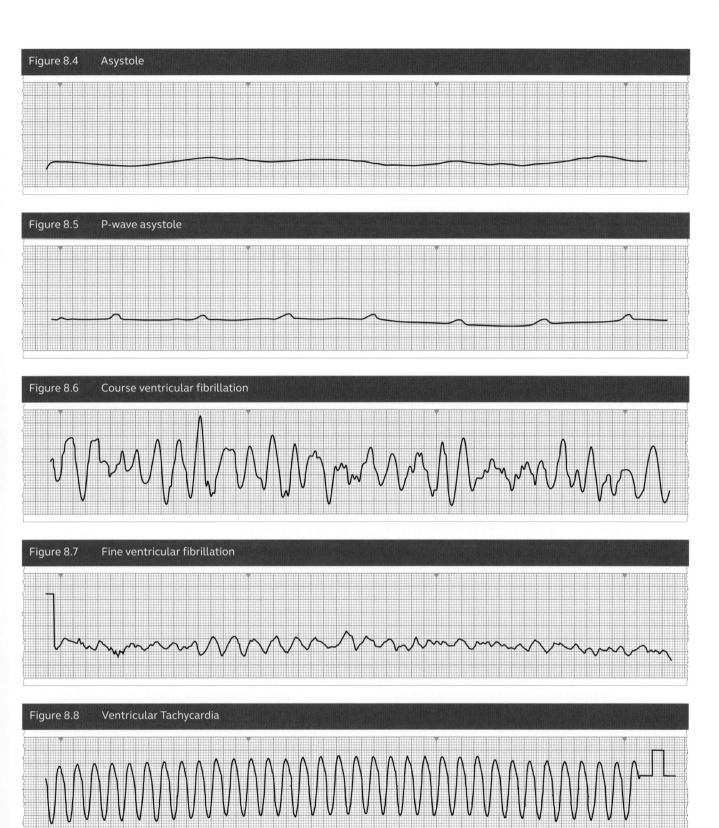

Figure 8.4   Asystole

Figure 8.5   P-wave asystole

Figure 8.6   Course ventricular fibrillation

Figure 8.7   Fine ventricular fibrillation

Figure 8.8   Ventricular Tachycardia

All the cardiorespiratory arrest rhythms may be due to an underlying reversible condition; identify and treat all reversible causes listed within the paediatric advanced life support algorithm (Figure 8.9).

Management of asystole and PEA

1. Perform continuous CPR

- Continue to ventilate with high concentration inspired oxygen 100%. Provide ventilation initially by bag-mask ventilation (BMV). Do not titrate the concentration of inspired oxygen during CPR. To provide an adequate seal of the mask, a two-person technique is advocated.

- If ventilating with a bag-mask use a ratio of 15 chest compressions to 2 ventilations

- Use a compression rate of 100–120 min^{-1}. Depth of compression is one-third of the depth of the chest, approximately 4 cm in an infant and 5 cm in a child.

- When performing chest compressions, choose a team member who will be able to deliver them most effectively and use a rigid surface/backboard so that chest compressions are more effective

- If BMV can be successfully performed, then continue with this mode of ventilation. A team member with the necessary skills to safely provide an advanced airway should be summoned but only intubate the trachea if this can be performed with minimal interruption to chest compressions. If BMV is unsuccessful and a team member with the necessary skills to safely intubate is not present, a competent provider may use a supraglottic airway (SGA) (e.g. i-gel) as an alternative. Intubation should also be considered if BMV is becoming more difficult as the resuscitation progresses. Always confirm tracheal tube (TT) placement by end-tidal CO_2 monitoring.

  If the patient is intubated, chest compressions can be continuous if this does not interfere with satisfactory ventilation.

- Once the child's trachea has been intubated, and compressions are uninterrupted (only pausing every 2 min for rhythm check) ventilations should approximate to the lower limit of normal rate for age:

  - **Infants:** 25 breaths per min
  - **Children 1–8 years old:** 20 breaths per min
  - **Children 8–12 years old:** 15 breaths per min
  - **Children over 12 years old:** 10–12 breaths per min.

- Note: Once there is ROSC, the ventilation rate should be a normal physiological age-dependent respiratory rate that may then be adjusted to meet the goals of post-resuscitation care. Measure end-tidal carbon dioxide (end-tidal CO_2) to monitor ventilation and ensure correct TT placement.

2. Give adrenaline as soon as possible

- If vascular access has been established, give adrenaline 10 micrograms kg^{-1} (0.1 mL kg^{-1} of a 1:10 000 solution).

- If there is no circulatory access, obtain intraosseous (IO) access.

- The first dose of adrenaline should be given as soon as possible, preferably within 3 min of identification of cardiorespiratory arrest (for non-shockable rhythms).

3. Continue CPR, only pausing briefly every 2 min to check for rhythm change

- Give adrenaline 10 micrograms kg^{-1} every 3–5 min (i.e. every other cycle) while maintaining effective chest compressions and ventilation without interruption.

- The aim is to maximise chest compression time, and the chest compression fraction (CCF) should be equal to or greater than 80%.

4. Change the person performing chest compressions at least every 2 min.

- Watch for fatigue and/or suboptimal compressions and switch rescuers earlier if necessary.

5. Consider and correct reversible causes:

- Consider the 4 H's and 4 T's.

6. After each 2 min of uninterrupted CPR, pause briefly to assess the rhythm:

- If asystole:
  - Continue CPR using the non-shockable side of the algorithm.

- If VF/pVT:
  - Continue CPR and switch to the shockable (VF/pVT) side of the algorithm as below.

- If organised electrical activity is seen, check for signs of life and a pulse:
  - If there is ROSC, continue post-resuscitation care.
  - If there is no pulse (or a pulse rate of <60 min^{-1}), and there are no other signs of life, continue CPR and continue with the non-shockable sequence above.
  - Feeling for a pulse:

    In an infant: feel for the brachial pulse on the inner aspect of the upper arm.

    In a child aged over 1 year: feel for the carotid pulse in the neck.

    For both infants and children: the femoral pulse in the groin (mid-way between the anterior superior iliac spine and the symphysis pubis) can also be used.

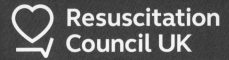

Paediatric advanced life support

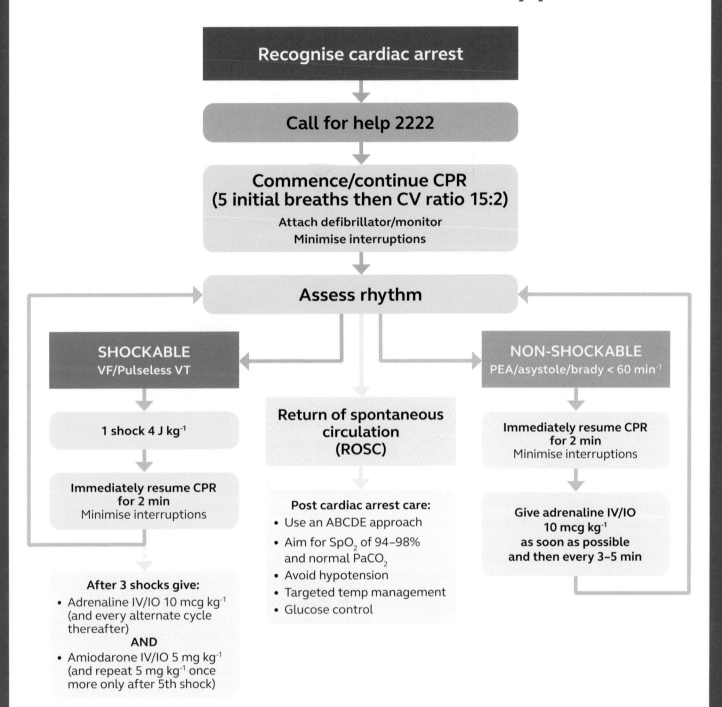

Recognise cardiac arrest

Call for help 2222

Commence/continue CPR
(5 initial breaths then CV ratio 15:2)
Attach defibrillator/monitor
Minimise interruptions

Assess rhythm

SHOCKABLE
VF/Pulseless VT

1 shock 4 J kg^{-1}

Immediately resume CPR
for 2 min
Minimise interruptions

After 3 shocks give:
- Adrenaline IV/IO 10 mcg kg^{-1} (and every alternate cycle thereafter)
AND
- Amiodarone IV/IO 5 mg kg^{-1} (and repeat 5 mg kg^{-1} once more only after 5th shock)

Return of spontaneous circulation (ROSC)

Post cardiac arrest care:
- Use an ABCDE approach
- Aim for SpO$_2$ of 94–98% and normal PaCO$_2$
- Avoid hypotension
- Targeted temp management
- Glucose control

NON-SHOCKABLE
PEA/asystole/brady < 60 min^{-1}

Immediately resume CPR
for 2 min
Minimise interruptions

Give adrenaline IV/IO
10 mcg kg^{-1}
as soon as possible
and then every 3–5 min

During CPR
- **Ensure high quality chest compressions are delivered:**
  – Correct rate, depth and full recoil
- Provide BMV with 100% oxygen (2 person approach)
- Provide continuous chest compressions when a tracheal tube is in place.
- Competent providers can consider an advanced airway and capnography, and ventilate at a rate (breaths minute^{-1}) of:

Infants: 25	1–8 years: 20	8–12 years: 15	> 12 years: 10–12

- Vascular access IV/IO
- Once started, give Adrenaline every 3-5 min
- Maximum single dose Adrenaline 1 mg
- Maximum single dose Amiodarone 300 mg

Identify and treat reversible causes
- Hypoxia
- Hypovolaemia
- Hyperkalaemia, hypercalcaemia, hypermagnesemia, hypoglycaemia
- Hypo-/hyperthermia
- Thrombosis – coronary or pulmonary
- Tension pneumothorax
- Tamponade – cardiac
- Toxic agents

Adjust algorithm in specific settings (e.g. special circumstances)

Figure 8.9   Paediatric advanced life support algorithm

119

Shockable rhythms (VF and pVT)

Ventricular fibrillation

This rhythm shows rapid, chaotic, irregular waves of varying frequency and amplitude. VF is sometimes classified as 'coarse or fine' depending on the amplitude (height) of the complexes (Figures 8.6 and 8.7). As soon as identified, defibrillation should immediately be attempted (regardless of the ECG amplitude). If in doubt, consider the rhythm to be shockable. Shockable rhythms are less common in children but may occur as a secondary event and are more likely when there has been a witnessed and sudden collapse. It is seen more often in the intensive care unit and cardiac ward or in adolescents on the sporting field.

Pulseless ventricular tachycardia (pVT)

This rhythm is a broad complex tachycardia (Figure 8.8). It is rare in children and is managed in the same way as VF (i.e. defibrillation).

Management of VF/pVT

1. **Continue CPR until a defibrillator is available.**
2. **Apply defibrillation pads (self-adhesive pads are standard) in the antero-lateral or antero-posterior position if not yet in place.**
3. **Defibrillate the heart (as soon as possible):**
   - Charge the defibrillator while another rescuer continues chest compressions.
   - Once the defibrillator is charged, pause the chest compressions, quickly ensure that all rescuers are clear of the patient and then deliver the shock. Minimise the delay between stopping chest compressions and delivery of the shock (< 5 s).
   - Give 1 shock of 4 J kg^{-1} if using a manual defibrillator. It seems reasonable not to use doses above those suggested for adults.
   - If using an AED for a child of less than 8 years, preferably use a paediatric attenuated shock energy (50–75 J) if an attenuator is available. If one is not available use a standard AED which will deliver adult shock energy doses.
   - If using an AED for a child over 8 years, use the adult shock energy.
   - If using paddles, charging should be done with paddles on the chest, pausing compressions at that stage.

4. **Resume CPR:**
   - Without reassessing the rhythm or feeling for a pulse, resume CPR immediately, starting with chest compressions.
   - Good quality CPR is maximised if a feedback device is used.
5. **Continue CPR for 2 min, then pause briefly to check the monitor:**
   - If still VF/pVT, give a second shock (with the same energy level 4 J kg^{-1}) and strategy for delivery as the first shock.
6. **Resume CPR:**
   - Without reassessing the rhythm or feeling for a pulse, resume CPR immediately, starting with chest compressions.
7. **Continue CPR for 2 min, then pause briefly to check the monitor.**
8. **If still VF/pVT:**
   - Give a third shock with the same energy level 4 J kg^{-1} and strategy for delivery as the previous shock.
9. **Resume CPR:**
   - Without reassessing the rhythm or feeling for a pulse, resume CPR immediately, starting with chest compressions.
   - Give adrenaline 10 micrograms kg^{-1} (0.1 mL kg^{-1} of 1:10 000 solution) and amiodarone 5 mg kg^{-1} (or lidocaine 1 mg kg^{-1} may be used as an alternative to amiodarone for providers competent in its use) after the third shock and after chest compressions have resumed.
   - Repeat adrenaline 10 micrograms kg^{-1} (0.1 mL kg^{-1} of 1:10 000 solution) every alternate cycle (every 3–5 min) until ROSC.
   - Repeat amiodarone 5 mg kg^{-1} one further time, after the fifth shock if still in a shockable rhythm.

10. **Continue giving shocks every 2 min, continuing compressions during charging of the defibrillator and minimising the breaks in chest compressions as much as possible.**
   - Change the person performing chest compressions at least every 2 min. Watch for fatigue and/or suboptimal compressions and switch rescuers earlier if necessary.
   - Consider and correct reversible causes (4 H's and 4 T's).

- After each 2 min of uninterrupted CPR, pause briefly to assess the rhythm.
- If still VF/pVT:
  - Continue CPR with the shockable (VF/pVT) sequence.
  - Consider escalating energy doses after seeking expert help for the 6th shock in refractory VF/pVT.
- If asystole:
  - Continue CPR and switch to the non-shockable (asystole or PEA) side of the algorithm.
- If organised electrical activity is seen, check for signs of life and a pulse:
  - If there is ROSC, continue post-resuscitation care.
  - If there is no pulse (or a pulse rate of <60 min^{-1}), and there are no other signs of life, continue CPR and continue as for the non-shockable side of the algorithm.

11. If defibrillation was successful but VF/pVT recurs:

- Resume the CPR sequence and defibrillate. Give an amiodarone bolus (unless two doses have already been given) and start a continuous infusion.

12. CPR should be continued unless:

- An organised perfusing rhythm is recognised and confirmed by a clinical assessment indicating signs of life (ROSC).
- There are criteria for withdrawing resuscitation.

13. After the event:

- Debriefing of the team should be conducted to express any concerns and to allow the team to reflect on their clinical practice in a supportive environment (this has been shown to improve practice).

Important notes

Good team planning before each action will minimise hands-off time and improve the quality of CPR.

Studies show that visual assessment of depth of compressions is inaccurate; therefore, feedback devices should be utilised where possible. When correct chest compression depth and rate are achieved, the chances of survival are markedly improved.

The interval between stopping chest compressions and delivering a shock must be minimal; longer interruptions reduce the likelihood of a shock restoring a perfusing rhythm.

Chest compressions are resumed immediately after a shock without reassessing the rhythm or feeling for a pulse because, even if the defibrillation attempt is successful in restoring a rhythm, it is unlikely that the heart will immediately pump effectively. Giving further chest compressions does not increase the chance of VF recurring.

If an organised rhythm is observed during a 2 min cycle of CPR, do not interrupt chest compressions to palpate a pulse unless the patient shows signs of life demonstrating a return of spontaneous circulation (ROSC).

Airway and ventilation

The vast majority of children can be adequately ventilated with BMV in the initial stages of resuscitation. It is often better to continue with this until ROSC rather than attempt tracheal intubation and temporarily interrupt chest compressions and oxygenation during laryngoscopy.

If BMV is unsuccessful and a team member with the necessary skills to safely intubate the child or infant is not yet present, a suitably trained provider may use a supraglottic airway (SGA) as an alternative .

A tracheal tube (TT) provides the most reliable airway. As soon as the airway is secured with a TT, chest compressions should be performed continuously unless this compromises the delivery of adequate tidal volumes.

If laryngoscopy is to be performed during CPR, it should be attempted without interruption of chest compressions, although there may need to be a brief pause as the TT is passed through the vocal cords.

End-tidal CO_2 should be continuously monitored once a TT or SGA is in place:

- The absence of exhaled CO_2 during CPR should prompt providers to check tracheal tube placement, remember **'no trace, wrong place'**. An attenuated CO_2 waveform, however, may reflect low or absent pulmonary blood flow; providers should check the quality of chest compressions delivered.
- Try to improve chest compression quality if the end-tidal CO_2 remains below 2 kPa. This may indicate low cardiac output and low pulmonary blood flow; a sudden rise in the end-tidal CO_2 can be an early indication of ROSC.
- Be careful when interpreting end-tidal CO_2 values after giving adrenaline or other vasoconstrictor drugs when there may be a transient decrease in end-tidal CO_2, or after the use of sodium bicarbonate when there may be a transient increase in the end-tidal values.
- Current evidence does not support the use of a threshold end-tidal CO_2 value as an indicator for stopping the resuscitation attempt.

08

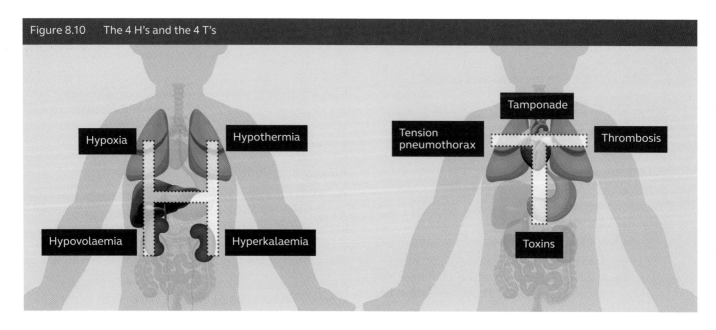

Figure 8.10   The 4 H's and the 4 T's

For children or infants already on a mechanical ventilator at the time of cardiac arrest, either continue to ventilate with the ventilator or disconnect and ventilate by means of a self-inflating bag. In the former case, ensure that the ventilator is in a volume-controlled mode, that triggers and limits are disabled, and ventilation rate, tidal volume and fraction of inspired oxygen (FiO_2) are appropriate for CPR. There is no evidence to support any specific level of positive end-expiratory pressure (PEEP) during CPR. Ventilator dysfunction can itself be a cause of cardiorespiratory arrest.

Once there is a sustained return of spontaneous circulation (ROSC), titrate the FiO_2 to SpO_2 of 94–98%.

In children and infants who do not regain consciousness or for other clinical indications, an advanced airway may be required. Team members with the necessary skills to insert an advanced airway will be required (drugs may be needed at this point to assist).

History and reversible causes

Obtaining relevant information about the child's underlying medical condition and any predisposing events can help determine likely causes and potential outcome from the cardiorespiratory arrest. The early identification and proper treatment of any identifiable reversible cause during CPR is a priority for all ALS providers.

The 4 H's and the 4 T's

Use the mnemonic 4 H's and 4 T's to remember what to actively look for (Figure 8.10 and Table 8.1).

- Hypoxia
- Hypovolemia
- Hypo or hyperkalaemia / -calcaemia / -magnesaemia and hypoglycaemia
- Hypo or hyperthermia
- Tension pneumothorax
- Tamponade
- Thrombosis (cardiac or pulmonary)
- Toxic agents.

Unless otherwise specified, the specific treatment for each of these causes is the same in cardiorespiratory arrest as in acute life-threatening disease.

Hypoxia

This is a frequent cause of paediatric cardiorespiratory arrest. The risks of it occurring, or persisting, during resuscitation should be minimised by ensuring effective ventilation with 100% oxygen. It is essential to ensure that there is adequate bilateral chest movement.

Hypovolaemia

Loss of circulating volume can often result in cardiorespiratory arrest. When a child shows signs of circulatory failure, controlled volume administration is indicated. Hypovolaemia may be due to many different causes (e.g. haemorrhage from trauma, diarrhoea and vomiting, anaphylaxis, severe sepsis), and these need to be identified and treated appropriately. If a clinical presentation or history suggests hypovolaemia, start rapid circulatory volume replacement with an initial bolus of isotonic balanced crystalloid or 0.9% sodium chloride solution; volume and frequency of boluses are discussed in Chapter 5.

Hypo/hyperkalaemia, metabolic causes

Electrolyte and metabolic disorders may be suggested by the child's medical history and/or biochemical tests.

Specific treatment should be given to correct these problems. An estimation of blood glucose level should be obtained early as both hypo and hyperglycaemia are common and associated with increased morbidity and mortality.

Hypothermia and Hyperthermia

Low body temperature may be an unlikely problem in hospitalised children, but it should always be considered, particularly in small or premature infants or in children being managed in the emergency department. A low-reading thermometer should be used to record a core temperature when hypothermia is considered a possibility. If the child's temperature is > 34°C, they should not be actively rewarmed.

Hyperthermia should initially be treated with physical methods, such as tepid sponging, cooling mattresses and cool IV fluids. However, since it may be caused by many different aetiologies (e.g. poisonings, anaesthesia, heatstroke), further management should be directed by the specific cause.

Tension pneumothorax

Signs of a tension pneumothorax (e.g. decreased chest movement and air entry, hyperresonance on the affected side, tracheal deviation away from the affected side) should be sought, particularly in children who have suffered trauma, following thoracic surgery or jugular or subclavian vein central line insertion. If a tension pneumothorax is thought to be present, rapid needle decompression is required (or thoracostomy in a trauma setting), followed by chest drain insertion.

Tamponade (cardiac)

This is not a common cause of cardiorespiratory arrest in children but may occur following cardiothoracic surgery, penetrating chest trauma or some viral illnesses. It can be difficult to diagnose as typical signs (e.g. distended neck veins and hypovolaemia) are often masked by the cardiorespiratory arrest. If there is a strong history, thoracotomy or needle pericardiocentesis is indicated.

Toxins

In the absence of a confirmed history, accidental or deliberate poisoning with toxins (therapeutic or toxic substances (e.g. digoxin toxicity, tricyclic antidepressant overdose)) may only be discovered after laboratory analysis. Appropriate antidotes should be administered as soon as possible when indicated and available (e.g. sodium bicarbonate in tricyclic poisonings). Seek advice from a poisons centre for up-to-date guidance for severe or uncommon poisonings. However, the management of these children is frequently based on measures to support their vital organs. Remember to also check the child's drug chart.

Thrombosis (coronary or pulmonary)

It is unusual for children to suffer from thromboembolic complications, but they can occur. If suspected, appropriate thrombolysis would be needed (e.g. alteplase as per local guidelines).

Table 8.1 Reversible causes of cardiorespiratory arrest

Consider	Identification:	Treatment
Hypoxia	History/clinical exam +/-oxygen saturation (if trace picked up)	Ventilation with 100% FiO_2
Hypovolaemia	History +/- POCUS*	Fluid bolus 10 mL kg^{-1} isotonic crystalloid; blood products (major haemorrhage)
Hyper/hypokalaemia	History + blood gas analysis	Correction/reduction of metabolic derangement
Hypothermia/ Hyperthermia	History + core temperature	External (e.g. blanket), internal (e.g. cold/warm fluids, extracorporeal circuit) techniques
Thromboembolism	History +/- POCUS * (e.g. dilated right ventricle)	IV thrombolysis
Tension pneumothorax	Examine symmetrical air entry +/- POCUS*	Needle thoracocentesis/ thoracostomy (trauma)
Tamponade (cardiac)	History +/- POCUS * (e.g. pericardial fluid collection)	Needle pericardiocentesis/ thoracotomy (trauma)
Toxic	History / ECG	Specific toxic treatment (e.g. sodium bicarbonate for tricyclic drug poisoning)
*POCUS: point of care ultrasound – if competent operator available.		

Stopping resuscitation

Cardiopulmonary resuscitation efforts are less likely to be successful in achieving ROSC if there have been no signs of cardiac output, despite at least 30 min of continuous, good quality CPR in children. However, occasionally good quality survival has been reported for longer durations of CPR, so the circumstances of the cardiorespiratory arrest and presenting rhythm must all be taken into consideration when making the decision to stop resuscitation. CPR is more often successful in children < 1 year of age and in those presenting with VF or pVT.

It would be appropriate to prolong resuscitation attempts in children with the following conditions:

- hypothermia
- poisoning
- persistent VF/ pVT
- thrombolysis.

The resuscitation team may also consider that specific circumstances (e.g. awaiting the arrival of family members) may make it appropriate to maintain resuscitation efforts.

After the event, debriefing of the event should be conducted, to express any concerns and to allow the team to reflect on their clinical practice in a supportive environment.

A record of the event should be written in real-time. This should be completed by a senior member of the resuscitation team and allocated by the team leader. The scribe notes should then be added to, if necessary, and countersigned by all team members who took an active part in the event (e.g. anaesthetist, ICU medic, nurses etc.).

Presence of parents during resuscitation

The opportunity to be present during at least part of the resuscitation of their child should be offered to parents/carers. Evidence suggests that most parents want to be present during a resuscitation attempt, which can aid with their grieving process (less anxiety and depression when assessed several months later). Reports show that being at the child or infant's side is comforting to the parents or careers and helps them gain a realistic view of attempted resuscitation and death.

The following should be considered (whether the parent is actually in the room beside their child or elsewhere in the ward/department):

- A specific member of staff should be delegated to remain with the parents throughout to offer empathetic but realistic support. They can also ensure the parents do not distract the resuscitation team.

- If necessary, an appropriate interpreter must be present to facilitate accuracy of communication between parents and the resuscitation team leader.
- When appropriate, physical contact with their child during the event should be allowed.
- Time to say 'goodbye' (in unsuccessful resuscitation attempts) should be encouraged.
- The resuscitation team leader decides when to stop resuscitation efforts and not the parents.
- Appropriate referrals and counselling should be organised for the parents to ensure they receive adequate support.

08: Summary learning

The optimal management of in-hospital cardiorespiratory arrest is always based on the rapid initiation of effective ventilation, oxygenation and good quality chest compressions.

The paediatric advanced life support algorithm provides a framework for cardiopulmonary arrest management with an emphasis on providing good quality CPR with minimal interruptions in chest compression delivery.

Asystole and PEA are non-shockable arrhythmias, and their management is based on effective CPR, adrenaline administration and treatment of reversible causes.

VF and pVT are shockable arrhythmias, and their management is based on effective CPR, early defibrillation and treatment of reversible causes.

The parents/carers should be supported and, ideally, be present during the resuscitation of their child.

My key take-home messages from this chapter are:

Further reading

Eppich WJ, Brannen M, Hunt EA: Team training: Implications for emergency and critical care pediatrics. Curr Opin Pediatr 2008;20:255-260.

Brady PW, Muething S, Kotagal U, Ashby M, Gallagher R, Hall D, Goodfriend M, White C, Bracke TM, DeCastro V, Geiser M, Simon J, Tucker KM, Olivea J, Conway PH, Wheeler DS. Improving situation awareness to reduce unrecognised clinical deterioration and serious safety events. Pediatrics. 2013 Jan;131(1):e298-308.

Weinstock P, Halamek LP: Teamwork during resuscitation. Pediatr Clin North Am 2008;55:1011-1024, xi-xii.

TIMMIS, V. 2020. Should family members be present at resuscitation? Arch Dis Child, 105, 506-508.

WALKER, W. & GAVIN, C. 2019. Family presence during resuscitation: A narrative review of the practices and views of critical care nurses. Intensive Crit Care Nurs, 53, 15-22.

Hunt EA, Duval- Arnould JM, Bembea MM, et al. Association between time to defibrillation and survival in pediatric in-hospital cardiac arrest with a first documented shockable rhythm. JAMA Netw Open 2018;1: e182643.

Skellett S, Orzechowska I, Thomas K, Fortune PM. The landscape of paediatric in-hospital cardiac arrest in the United Kingdom National Cardiac Arrest Audit. Resuscitation 2020;155:165-71.

Maconochie IK, Aickin R, Hazinski MF, et al. Pediatric life support: 2020 international consensus on cardiopulmonary resuscitation and emergency cardiovascular care science with treatment recommendations. Resuscitation 2020;156:A120-55.

Goto Y, Funada A, Goto Y. Duration of prehospital cardiopulmonary resuscitation and favorable neurological outcomes for pediatric out-of-hospital cardiac arrests: a nationwide, population-based cohort study. Circulation 2016;134:2046-59.

Early warning scores in Paediatrics: an overview. SM Chapman, IK Maconochie Archives of disease in childhood 104 (4), 395-399,2019

Effect of a Paediatric Early Warning System on All-Cause Mortality in Pediatric Patients: The EPOCH Randomised Clinical Trial. Christopher S Parshuram et al JAMA 2018

Smith GB. In-hospital cardiac arrest: Is it time for an in-hospital 'chain of prevention'? Resuscitation 2010:81:1209-11.

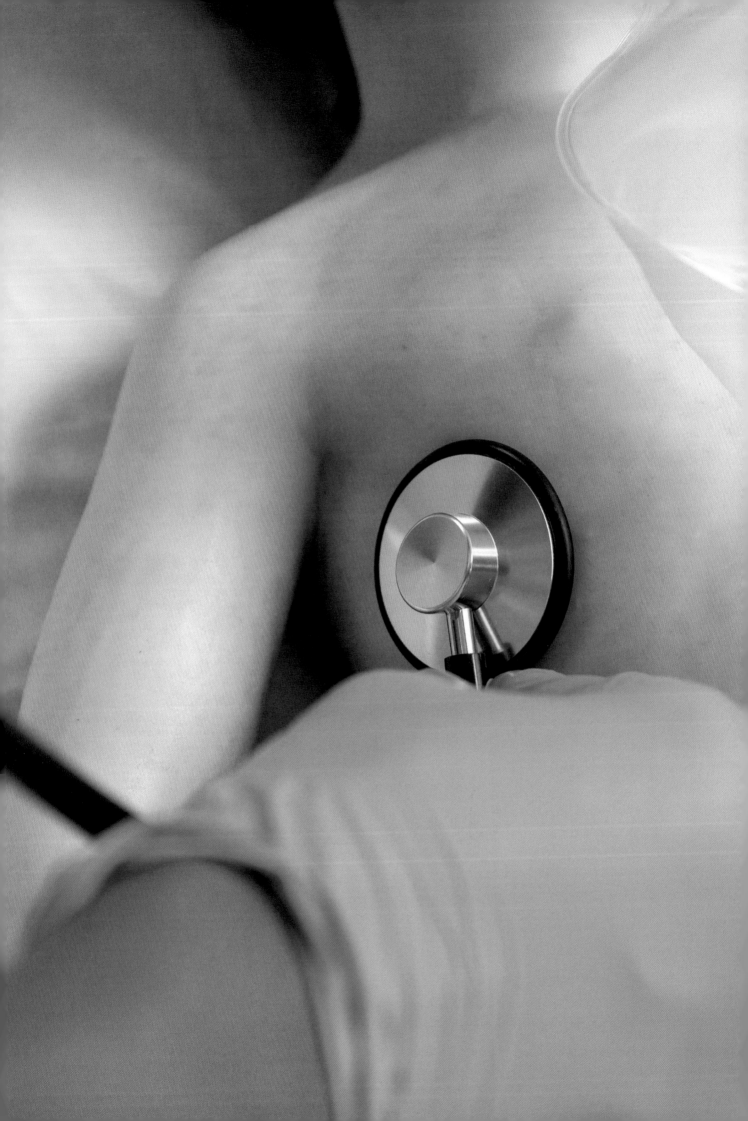

Post-resuscitation care, stabilisation and transfer

In this chapter

The learning outcomes will enable you to:

Understand the importance of post-resuscitation stabilisation and optimisation of organ function following cardiorespiratory arrest

Describe the specific investigations and monitoring indicated

Facilitate the safe transfer of a critically unwell child

Continued resuscitation

Cardiorespiratory arrest represents the most severe shock state during which delivery of oxygen and metabolic substrates to tissues is abruptly halted. Cardiopulmonary resuscitation (CPR) only partially reverses this process, achieving cardiac output and systemic oxygen delivery that is much less than normal.

The aim of post-resuscitation care is to restore oxygenation and perfusion to the vital organs as rapidly as possible to minimise the primary injury. For children and infants who have had a cardiorespiratory arrest, the initial step is the restoration of spontaneous circulation (ROSC), but this is only the first step in the continuous process of resuscitation management.

A child or infant who is successfully resuscitated from a cardiorespiratory arrest typically suffers from multiple organ system failure resulting from hypoxia, ischaemia and subsequent reperfusion injury. This is seen most often in children who remain comatose post ROSC; the effect to which each patient is affected depends on various factors, including pre-arrest co-morbidities, duration of the ischaemic insult and cause of the cardiorespiratory arrest.

A significant percentage of resuscitated children ultimately die or survive with serious neurological sequelae. Therefore, the main goal of post-resuscitation care is to maintain oxygenation and perfusion to vital organs to prevent secondary organ injury whenever possible.

Secondary organ damage may include:

- hypoxic-ischaemic brain injury
- ischaemic myocardial damage (global cardiac dysfunction)
- hypoxic pulmonary damage (acute lung injury (ALI) and acute respiratory distress syndrome (ARDS))
- acute kidney injury
- coagulopathy (disseminated intravascular coagulation (DIC))
- ischaemic hepatitis
- acute gastrointestinal lesions.

The ABCDE approach must be followed in the immediate post-resuscitation phase as it focuses on the management priorities. However, the ongoing care of the child requires the expertise of many healthcare professionals and is best delivered in a paediatric intensive care unit (PICU). This may require a specialist team to perform the critical care transfer.

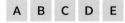

> The main goal of post-resuscitation care is to maintain oxygenation and perfusion to vital organs to prevent secondary organ injury whenever possible

A B Stabilisation of airway and breathing

The aim of respiratory management is to maintain ventilation, avoiding hypoxia, hyperoxia, hypocapnia and hypercapnia, which may worsen the child's prognosis.

If the child (or infant) has been resuscitated using BMV, a decision needs to be made whether they will need ongoing ventilation via the placement of a tracheal tube. Factors that may affect this decision include:

- if intubation is needed to maintain a safe airway in a child with a reduced level of consciousness
- the requirements for the safe transfer to a PICU
- if it is not possible to maintain ventilation and/or oxygenation by non-invasive means.

Vital signs, such as heart rate, blood pressure, SpO_2 and end-tidal CO_2, must be monitored post-resuscitation. Additionally, blood gases can be used to guide further management. Although 100% oxygen is used for resuscitation, prolonged administration of high oxygen concentrations can result in pulmonary and cerebral toxicity. Once the child is stable, titrate FiO_2 to achieve normoxaemia (PaO_2 10–13 kPa) or, if arterial blood gas is not available, maintain SpO_2 in the range of 94–98%. Maintain a high FiO_2 in presumed carbon monoxide poisoning or severe anaemia.

Once an advanced airway is in place, end-tidal CO_2 monitoring is mandatory. This will confirm the correct placement of a tracheal tube (no trace, wrong place), allow continuous CO_2 monitoring and support the optimisation of ventilation to maintain normocapnia. Provide a normal ventilatory rate and tidal volume for the child's age (5–7 mL kg^{-1}) to achieve a normal $PaCO_2$ (4.5–6 kPa). Avoid both hypocapnia and hypercapnia, as studies have shown that both are associated with increased mortality. In a few children, the usual values for $PaCO_2$ and PaO_2 may deviate from the population normal values for age (e.g. in children with chronic lung disease or congenital heart conditions); aim to restore values to that child's normal levels. Do not use end-tidal CO_2 as a surrogate for $PaCO_2$ when aiming for normocapnia as part of neuroprotective care unless there is a proven correlation.

BMV causes gastric distention, which will impede ventilation and may cause vomiting. A gastric tube is usually required to deflate the stomach if it has become distended following BMV and is required in children receiving mechanical ventilation.

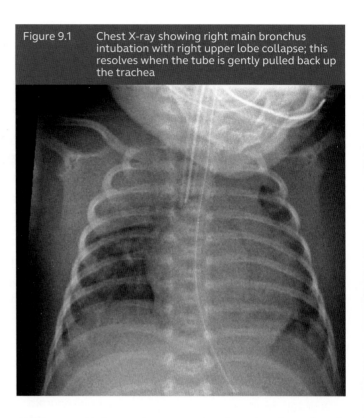

Figure 9.1   Chest X-ray showing right main bronchus intubation with right upper lobe collapse; this resolves when the tube is gently pulled back up the trachea

Children and infants who remain intubated and ventilated will need sedation and analgesia in most cases. If a resuscitated child has a tracheal tube in place and starts to make respiratory effort but remains unconscious, it is usually preferable to leave them intubated and ventilated (with appropriate sedation and analgesia) until after transfer and admission to PICU, since they can deteriorate rapidly, and reintubation during transfer is extremely hazardous.

A chest X-ray should be obtained to check the position of the tracheal tube, gastric tube and central line if inserted in the neck (Figure 9.1). The tracheal tube may need to be re-positioned so that it is in an optimal position. You should also look for any lung pathology and check for any rib fractures (very rare in children).

Following intubation, the most common post-resuscitation airway/breathing complications can be identified by considering the acronym DOPES (Table 9.1).

Table 9.1   Causes of sudden deterioration in an intubated patient

D	Displacement of the tracheal tube (e.g. oesophagus, right main bronchus)
O	Obstruction of artificial airway (accumulated secretions (e.g. bronchiolitis), kinking of the tracheal tube)
P	Pneumothorax (from excessive BMV pressure, rib fractures)
E	Equipment failure (e.g. disconnected oxygen supply)
S	Stomach distension (following expired air or bag-mask ventilation)

C Circulation

The aim of circulatory management is to ensure adequate organ perfusion and tissue oxygenation.

Haemodynamic function and cardiac rhythm are likely to be unstable in the immediate post-resuscitation phase. Global myocardial hypokinesis, systemic inflammation, disturbed vasoregulation and reperfusion injury all contribute to the clinical picture. Clinical assessment of the child's circulation (heart rate, blood pressure, capillary refill time, peripheral temperature, core temperature and urine output) is important and will aid in the evaluation of any treatment response. The minimum monitoring that should be in place includes ECG, SpO_2, BP and end-tidal CO_2 monitoring. Serial blood lactate levels can be monitored to assess the response to interventions.

The optimal haemodynamic targets in the post-resuscitation phase remain unclear, but studies have shown that hypotension (blood pressure < 5th centile for age) is associated with lower survival to hospital discharge. Therefore, the mean or systolic arterial pressure (SBP/MAP) should be targeted between the 5th and 50th centile for the child and never allowed to drift below the 5th centile (Table 9.2). Blood pressure is often labile in the post–cardiorespiratory arrest period, and continuous arterial pressure monitoring is recommended.

Table 9.2 Blood pressure 5th and 50th centile by age

Blood pressure for age (mmHg)	1 month	1 year	5 year	10 year
50th centile for Systolic BP	75	95	100	110
5th centile for Systolic BP	50	70	75	80
50th centile for mean arterial pressure (MAP)	55	70	75	75
5th centile for mean arterial blood pressure (MAP)	40	50	55	55

Optimising circulation and hence organ perfusion may require both restoration of the circulating volume and vasoactive treatment to achieve haemodynamic goals. Resuscitation boluses of 10 mL kg^{-1} balanced isotonic crystalloids or 0.9% sodium chloride may be required to optimise circulating volume with reassessment after each bolus to avoid fluid overload (i.e. look for advancing liver edge, bilateral basal crepitations and in older patients a raised jugular venous pressure). Crystalloids can be safely used in the peri-resuscitation period, but some patients may require blood products (red cells, fresh frozen plasma, cryoprecipitate or platelets). Coagulopathy either from DIC or liver dysfunction may develop as part of the post-cardiac arrest syndrome following hypoxic injury.

If the child has signs of fluid overload or is becoming less fluid responsive, then an early echocardiogram may be useful in assessing cardiac function and guide further management with vasoactive medications, such as inotropes or vasoconstrictors. Commonly used vasoactive drugs include adrenaline and noradrenaline but consensus guidelines for specific conditions should be followed (e.g. sepsis guidelines for children). Vasoactive medications are preferably administered via dedicated central venous catheters but can be administered peripherally in the short-term. Having a central line with multiple lumens ensures that these drugs are not interrupted to deliver other medications and fluids, and avoids incompatibilities. A central line in the neck may allow measurement of central venous pressure (CVP), a measure of preload (i.e. the filling volume of the heart); this may be appropriate in some children and will help prevent excessive fluid administration or detect a failing heart.

Measuring urine output, which should be > 1 mL kg^{-1} h^{-1} in children and > 2 mL kg^{-1} h^{-1} in infants, is a marker of end-organ perfusion and therefore, circulatory adequacy.

Maintenance fluids should be based on biochemistry evaluations, and blood glucose should be measured. Glucose should be administered judiciously to avoid hypoglycaemia or hyperglycaemia as both conditions can have a harmful effect on neurological outcome in critically unwell children. Careful monitoring is required.

D Disability

The main cause of death after ROSC in children is brain injury. Protection of the brain against secondary injury is therefore essential. The brain is highly vulnerable to hypoxia and ischaemia. It can also be injured by direct trauma, infection, hyperglycaemia, hypoglycaemia, hypocapnia, hypercapnia, seizures or raised intracranial pressure.

Secondary brain injury can be minimised by:
- avoiding hypoxia, hypocapnia and hypercapnia by closely monitoring SpO_2, end-tidal CO_2, blood gases and providing adequate oxygen and ventilation
- avoiding and treating hypotension with fluids and vasoactive medications; keep the BP between the 5–50th centile the patient's age
- recognising and promptly treating seizures
- correcting glucose and electrolyte abnormalities
- close monitoring, treatment and diagnosis of signs of raised ICP.

An assessment of neurological status should be performed early to obtain a post-resuscitation baseline, help identify neurological deficits and aid in predicting prognosis.

The conscious level should be assessed with either the AVPU or Glasgow Coma Scale scoring systems. Pupil reactivity, posturing and focal signs should also be noted and regularly recorded.

Neuroprotective care post-ROSC aims to avoid secondary brain injury and should start from the first minutes after ROSC.

Ventilation

Studies suggest that ventilation to normocapnia is appropriate (4.5–6.0 kPa) as the response of the cerebral circulation to changes in CO_2 appears preserved. Low levels of CO_2 may result in cerebral vasoconstriction, and reduced cerebral blood flow and high levels of CO_2 to cerebral vasodilation and high cerebral blood flow; both of these may aggravate any brain swelling which occurs after cardiorespiratory arrest.

Cerebral perfusion

Immediately following ROSC, there may be a period of unstable cerebral blood flow. Cerebral perfusion pressure (CPP) is dependent on mean arterial pressure (MAP) and intracranial pressure (CPP = MAP-ICP). Hypotension will compromise cerebral blood flow and may worsen any neurological injury, so it must be avoided.

Seizure control

The occurrence of seizures post-resuscitation is associated with a poorer outcome. For children who remain comatose after ROSC, it is recommended that they have continuous EEG monitoring and that this is employed as soon as possible (changes in EEG over time may also help with prognostication). Control of seizure activity (clinical or sub-clinical) is essential to prevent increased cerebral metabolism and potential neurological injury. As for all children with seizures, blood glucose levels should be checked. Commonly used treatments for seizure (e.g. levetiracetam, benzodiazepines, phenytoin) may cause hypotension, and the BP and ECG need to be closely monitored.

Signs of raised intracranial pressure

Signs of raised intracranial pressure (ICP) need to be reviewed, investigated, and treatment given (e.g. hypertonic sodium chloride, mannitol).

Targeted Temperature Management (TTM)

Post ROSC care involves strict control of temperature to avoid hyperthermia (> 37.5°C) and severe hypothermia (< 32°C) and is mandatory. Hyperthermia post cardiorespiratory arrest is common in the first 48 h and is known to worsen brain injury with an increase in morbidity for every 1°C above 37°C; hence fever should be treated aggressively with antipyretics and active cooling. Two

large paediatric randomised controlled trials (THAPCA trials) have been published looking at temperature control for patients after cardiorespiratory arrest. These compared mild therapeutic hypothermia (TH) (32–34°C) with therapeutic normothermia (TN) (36.8°C, controlled to prevent temperatures above 37.5°C) following in-hospital and out-of-hospital cardiorespiratory arrest. In both the out-of-hospital and in-hospital groups, there was no significant difference in survival or one-year functional outcome between the two different temperature groups (TH and TN). There were no differences in complications between the two groups, and it was concluded that TH appeared a safe therapy. It may be that the avoidance of fever confers a better outcome and is the important goal in TTM for patients following cardiorespiratory arrest. Children post ROSC can therefore be managed with either TN or TH, but TH should only be done at centres with equipment and expertise to manage this therapy. Note that the successfully resuscitated child with hypothermia and ROSC should not be immediately rewarmed actively unless the temperature is less than 32°C. The optimal duration of TTM is unknown, and different centres use 24, 48 or 72 h.

Blood glucose

Hypoglycaemia (< 3 mmol L⁻¹) and hyperglycaemia are associated with worse neurological outcome. Studies have not shown that tight control of blood glucose levels confers any benefit for paediatric patients, and it carries the risk of inadvertent hypoglycaemia, so it is not recommended. Glucose should be delivered as a continuous infusion rather than as boluses, and blood glucose levels should be monitored frequently.

Maintenance fluids

Maintenance fluids should be started in children with a choice of fluid directed by electrolyte and blood glucose measurements; usually balanced isotonic crystalloids or 0.9% sodium chloride, with or without 5 or 10% dextrose can be used. Maintenance requirements are best prescribed at 70% of normal values in critically unwell children.

Analgesia, sedation and neuromuscular blockers

If children do not show adequate signs of awakening within the first 10 min after ROSC, mechanical ventilation and ongoing analgesia and sedation will be required. Adequate analgesia and sedation will reduce oxygen consumption, facilitate ventilation and prevent complications. Neuromuscular blockade is not routinely used but may be needed to facilitate ventilation and prevent shivering during targeted temperature management. Therefore, the prevention and treatment of pain and the maintenance of an adequate level of sedation are a priority. There are many sedatives, analgesics and neuromuscular blockers available, but it is best to become familiar with the use of a small range, knowing their indications, beneficial actions and adverse effects. Never administer a neuromuscular blocker without ensuring that the child is deeply sedated and will remain so. Sedation and neuromuscular blockers may not be necessary in a profound coma and may interfere with neurological evaluation; always discuss such cases with the local transport team and/or PICU for guidance.

E Exposure

Exposure and a full examination to detect any lesions (e.g. rashes, wounds) should be undertaken and may help in making the diagnosis, informing specific management of the child (e.g. the purpuric rash of meningococcaemia may prompt treatment with broad-spectrum antibiotics if not already given). Care should be taken to respect the child's dignity, and excessive hypothermia avoided especially in infants.

Other organs

Kidneys

Renal function should be monitored by measuring urine output and the serum urea and creatinine levels. Insertion of a urinary catheter may be necessary. Treatment is directed towards maintaining an adequate circulating volume, which sustains renal perfusion. Hence diuretics are only indicated if decreased urine output persists after adequate fluid resuscitation. Additionally, after ROSC, some patients, particularly those after a prolonged cardiorespiratory arrest, may develop acute kidney injury secondary to hypoxia and hypoperfusion. This may lead to anuria, causing fluid overload and electrolyte disturbances, particularly hyperkalaemia, so monitoring is essential.

Gastrointestinal

The gastrointestinal mucosa and liver can also be affected by hypoxia and ischaemia. Liver dysfunction may be reflected by raised transaminases and or reduced coagulation factors. Monitoring of liver function tests and support of coagulation by replacement of clotting factors may be required. Gastrointestinal mucosal injury can contribute to multi-organ failure due to leakage of toxins and bacteria into the circulation. Treatment is aimed at maintaining adequate circulating volume and gut perfusion.

Haematological

Full blood count and coagulation studies should be sent and regularly monitored. Red blood cell transfusions to maintain haemoglobin > 70 g L^{-1} should be given to optimise oxygenation. Plasma products and platelets may be needed if DIC has developed post hypoxic insult.

Further assessment

History

An essential part of post-resuscitation care is the identification and treatment of the precipitating cause of cardiorespiratory arrest to prevent further episodes. A comprehensive history should be taken, and this should include relevant details about the past medical history, previous health/ill health and medications, as well as precipitating events. Details about the initial management of the current event (e.g. delay in starting resuscitation) should also be sought, as these may influence ongoing management.

Investigations

The child's physiological parameters are likely to be deranged in the immediate post-resuscitation period; urgent haematological, biochemical, radiological and cardiological investigations may all be indicated (Table 9.3).

Table 9.3   Post-resuscitation investigations

Investigation	Rationale
Arterial and/or venous blood gas (plus lactate)	Ensure adequate ventilation Assess tissue perfusion
Biochemistry	Assess renal function Maintain normoglycaemia Assess electrolyte balance (especially Na$^+$, K$^+$, Mg2$^+$, Ca$^+$) Liver function tests to look for ischaemic injury
Full blood count Clotting screen Group and Save Cultures (blood, urine etc.)	Assess haemoglobin level and exclude anaemia Monitor infection markers (e.g. white cell count, CRP etc.) Identify underlying blood disorders Assess any coagulopathy from sepsis or ischaemia Allows for urgent crossmatch
Chest X-ray	Establish position of tracheal tube, central venous lines, gastric tube (as appropriate) Detect underlying pathology (primary respiratory or cardiac disease, aspiration) Exclude pneumothorax/rib fractures Estimate heart size

Other investigations as indicated (e.g. head CT or pelvis X-rays, cardiac echography, 12-lead ECG, serum and urine toxicology)

Blood gas interpretation

The ability to interpret a blood gas can give important information about the patient to help guide further management. The following is a simple guide to basic blood gas analysis.

The parameters commonly measured are: pH, PaO_2, $PaCO_2$, standard bicarbonate (SB), base excess (BE) and lactate. Directly measured values are: pH, $PaCO_2$, PaO_2, glucose and lactate. Calculated values are SB, BE and O_2 saturation (unless a co-oximeter is used).

The pH is the negative logarithm of hydrogen ion concentration in the blood (a decrease in pH from 7.0 to 6.0 indicates a ten-fold increase in the concentration of H^+ ions). It is a scale that measures the acid-base balance. Its normal range in the human body is 7.35 to 7.45. Staying within this normal range is important for the body's enzymes and biological processes to work optimally.

The body, therefore, regulates its acid-base balance tightly by means of both the kidney and the respiratory systems. Acid is produced by almost all biological processes in the body. This is initially buffered in the blood by a number of systems, the most important being the bicarbonate/carbonic acid system (Table 9.4).

- The kidneys can excrete excess acid in the urine and can also generate bicarbonate ions; these responses usually take hours.
- Carbon dioxide partially dissolves in plasma, forming carbonic acid. High carbon dioxide levels (hypercapnia, as in hypoventilation) result in an acid load and a fall in pH. Low carbon dioxide levels (hypocapnia, as in hyperventilation) can cause a rise in pH; these (ventilatory) responses usually take minutes.

Table 9.4   Blood gas interpretation

pH	CO_2	HCO_3	Interpretation
< 7.35	↑		Respiratory acidosis
< 7.35		↓	Metabolic acidosis
> 7.45	↓		Respiratory alkalosis
> 7.45		↑	Metabolic alkalosis
< 7.35	↑	↓	Combined respiratory and metabolic acidosis
> 7.45	↓	↑	Combined respiratory and metabolic alkalosis

Simple blood gas analysis

STEP 1: Is the pH normal?
- If the pH is < 7.35 this is this called acidaemia
- If the pH is > 7.45 this is this called alkalaemia

STEP 2: Is there a metabolic or respiratory abnormality or both?
- Metabolic acidosis is defined as SB ≤ 22 mmol L^{-1}
- Metabolic alkalosis is defined as SB > 26 mmol L^{-1}
- Respiratory acidosis is defined as $paCO_2$ > 6 kPa (45 mmHg)
- Respiratory alkalosis is defined as $paCO_2$ < 4.5 kPa (35 mmHg)

STEP 3: Is the metabolic or respiratory abnormality compensated, partially compensated or uncompensated?
- A respiratory or metabolic abnormality can exist with or without an acidaemia or alkalaemia. This is because the body will try and compensate for any abnormality and correct the pH.

Example 1

If there is a metabolic acidosis, then the respiratory centre will be stimulated, and the patient will hyperventilate, causing the carbon dioxide level to fall, resulting in a respiratory alkalosis. In this scenario, the pH will initially be normal as the respiratory system compensates, but eventually, the compensatory mechanisms will fail, and the pH will start to fall, resulting in an acidaemia.

Example 2

A child with profound shock who is unconscious may be unable to mount a respiratory response to the metabolic acidosis and may present with a metabolic and respiratory acidosis with no compensation.

Consequences of an abnormal blood gas

Once a blood gas has been interpreted, the causes of the abnormalities can be sought. Metabolic or respiratory acidosis with or without an acidaemia are the commonest abnormalities seen in the acutely unwell child. An alkalosis in an acute illness may be due to poisonings (e.g. salicylate overdose).

Causes of respiratory acidosis include, for instance, pneumonia, asthma, neuromuscular disorders and coma.

Causes of metabolic acidosis include among others, diarrhoea and vomiting, sepsis, heart failure, diabetic ketoacidosis and/or any form of shock (causing hypoperfusion and tissue hypoxia with lactic acidosis).

To help determine the cause of a metabolic acidosis, various further tests can be performed, such as chloride levels and anion gap, but these are outside the scope of this discussion.

Measuring the pH of the blood gives information about the severity of the child's condition, but it is also important as it in itself affects the circulation and oxygen delivery in different organs and tissues.

Changes in pH affect the oxyhaemoglobin dissociation curve. A rise in $PaCO_2$ and drop in pH causes pulmonary vascular resistance to rise affecting blood flow to the lungs.

The cerebral circulation is also affected by pH and $PaCO_2$: when the $PaCO_2$ rises, and the pH drops, the cerebral blood vessels dilate and cerebral blood flow increases; this may not be desirable in children who have cerebral oedema. When $PaCO_2$ drops and pH increases, there is cerebral vasoconstriction which may potentiate any cerebral ischaemia.

Facilitating safe patient transfer

Following stabilisation after ROSC, the child or infant should be safely transferred to an appropriate PICU for definitive and ongoing medical support. The decision to transfer should be made after discussion between senior members of the transport/PICU team, the clinical emergency team leader and the child's primary team. Other considerations pre-transfer are listed in Figure 9.5.

The transfer team, whether in-hospital or between hospitals, must be sufficiently experienced to be able to deliver any life-saving emergency interventions during the transfer period in any location (e.g. in an ambulance). In the UK, a dedicated paediatric transfer team will usually be involved. There are some circumstances, for example, intracranial bleeds and blocked VP shunts which require rapid transfer for urgent neurosurgical intervention, which will be done by the most experienced available local team (most commonly the anaesthetic/emergency medicine/intensive care consultants).

Table 9.5 Pre-transfer considerations

	Stabilise the child (ongoing or recurrent cardiorespiratory arrest precludes transfer).
	Arrange the most appropriate mode of transport.
	Inform the paediatric consultant and any other speciality lead involved in the immediate care of the child (e.g. anaesthetist, surgeon, department nurse in charge, child protection lead if appropriate).
	Inform the child's parents of transfer details and ensure they have appropriate means of transport to the PICU.
A	Ensure a secure airway (aspirate any endotracheal tube secretions prior to transfer).
B	Ensure appropriate settings on transport ventilator, adequate portable oxygen supplies for the length of the journey, and alternative means of ventilating the child (manual ventilation circuit that can be used either with or without oxygen supply). Deflate the stomach with a gastric tube.
C	Ensure adequate intravenous access.
D	Ensure adequate sedation and analgesia being delivered +/- neuromuscular blocker and that sufficient drugs are available for the journey. Reassess pupillary reaction and conscious level.
E	Ensure heat loss during transfer is kept to a minimum (unless intentionally cooling the patient) with insulation blankets and warming devices.
	Fluids: Ensure maintenance fluids are running, and blood glucose levels are monitored. Consider a urinary catheter prior to transfer. Monitor urine output. Transfer all medication/fluid infusions and monitoring to portable transport devices.
	Contact PICU to update them of the child's clinical status and provide an estimated time of arrival before departure.
	Prepare full and clear records of the event, including all interventions (copies of notes, drug charts, X-rays is ideal).
	Just prior to moving the child run through the ABCDE assessment aloud with all team members involved. Request any suggestions or comments from the team and then confirm with all team members that they are in agreement to move the patient.

Information required by the paediatric transport team

If an inter-hospital transfer is required, then a referral to a dedicated paediatric transport service may be required. Even if the transfer is time-critical and the in-house team will be transferring the child, then the paediatric transport team should still be contacted as they will assist in locating the nearest appropriate available bed and help with emergency medical advice.

Certain information is required for this referral as detailed below:

- Child's details: (name, date of birth, gender, weight – actual or estimated).

- Referrers details: your name, position, attending consultant paediatrician and whether they have been informed of the transfer yet.

- Child's medical details: presenting complaint, past medical history including gestational age at birth, immunisation history, risk of contagious disease stratification and HPA involvement (recent travel, recent contagious contacts), family information that may be relevant and any child protection concerns.

- Details of any cardiorespiratory arrest: onset time of cardiorespiratory arrest, time of ROSC, location of arrest, special circumstances (i.e. submersion, hypothermia).

- Status currently: stable/unstable; compensated/decompensated.

- Treatment delivered so far: number of resuscitation cycles given and medications delivered before ROSC. Type and amount of fluid given, other medications given. Airway type, mode of ventilation, type of venous access or intraosseous access, neurological status and sedation muscle relaxant being delivered, body temperature and cooling or warming required, fluids being given, presence of anuria, suspicion of intra-abdominal or intra-thoracic mass.

- Investigation results: blood results, blood gases, any imaging performed.

09: Summary learning

ROSC following cardiopulmonary resuscitation is merely the first step in the continuous process of resuscitation management.

The ongoing management of seriously ill children includes appropriate vital sign monitoring, supportive therapies based on continuous ABCDE assessment and safe transfer to a PICU facility.

The prognosis for children following cardiorespiratory arrest depends on many factors, including the quality of post-resuscitation care.

The ability to predict the neurological outcome of children following cardiopulmonary resuscitation remains limited.

My key take-home messages from this chapter are:

Further reading

Macrae D, Grieve R, Allen E et al. A Randomised Trial of Hyperglycemic Control in Pediatric Intensive Care. New England Journal of Medicine. 2014. 370; 107-118.

Laverriere EK, Polansky M, French B, Nadkarni VM, Berg RA, Topjian AA. Association of Duration of Hypotension With Survival After Pediatric Cardiac Arrest. Pediatr Crit Care Med. 2020; 21:143–149. doi: 10.1097/PCC.0000000000002119

Topjian AA, Telford R, Holubkov R, Nadkarni VM, Berg RA, Dean JM, Moler FW; on behalf of the Therapeutic Hypothermia after Pediatric Cardiac Arrest (THAPCA) Trial Investigators. The association of early post-resuscitation hypotension with discharge survival following targeted temperature management for pediatric in-hospital cardiac arrest. Resuscitation. 2019; 141:24–34. doi: 10.1016/j.resuscitation.2019.05.032

Del Castillo J, López-Herce J, Matamoros M, Cañadas S, Rodriguez-Calvo A, Cechetti C, Rodriguez-Núñez A, Alvarez AC; Iberoamerican Pediatric Cardiac Arrest Study Network RIBEPCI. Hyperoxia, hypocapnia and hypercapnia as outcome factors after cardiac arrest in children. Resuscitation. 2012; 83:1456–1461. doi: 10.1016/j.resuscitation.2012.07.019

Moler FW, Silverstein FS, Holubkov R et al. Therapeutic Hypothermia after Out-of-Hospital Cardiac Arrest in Children. New England Journal of Medicine. 2015. 372. 1898-1908.

Moler FW, Silverstein FS, Holubkov R et al. Therapeutic Hypothermia after In-Hospital Cardiac Arrest in Children. New England Journal of Medicine 2017;376:318-329.

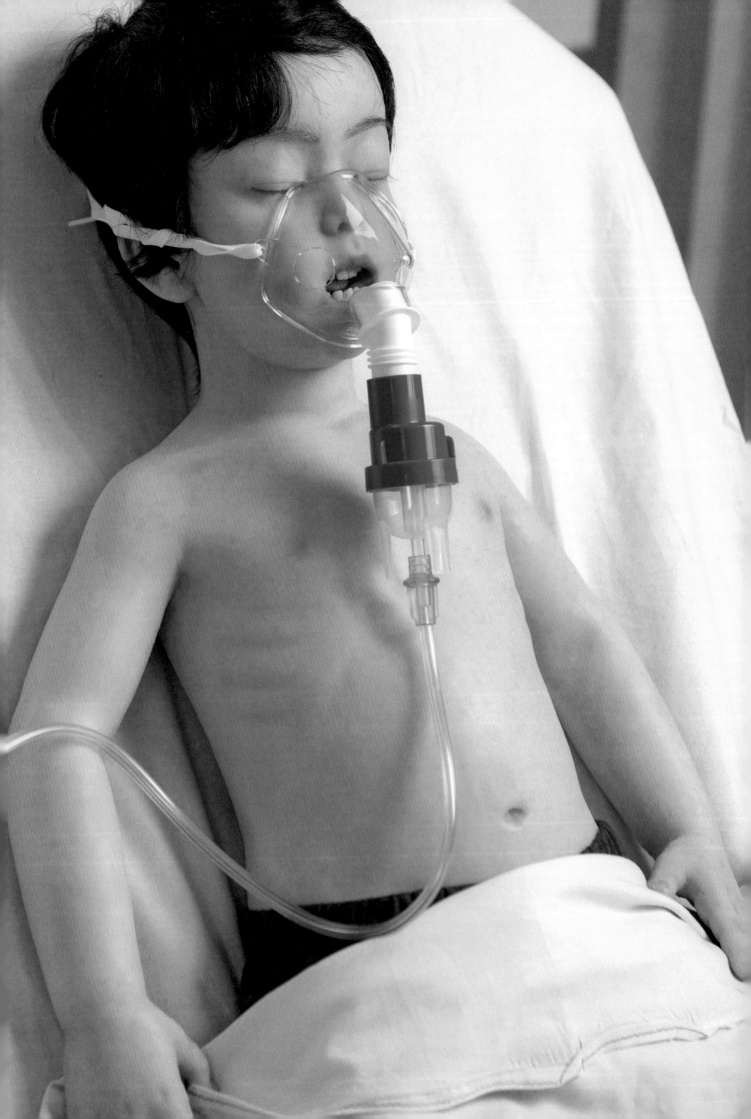

Paediatric emergencies

The learning outcomes will enable you to:

Identify common paediatric illnesses

Modify the ABCDE approach in certain paediatric illnesses

Describe the management of some electrolyte disturbances encountered in critically ill children

Introduction

In childhood, cardiorespiratory arrest is mainly secondary to injury or illness, and its outcome is poor; therefore, strategies to recognise and manage diseases early may prevent progression to organ failure and cardiorespiratory arrest.

Initially, recognition of respiratory and/or circulatory failure are more important than making a precise diagnosis of the disease. However, in certain circumstances, knowledge of specific disease processes enables appropriate management.

> Initially, recognition of respiratory and/ or circulatory failure are more important than making a precise diagnosis of the disease

Illnesses affecting the airway

Laryngotracheitis (croup)

Croup is an acute clinical syndrome of inspiratory stridor, barking cough, hoarseness, and variable degrees of respiratory distress. Acute viral laryngotracheobronchitis (viral croup) is the most common form of croup and accounts for over 95% of laryngotracheal infections.

Parainfluenza viruses are the most common pathogens, but other respiratory viruses (e.g. respiratory syncytial virus (RSV) and adenoviruses) produce a similar clinical picture.

The majority of children with croup are managed at home, whilst those in moderate to severe respiratory distress may need admission and supportive treatment.

Steroids may be used to reduce laryngeal oedema. An oral steroid, dexamethasone, shows clear benefit even in mild cases of croup in reducing airway oedema; improvement in symptoms is seen within 2 to 3 h. One to two doses may be given, and a third dose may be given after 12 h if required. A few children may require intubation owing to a combination of exhaustion and respiratory failure.

A Airway

Signs of upper airway obstruction are present with stridor and barking cough. There is a risk of marked swelling of the larynx and trachea, which can lead to partial or complete obstruction of the airway if the oedema progresses. If the child is conscious and breathing, manipulation or agitation will likely increase respiratory effort and obstruction, so it is recommended to allow the child to adopt a comfortable body position. However, if the infant/child is decompensating, open the airway, give 100% oxygen and start bag-mask ventilation (BMV) if required. Advanced airway management is needed in only a few severe cases, but it may be a challenge, and inexperienced interference may worsen the situation. Help should be called in the form of an experienced team, including an anaesthetist. Be aware that a narrower diameter tracheal tube than would normally be suitable for the child's size may be required.

B Breathing

Respiratory rate and work of breathing increase with progressive airway obstruction, but the rate may start to fall when the obstruction is more severe, and decompensated respiratory failure occurs. Reliable respiratory monitoring should be established, and oxygen given in a non-threatening manner. Nebulised adrenaline can be given to reduce airway oedema (3–5 mL of 1:1000 adrenaline) for children in severe respiratory distress. Improvement is seen in minutes but wears off after 1 to 2 h, after which there may be rebound laryngeal and tracheal oedema. Nebulised steroids such as budesonide can be given with nebulised adrenaline if the child is vomiting and unable to take dexamethasone. Nebulised budesonide is equivalent to but not superior to dexamethasone in effectiveness. Rarely, BMV will be needed in preparation for an advanced airway (in this case, the two-person technique may be required). Respiratory failure is due to upper airway obstruction and will improve when the airway is adequately managed, and patency is restored.

C Circulation

This is normal until decompensated respiratory failure develops.

D Disability

Exhaustion is an ominous sign, indicating decompensated respiratory failure.

Epiglottitis

This is an intense swelling of the epiglottis and surrounding tissues caused by a bacterial infection, almost exclusively Haemophilus influenzae type B. It is predominantly seen in children aged one to six years. It is now extremely uncommon owing to the widespread uptake of Hib vaccination for children in the UK. Typically, the child suddenly develops a high fever and is lethargic, pale and toxic. They are usually sitting immobile with their mouth open and chin raised. There may be excessive drooling owing to an inability to swallow saliva as it is painful to do so.

The key issue in managing the child with suspected epiglottitis is not to look in the throat nor perform a lateral X-ray of the neck (which may make the situation worse) until a senior team is available to secure an advanced airway if needed.

Bacterial tracheitis

This is a bacterial infection of the trachea, resulting in the formation of mucopurulent exudates (that can form 'membranes'), which may acutely obstruct the upper airway; this can be life-threatening. It is most common in children between the ages of three and eight years and should be considered in any child with signs of upper airway obstruction not responding to croup management. The presentation can be acute or subacute with a barking cough, stridor, and fever.

A Airway

Signs of upper airway obstruction are present with stridor and barking cough. Don't agitate the child and call early for senior help. If the child deteriorates acutely, BMV should be effective. Many children will need intubation. It should be anticipated that a smaller diameter TT may be needed due to airway narrowing, secondary to airway oedema, and to prevent further trauma to the inflamed subglottic area. Frequent suctioning and high humidity of inspired air and oxygen will be needed to prevent tube obstruction.

B Breathing

There is tachypnoea and increased respiratory effort, respiratory stridor and cough. Respiratory failure is due to the upper airway obstruction.

C Circulation

This is normal until decompensated respiratory failure develops. Inappropriate management can lead to sudden cardiorespiratory arrest because of complete airway obstruction.

Disease specific management

Once the airway has been stabilised, intravenous access should be obtained for intravenous antibiotics. Broad-spectrum antibiotics effective against staphylococcus and streptococcus species are indicated. Frequent airway toilet will be required for children who have been intubated.

Illnesses affecting breathing

Bronchiolitis

Bronchiolitis is a common respiratory infection of infancy caused by RSV in 75% of cases; the remainder are due to parainfluenza, influenza and adenoviruses. Typically, the infant has a coryzal prodrome lasting
1 to 3 days with a persistent cough, raised respiratory rate (there may be chest recession), wheeze, crackles or both. It occurs mainly in the autumn and winter and is the reason for 1–2% of all infant admissions to hospital. 90% of patients are aged one to nine months, and it is uncommon after one year. A subset of infants is at higher risk of developing more severe disease: infants less than three months old; infants with congenital heart disease; ex-premature infants; infants with chronic lung disease and infants with immunodeficiency. As there is no specific treatment for bronchiolitis, management is supportive.

Admission to hospital is recommended if:

- apnoea (observed or reported)
- persistent oxygen saturation of less than 92% when breathing air
- inadequate oral fluid intake (50–75% of usual volume, taking account of risk factors and using clinical judgement)
- severe respiratory distress, for example, grunting, marked chest recession, or a respiratory rate of over 70 breaths min^{-1}.

Most children can be discharged from ED with safety netting advice, the peak time for symptoms being between 3 and 5 days after onset, whilst the cough resolves in 90% of infants within 3 weeks.

Management of bronchiolitis

The approach to those who are severely affected by bronchiolitis is indicated as follows:

A Airway

Nasal obstruction from secretions can occur. In the hospital setting, gentle suction of the nose will remove secretions if nasal obstruction impairs air entry.

B Breathing

The inflammatory process causes oedema of the small airways and copious secretions, which can lead to hypoxia and hypercapnia; a ventilation-perfusion mismatch occurs. Apnoea and exhaustion can also occur.

The ventilation-perfusion mismatch may necessitate mechanical ventilation, although many children may be managed by continuous positive airway pressure (CPAP) or humidified high-flow nasal cannula (HFNC) oxygen. Non-invasive ventilation is the first choice of management for respiratory failure in infants with bronchiolitis. Mechanical ventilation is required in 3% of hospitalised infants overall. This can be due to recurrent apnoea, exhaustion or progressive respiratory failure.

C Circulation

This is normal until decompensated respiratory failure occurs.

D Disability

Tiredness, irritability and agitation reflect failing respiratory compensation. Decreasing responsiveness is an ominous sign, and exhaustion is a pre-terminal event.

Asthma

The UK continues to have the highest prevalence of childhood asthma in Europe, with significant related morbidity and mortality when compared to our European counterparts. 1.1 million children in the UK are currently receiving treatment for asthma (1 in 11 children), and 40 children die each year in the UK from asthma. The majority of asthma-related deaths occur before hospital admission. Cardiac arrest can be caused by hypoxia, tension pneumothorax, dynamic hyperinflation or secondary arrhythmias (caused by drugs or electrolyte disorders).

The following management relates to those children who present with moderate to severe or life-threatening asthma:

A Airway

The airway is normally open but can become obstructed when consciousness decreases.

B Breathing

Expiratory wheezing is found as a sign of lower airway obstruction. This can be caused by other conditions as well as asthma, including foreign body inhalation, anaphylaxis and bronchiolitis.

Respiratory monitoring should be established and supplemental oxygen administered. As long as there is compensated respiratory failure, avoid distressing the child, being aware that agitation may also be a sign of ongoing hypoxaemia. The volume of the wheeze is not directly related to severity as the absence of wheezing may indicate a critical obstruction, whereas increased wheezing may indicate a positive response to bronchodilation.

The severity of the asthma attack can be evaluated by monitoring oxygen saturations and the child's clinical status (especially respiratory rate and work of breathing), and response to treatment. If there are clinical signs of decompensation or exhaustion with decreasing consciousness, an arterial blood gas is indicated. In the case of decompensated respiratory failure, it might become necessary to support ventilation. Indications for intubation in asthma include a rapid deterioration in conscious level, severe hypoxia, cardiac or respiratory arrest. In severe asthma, intubation might be very challenging, as is mechanical ventilation, even when an advanced airway is established. In severe asthma, pneumothorax must be considered.

C Circulation

Circulation might be normal, but equally, dehydration or obstructive shock (caused by pneumothorax or dynamic hyperinflation) can occur.

Management of asthma

The early management of asthma is detailed in Table 10.1.

- Nebulised/inhaled beta-2 agonists are first line agents for an acute asthma attack and should be administered as early as possible.

- Doses can be repeated at regular intervals. Severe attacks may even necessitate continuous nebulised short-acting beta-2 agonists (e.g. salbutamol). Use oxygen to drive the nebuliser unit (there will be an optimal flow rate to drive the nebuliser to generate the optimal particle size, often 6 to 8 L min^{-1}). Alternatively, salbutamol can also be given by a metered-dose inhaler (pMDI) and a large volume spacer +/- a face mask (for children with moderate asthma, this may be equally effective). In life-threatening asthma, hypoventilation may prevent effective delivery of nebulised drugs, necessitating the use of intravenous infusion.

- Steroids: asthma is an inflammatory disorder, and steroids are mandatory for treatment. Give steroids early, either intravenous or oral.

- Nebulised anticholinergics: (e.g. ipratropium) may produce additional bronchodilation.

- Magnesium: a single dose of IV magnesium sulfate can be given in acute severe asthma not responding to inhaled bronchodilator therapy. Give IV magnesium as a slow bolus to diminish the risk of hypotension.

- Aminophylline: IV aminophylline may give additional benefit for children with severe or life-threatening asthma. It is given as a loading dose, followed by a continuous infusion. Serum concentrations must be monitored.

Table 10.1 Early management of asthma – September 2019. Based on the British Thoracic Society, Scottish Intercollegiate Guidelines Network, British guideline on the management of asthma revised 2019

Recognition of asthma	
These clinical features increase the probability of a diagnosis of asthma	More than one of the following: wheeze, cough, difficulty breathing and chest tightness. The risk is increased if these symptoms are recurrent, worse at night or in the early morning, occur during or after exercise or trigger dependent (e.g. with exposure to pets, cold, humidity, heightened emotions or occurring independent of upper respiratory tract infections).
	Personal history of atopic disorder.
	Family history of atopic disorder and/or asthma.
	Widespread wheeze heard on auscultation.
	History of improvement in symptoms or lung function in response to adequate therapy.

Acute asthma in children under 2 years	
The assessment of acute asthma in early childhood can be difficult	Intermittent wheezing attacks are usually due to viral infection and the response to asthma medication is inconsistent.
	Prematurity and low birth weight are risk factors for recurrent wheezing.
	The differential diagnosis of symptoms includes, aspiration pneumonitis, pneumonia, bronchiolitis, tracheomalacia, complications of underlying conditions such as congenital anomalies and cystic fibrosis.

Classification of severity of acute presentation

Moderate	Acute Severe	Life-threatening
Normal mental state.	Agitated, distressed.	Confused, drowsy, exhausted.
Ability to talk in sentences or vocalise as normal.	Can't complete sentences in one breath.	Unable to talk.
Some accessory muscle use.	Moderate to marked accessory muscle use.	Maximal accessory muscle use (poor respiratory effort is pre-terminal).
PEF ≥ 50% of best or predicted.	PEF 33–50% of best or predicted.	Marked tachycardia (sudden fall in HR is pre-terminal).
O_2 saturations > 92% in air.	O_2 saturations < 92% in air.	PEF < 33% of best or predicted.
Moderate tachycardia.	HR > 125 min^{-1} (> 5 years).	O_2 saturations < 92% in air.
HR ≤ 125 min^{-1} (> 5 years).	HR > 140 min^{-1} (2–5 years).	Silent chest.
HR ≤ 140 min^{-1} (2–5 years).	RR > 30 min^{-1} (> 5 years).	Cyanosis.
RR ≤ 30 min^{-1} (> 5 years).	RR > 40 min^{-1} (2–5 years).	Hypotension.
RR ≤ 40 min^{-1} (2–5 years).		

Management of asthma

Moderate	Acute Severe	Life-threatening
Continuous O_2 saturation monitoring.	Continuous O_2 saturation monitoring.	Continuous O_2 saturation monitoring.
High-flow O_2 via face mask titrated to achieve O_2 saturations 94–98%.	**High-flow** O_2 via face mask titrated to achieve O_2 saturations 94–98%.	**High-flow** O_2 via face mask titrated to achieve O_2 saturations 94–98%.
ß2 agonist 2–10 puffs via pMDI + spacer. +/- face mask, repeat dose every 20 min reviewing effect; no improvement in 1 h treat as acute severe.	**ß2 agonist** nebulised (salbutamol 2.5–5 mg) every 20 min with **Ipratropium bromide** (250 mcg) for first 2 h; review frequently.	Refer to PICU.
Ipratropium bromide given early via pMDI. + spacer +/- face mask, particularly if poorly responsive to ß2 agonist.	**Oral steroids:** 20 mg prednisolone for children aged 2 to 5 years; 30 to 40 mg for children > 5 years.	**ß2 agonist** nebulised (salbutamol 2.5–5 mg) every 20 min with **Ipratropium bromide** (250 mcg) for first 2 h; review frequently.
Oral steroids: 20 mg prednisolone for children aged 2 to 5 years; 30 to 40 mg for children > 5 years.	Consider intravenous **magnesium** and **aminophylline** if the child is unresponsive to maximal doses of bronchodilators and steroids.	**Oral steroids:** 20 mg prednisolone (2 to 5 years); 30 to 40 mg (> 5 years). Repeat dose if vomiting or consider intravenous **steroids** (hydrocortisone 4 mg kg^{-1} every 4 h).
	Consider ABG if poor response to early treatment.	Give bolus of **intravenous magnesium**.
	Refer to PICU.	Consider early single bolus dose of **intravenous salbutamol** where the child has responded poorly to inhaled therapy followed by an infusion.
		Consider **aminophylline** if the child is unresponsive to maximal doses of bronchodilators and steroids.
		Consider ABG if poor response to early treatment.

Note: Evidence is unclear which of intravenous salbutamol, aminophylline or magnesium should be first line in severe asthma.

Illnesses affecting the circulation

Anaphylaxis

Anaphylaxis is a potentially life-threatening allergic reaction. The overall prognosis of anaphylaxis is good, with a case fatality rate of under 1% in those presenting to hospitals in the UK. The risk of death may be increased in those with pre-existing asthma, particularly if this is poorly controlled or treatment with adrenaline is delayed.

Where anaphylaxis is fatal, death usually occurs very soon after exposure to the trigger. Fatal food reactions typically cause respiratory arrest after approximately 30 min; insect stings cause collapse from shock after 10–15 min and deaths caused by intravenous medication occur most commonly within 5 min. Food is the most common cause of anaphylaxis in young people, and preschool-aged children have the highest rate of hospitalisation due to food-anaphylaxis (but a disproportionately low rate of fatal outcomes). The greatest risk from fatal food allergy appears to be in teenagers and adults up to age 30 years. In contrast, fatal anaphylaxis due to drugs is rare in children.

The most common triggers are:

- food: peanut, tree nuts, cow's milk
- medications: Neuromuscular blocking agents, antibiotics (penicillins, cephalosporins, teicoplanin), contrast media, non-steroidal anti-inflammatory drugs (NSAIDs)
- insect stings.

Pathophysiology

In anaphylaxis, there is activation of multiple inflammatory pathways causing:

- Tissue oedema and smooth muscle contraction in the airways (causing bronchospasm and wheeze). This is the most common presentation for food-induced anaphylaxis.
- Fluid extravasation (tissue oedema, hypovolemia) and a profound reduction in venous tone.
- Depressed myocardial function has been reported, which can cause cardiogenic shock.
- Fluid redistribution into the bowel and smooth muscle (resulting in abdominal pain).

Recognition of anaphylaxis

Anaphylaxis is a clinical diagnosis and is likely when the following criteria are met:

- sudden onset and rapid progression of symptoms (minutes to several hours)
- Airway and/or Breathing and/or Circulation problems
- usually skin and/or mucosal changes (flushing, urticaria, angioedema)
- exposure to a known allergen for the patient helps supports the diagnosis.

Skin or mucosal changes alone are not a sign of anaphylaxis and can be subtle or absent in up to 20% of reactions (some patient may have only bronchospasm or a decrease in blood pressure (i.e. a circulation problem). There can also be gastrointestinal symptoms (e.g. vomiting, abdominal pain, incontinence). These are more significant where the route of exposure is non-oral (e.g. venom sting).

A Airway problems

- Airway swelling, e.g. throat and tongue swelling (pharyngeal/laryngeal oedema). The patient has difficulty in breathing and/or swallowing and may complain that their throat is closing up.
- Hoarse voice.
- Stridor (a high-pitched inspiratory noise caused by upper airway obstruction).

B Breathing problems

- Shortness of breath – increased respiratory rate.
- Wheeze and/or persistent cough.
- Patient becoming tired with the effort of breathing.
- Confusion caused by hypoxia.
- Cyanosis (mucous membranes appear blue) – this is usually a late sign.
- Respiratory arrest.

Respiratory presentations can vary from anaphylaxis with mild bronchospasm to life-threatening asthma with no other features to suggest anaphylaxis. Anaphylaxis can present primarily as respiratory arrest. Consider anaphylaxis in a person with sudden onset breathing difficulties, especially if known to be allergic to a food or insect sting.

C Circulation problems

- Signs of shock:
  - pale, cool peripheries
  - prolonged CRT.
- Significant increase in heart rate (tachycardia).
- Low blood pressure (hypotension):
  - feeling faint (dizziness)
  - collapse.
- Decreased conscious level or loss of consciousness
- Cardiac arrest.

Circulation problems (often referred to as anaphylactic shock) can be caused by direct myocardial depression, vasodilation and capillary leak with loss of fluid from the circulation. Characteristically, this results in a compensatory tachycardia. Bradycardia (a slow pulse) is usually a late feature, often preceding cardiac arrest.

D Disability problems

- Confusion.
- Agitation.
- Loss of consciousness.

E Exposure

- Skin and/or mucosal changes:
    - These are often the first feature of allergic reactions and present in over 80% of patients with anaphylaxis.
    - They can be subtle (e.g. patchy erythema) or dramatic (generalised rash).
    - They may involve just the skin, the mucosal membranes (e.g. lips), or both.
    - There may be urticaria, which can appear anywhere on the body. Wheals may be pale, pink or red, can be of different shapes and sizes, and are often surrounded by a red flare. They are usually itchy.
    - Angioedema involves swelling of deeper tissues, most commonly in the eyelids and lips, and sometimes the tongue and in the throat.

Management of anaphylaxis

1. Remove the suspected allergen (e.g. antibiotics, blood transfusion) if possible.

2. Treat life-threatening features using the ABCDE approach and call for help early (Figure 10.1).

    ### A Airway
    Open the airway.

    ### B Breathing
    Give 100% O_2 via a non-rebreathe mask with reservoir or BMV if required to maintain an SpO_2 94-98%. Prompt administration of intramuscular (IM) adrenaline may prevent the need for intubation. However, consider early intubation, particularly in children with tongue, lips and/or oropharyngeal swelling, and/or hoarseness. Early involvement of an experienced anaesthetist is important, as it may be a progressive condition; hence airway management before the total obstruction is an absolute must.

    ### C Circulation
    Lying flat with or without leg elevation is helpful for patients with a low blood pressure. If the child's clinical manifestations do not promptly respond to IM adrenaline, secure IV or IO access and give a fluid bolus 10 mL kg^{-1} IV balanced isotonic crystalloid or 0.9% sodium chloride and re-assess. Repeat bolus therapy as required to restore an adequate circulation; large volumes may be required (Chapter 5). Ensure IM adrenaline is administered every 5 min while attempting to secure intravenous or intraosseous access.

3. Give intramuscular (IM) adrenaline early to all children with signs of airway swelling, breathing difficulty or circulatory failure. Adrenaline is the first-line treatment for anaphylaxis (Table 10.2).
    - A single dose of IM adrenaline is well-tolerated and poses minimal risk in the context of an individual having an allergic reaction. If in doubt, give IM adrenaline.
    - Repeat IM adrenaline every 5 min if features of anaphylaxis do not resolve.

4. The majority of anaphylaxis reactions respond to initial treatment with intramuscular adrenaline, although around 10% will require more than 1 dose. Intravenous (IV) adrenaline must only be used in certain specialist settings and only by those skilled and experienced in its use.

5. Patients who require ongoing treatment for anaphylaxis despite 2 or more doses of IM adrenaline have refractory anaphylaxis.

6. Antihistamines are not recommended for the treatment of acute anaphylaxis. They are of no benefit in treating life-threatening symptoms, and their administration may delay more appropriate interventions such as further doses of adrenaline. Antihistamines may be helpful in alleviating cutaneous symptoms but should only be given after the patient has been stabilised. In this context, use a non-sedating oral antihistamine, such as cetirizine.

Table 10.2   Anaphylaxis IM adrenaline dose

Age	Intramuscular adrenaline dose
< 6 months	100–150 microgram IM (0.1–0.15 mL of 1 mg mL (1:1000) adrenaline
6 months–6 years	150 microgram IM (0.15 mL of 1 mg mL (1:1000) adrenaline
6–12 years	300 microgram IM (0.3 mL of 1 mg mL (1:1000) adrenaline
12+ years	500 microgram IM (0.5 mL of 1 mg mL (1:1000) adrenaline
Caution: do not give adrenaline as an intravenous bolus	

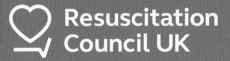
Anaphylaxis

Anaphylaxis?

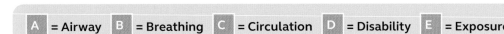
A = Airway   B = Breathing   C = Circulation   D = Disability   E = Exposure

Diagnosis – look for:
- Sudden onset of Airway and/or Breathing and/or Circulation problems[1]
- And usually skin changes (e.g. itchy rash)

Call for HELP
Call resuscitation team or ambulance

- Remove trigger if possible (e.g. stop any infusion)
- Lie patient flat (with or without legs elevated)
  - A sitting position may make breathing easier
  - If pregnant, lie on left side

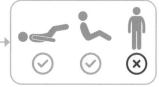

Give intramuscular (IM) adrenaline[2]

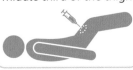
Inject at **anterolateral aspect** – middle third of the thigh

- Establish airway
- Give high flow oxygen
- Apply monitoring: pulse oximetry, ECG, blood pressure

If no response:
- Repeat IM adrenaline after 5 minutes
- IV fluid bolus[3]

If no improvement in Breathing or Circulation problems[1] despite TWO doses of IM adrenaline:
- Confirm resuscitation team or ambulance has been called
- Follow REFRACTORY ANAPHYLAXIS ALGORITHM

---

1. Life-threatening problems

Airway
Hoarse voice, stridor

Breathing
↑work of breathing, wheeze, fatigue, cyanosis, SpO_2 < 94%

Circulation
Low blood pressure, signs of shock, confusion, reduced consciousness

2. Intramuscular (IM) adrenaline
Use adrenaline at 1 mg/mL (1:1000) concentration

Adult and child > 12 years:	500 micrograms IM (0.5 mL)
Child 6–12 years:	300 micrograms IM (0.3 mL)
Child 6 months to 6 years:	150 micrograms IM (0.15 mL)
Child < 6 months:	100–150 micrograms IM (0.1–0.15 mL)

The above doses are for IM injection **only**.
Intravenous adrenaline for anaphylaxis to be given **only by experienced specialists** in an appropriate setting.

3. IV fluid challenge
Use crystalloid

Adults: 500–1000 mL
Children: 10 mL/kg

Figure 10.1   Anaphylaxis algorithm

7. The routine administration of corticosteroids is NOT recommended. However, consider giving steroids after initial resuscitation for refractory reactions or ongoing asthma/shock.

8. The specific test to help confirm a diagnosis of anaphylaxis is the measurement of mast cell tryptase; however, measuring blood tryptase levels must not delay initial resuscitation. Serial samples should be taken: first as soon as possible after resuscitation; the second at 1–2 h; third at 24 h after complete resolution of symptoms.

9. Follow the NICE guideline for the assessment and referral of patients suspected to have had anaphylaxis, specifically:

   - All patients should be referred to a specialist allergy clinic.

   - Consider whether to prescribe an adrenaline auto-injector. These are usually indicated in individuals with suspected anaphylaxis to an insect sting or food, which cannot be easily avoided.

   - Individuals prescribed adrenaline auto-injectors must receive training in their use.

10. Further research is needed to better identify and manage patients at the greatest risk of severe anaphylaxis.

    - Anaphylaxis reactions should be reported at the UK Anaphylaxis Registry (anaphylaxie.net).

    - Follow local guidance for reporting and debriefing of adverse events.

Management of refractory anaphylaxis

IV adrenaline infusions form the basis of treatment for refractory anaphylaxis (Figure 10.2), and expert help should be sought early. Dilute adrenaline can be infused via a peripheral cannula or IO needle until central venous access is obtained.

A Airway

If tracheal intubation is indicated, it should be performed by the most experienced clinician available, following a difficult airway protocol. Nebulised adrenaline can be used to treat upper airways obstruction but should not be prioritised over an adrenaline infusion or delay tracheal intubation in cases of critical upper airways obstruction.

B Breathing

Severe bronchospasm is common in food-induced anaphylaxis in children; in these cases, cardiac arrest is usually secondary to hypoxia. Treat severe respiratory symptoms with an adrenaline infusion as first-line therapy, in addition to nebulised and intravenous bronchodilator therapy (magnesium sulfate is not recommended as it causes significant vasodilation).

C Circulation

An adrenaline infusion should be the first-line treatment alongside a fluid bolus. Give further fluids as necessary. Large volumes may be needed for severe anaphylactic shock. Use a non-glucose containing crystalloid (e.g. Hartmann's and Plasma-Lyte) rather than 0.9% sodium chloride to reduce the risk of hyperchloraemia.

- It is reasonable to consider corticosteroids (such as hydrocortisone) for refractory reactions after initial resuscitation.

Cardiac arrest following anaphylaxis

Cardiac arrest following anaphylaxis is a situation when prolonged CPR should be considered (including extra-corporeal CPR). This is because the patients have usually arrested rapidly from a previously well state and a potentially reversible cause.

- Recognise cardiorespiratory arrest has occurred if the child becomes unresponsive or unconscious and breathing is absent or abnormal.

- Start CPR immediately. Good quality CPR with minimal interruption for other interventions improves the chances of survival from cardiac arrest, and follow the standard ALS algorithm.

Refractory anaphylaxis

No improvement in respiratory or cardiovascular symptoms
despite 2 appropriate doses of intramuscular adrenaline

A = Airway

Partial upper airway obstruction/stridor:
Nebulised adrenaline (5 mL of 1 mg/mL):

Total upper airway obstruction:
Expert help needed, follow difficult airway algorithm

B = Breathing

Oxygenation is more important than intubation

If apnoeic:
- Bag mask ventilation
- Consider tracheal intubation

Severe/persistent bronchospasm:
- Nebulised salbutamol and ipratropium with oxygen
- Consider IV bolus and/or infusion of salbutamol or aminophylline
- Inhalational anaesthesia

C = Circulation

Give further fluid boluses and titrate to response:
Child 10 mL/kg per bolus
Adult 500–1000 mL per bolus
- Use glucose-free crystalloid (e.g. Hartmann's Solution, Plasma-Lyte®)
Large volumes may be required (e.g. 3–5 L in adults)

Place arterial cannula for continuous BP monitoring

Establish central venous access

IF REFRACTORY TO ADRENALINE INFUSION
Consider adding a second vasopressor **in addition**
to adrenaline infusion:
- Noradrenaline, vasopressin or metaraminol
- In patients on beta-blockers, consider glucagon

Consider extracorporeal life support

Cardiac arrest – follow ALS ALGORITHM
- Start chest compressions early
- Use IV or IO adrenaline bolus (cardiac arrest protocol)
- Aggressive fluid resuscitation
- Consider prolonged resuscitation/extracorporeal CPR

**Establish dedicated
peripheral IV or IO access**

Give rapid IV fluid bolus
e.g. 0.9% sodium chloride

**Give IM* adrenaline
every 5 minutes until adrenaline
infusion has been started**

*IV boluses of adrenaline are
not recommended, but may be
appropriate in some specialist
settings (e.g. peri-operative) while
an infusion is set up

Give high flow oxygen
Titrate to SpO₂ 94–98%

**Monitor HR, BP, pulse oximetry
and ECG for cardiac arrhythmia**
Take blood sample
for mast cell tryptase

Seek expert[1] help early
Critical care support is essential

Start adrenaline infusion
Adrenaline is essential for treating
all aspects of anaphylaxis

&

Follow local protocol
OR

Peripheral low-dose IV adrenaline infusion:
- 1 mg (1 mL of 1 mg/mL [1:1000]) adrenaline in 100 mL of 0.9% sodium chloride
- Prime and connect with an infusion pump via a dedicated line

DO NOT 'piggy back' on to another infusion line
DO NOT infuse on the same side as a BP cuff as this will interfere with the infusion and risk extravasation

- In both adults and children, start at 0.5–1.0 mL/kg/hour, and **titrate according to clinical response**
- Continuous monitoring and observation is mandatory
- ↑↑ BP is likely to indicate adrenaline overdose

**Continue adrenaline infusion
and treat ABC symptoms**

Titrate according to clinical response

[1]Intravenous adrenaline for anaphylaxis to be given only by experienced specialists in an appropriate setting.

Figure 10.2   Refractory anaphylaxis algorithm

147

Children with cardiac problems

Cardiac problems are relatively common (6–8 per 1000 live births) and may present throughout childhood. These days, most congenital heart disease is diagnosed antenatally or in the immediate post-natal period but can be unexpected. Signs include the presence of a murmur, cardiac failure (tachypnoea, crackles on lung auscultation, hepatomegaly) and poor systemic perfusion such as prolonged CRT, poor or absent pulses and hypotension.

Cardiac problems can be classified as:

1. Congenital cardiac problems include:
   - cyanotic (e.g. transposition of great arteries)
   - obstructive (e.g. coarctation of the aorta)
   - hypoplastic (e.g. hypoplastic left heart) lesions.

   These tend to present earlier in life. In neonates, a prostaglandin infusion such as dinoprostone may be required to open and keep open the ductus arteriosus.

2. Other congenital non-cyanotic cardiac lesions include septal defects (e.g. ventricular septal defects, (VSD)), which may present with cardiac failure with signs including tachypnoea, tachycardia, poor perfusion, pallor, hepatomegaly, excessive weight gain or failure to thrive.

3. Later onset, acquired problems (e.g. myocarditis, cardiomyopathy) usually present with features of cardiac failure with signs including poor peripheral perfusion, tachycardia, tachypnoea and hepatomegaly, although arrhythmias are not uncommon as a mode of presentation (which can manifest as sudden collapse or potential seizure activity).

4. Rhythm disturbance (Chapter 6).

Recognition of cardiac conditions

A Airway
This is generally secure if consciousness is not compromised.

B Breathing
Several key clinical features include tachypnoea (cardiac failure) and low saturations (particularly in cyanotic congenital lesions). A cyanotic congenital cardiac problem is suspected if there is no improvement in saturations when oxygen is administered. In older children with an established cardiac diagnosis, it is helpful to establish and target their usual peripheral O_2 saturation values.

C Circulation
There may be signs of circulatory compromise or even shock, e.g. tachycardia, poor peripheral pulses, prolonged capillary refill time and possible hypotension. Other problems such as poor feeding or sepsis may lead to hypovolaemia; fluid boluses may be required, but these should be given with caution to avoid fluid overload.

D Disability
An abnormal conscious level may reflect impaired end-organ function due to respiratory or circulatory compromise.

E Exposure
Skin perfusion should be assessed by comparing both skin temperature gradients and central and peripheral CRT measurements. Consider the possibility of sepsis if fever is present.

Management of acute presentation of cardiac conditions

1. Get senior help immediately.

2. Give high-flow oxygen, especially when the diagnosis is uncertain. A brief period of oxygen is unlikely to close a patent ductus arteriosus. Start a prostaglandin infusion when a duct dependent problem is suspected (e.g. in cases of sudden unexplained deterioration in the first week or so after birth). Duct dependent lesions may be due to congenital cyanotic, obstructive or hypoplastic cardiac conditions. Prostaglandin infusions can be given peripherally or via a dedicated intraosseous line but should not be given by bolus. Higher doses may cause apnoea, requiring respiratory support.

3. Cautious use of diuretics may be helpful in cardiac failure (e.g. VSD). Additional respiratory support may be required.

4. Consider cautious fluid resuscitation using boluses of 5–10 mL kg⁻¹ of balanced crystalloid solution or 0.9% sodium chloride. Carefully re-assess after each bolus as worsening tachycardia or liver enlargement suggests fluid overload when diuretics rather than fluid resuscitation would be indicated.

5. Discuss further management with a paediatric cardiologist or intensivist as more sophisticated monitoring (e.g. invasive blood pressure) and therapy (e.g. vasoactive drugs) as well as transfer to a specialist centre may be required.

Sepsis

Sepsis is a common cause of death in children. It may be accompanied by organ dysfunction (severe sepsis) or hypotension (septic shock). Prompt recognition and management are required (Table 10.3). All hospitals in the UK should implement systems to monitor both early recognition and prompt management (e.g. sepsis six system for the recognition and treatment). Sepsis is diagnosed if there is suspected or proven evidence of infection as the cause of the acute illness plus at least two of the following: core temperature < 36°C or > 38.5°C; inappropriate tachycardia; altered mental state; reduced peripheral perfusion; white blood cell count < 4 or > 12 x 10^9 L^{-1}.

Recognition of sepsis

A Airway

This may be compromised by a reduced level of consciousness (e.g. viral, bacterial, fungal meningitis, or any other infection causing shock).

B Breathing

Children may have respiratory distress (tachypnoea, increased work of breathing) or respiratory failure due to the underlying condition (pneumonia) or as a result of other processes (septic response). Ventilatory support may be required.

C Circulation

Children may have tachycardia, prolonged capillary refill time, poor peripheral pulses and possibly hypotension. Sometimes sepsis results in vasodilatation with warm peripheries and early hypotension. These two differing clinical pictures were previously used to differentiate warm shock and cold shock, but studies have shown that clinical parameters are unreliable, and now this distinction is only made once haemodynamic monitoring is in place. Fluid maldistribution is common and severe sepsis often additionally causes myocardial dysfunction. Compensated circulatory failure may mask the true severity of the illness and urgency required in management. Careful assessment and re-assessment after the use of fluid resuscitation and the judicious use of inotropes is required.

D Disability

An abnormal conscious level may reflect impaired end-organ function due to respiratory or circulatory compromise. However, abnormal neurological status may reflect the underlying condition itself (e.g. meningitis). Blood glucose should always be checked as hypoglycaemia is relatively common and should be rechecked if new problems (e.g. seizures) are encountered.

E Exposure

This can give clues to the diagnosis. Look for rashes (e.g. meningococcal disease, toxic shock) or other skin lesions (e.g. herpes simplex).

Management of sepsis

1. Get senior help immediately.

2. Give 100% oxygen initially. Consider early intubation by an experienced anaesthetist especially if > 40 mL kg^{-1} of IV fluid has been required. Intubation is safer if performed when cardiovascular stability has been achieved.

3. Antibiotics should be administered within 1 h of presentation. The choice depends on the suspected site of infection and organism (and resistance pattern if known) – refer to local antibiotic guidelines. Third generation cephalosporins (e.g. cefotaxime) are often appropriate. Consider the possibility of other organisms (e.g. herpes simplex).

4. Fluid resuscitation using boluses of 10 mL kg^{-1} of a balanced crystalloid solution or 0.9% sodium chloride initially. Do not hesitate to use the intraosseous (IO) route. Large quantities of fluid may be required.

5. Carefully re-assess after each bolus to assess the effect of the intervention and to look for signs of fluid overload. If there are signs of fluid overload with persistent signs of circulatory failure, the child or infant is no longer fluid responsive and may need vasoactive drugs. Children with fever but without signs of circulatory failure **do not need** volume resuscitation. A tachycardia or fever alone is not enough to diagnose circulatory failure.

6. Vasoactive drugs may be required. These IV infusions optimise cardiac output by:
   - improving contractility, for example adrenaline, which is the first line inotrope in sepsis
   - raising systemic vascular resistance (vasoconstriction), such as noradrenaline in 'warm shock'
   - raising the heart rate (chronotropes) e.g. adrenaline.

7. Seek specialist advice early as more sophisticated monitoring (e.g. invasive blood pressure), management decisions (blood product use), and adjunctive treatments may be required.

Table 10.3   Surviving sepsis campaign international guidelines for the management of septic shock and sepsis-associated organ dysfunction in children

Time	Management
Recognition Sepsis **0 min**	**A, B assessment** Airway, RR, work of breathing, oxygen saturations, breath sounds, recognition respiratory distress/failure. Open airway and start high flow O_2 15 L min^{-1} or BMV as appropriate. **C assessment** HR, CRT, BP, peripheral and central perfusion, rhythm recognition; recognition circulatory failure/shock. Establish IV/IO access (take blood cultures, full blood count, blood glucose, urea and electrolytes, lactate*, blood gas and other bloods as indicated**) and give fluid resuscitation as below. **D assessment** AVPU score; recognition of altered mental status secondary to poor perfusion. **E assessment** Rash, temperature (high or low). Sepsis is diagnosed if there is evidence of infection as cause of the acute illness (suspected or proven) plus at least two of the following: core temperature < 36°C or > 38.5°C; white cell count elevated or depressed for age; inappropriate tachycardia; altered mental state; reduced peripheral perfusion.
Initial resuscitation **5–15 min**	• If no signs fluid overload (hepatomegaly, crackles at lung bases) then give 10 mL kg^{-1} balanced crystalloids*** IV bolus over 5–10 min and re-assess after each bolus up to 40–60 mL kg^{-1} or until perfusion improved. • Therapeutic end points: CRT < 2 s; normal BP for age; UO > 1 mL kg^{-1} h^{-1}, normal pulses, normal mental state. • Watch for signs of fluid overload; if present stop bolus therapy and start inotropic support. • Correct hypoglycaemia and hypocalcaemia. • Start broad-spectrum antibiotics; seek and aggressively control any infection source. • Call for more senior help and an anaesthetist urgently; call PICU for bed +/-PICU transfer team. • If mechanical ventilation is required, then cardiovascular instability during intubation is less likely after appropriate cardiovascular resuscitation.
Fluid refractory shock?	
Fluid refractory shock **15–60 min**	Start IV/IO inotrope infusion; central (preferable) or peripheral IV (clinical signs unreliable at differentiating 'warm' and 'cold' shock in children) **Adrenaline** 0.05–0.3 mcg kg^{-1} min^{-1} (use more dilute infusion if peripheral) **and/or** **Noradrenaline** via central IV or IO, starting infusion rate 0.05 mcg kg^{-1} min^{-1} Titrate inotropes upwards according to clinical response and haemodynamic effects using haemodynamic monitoring (where possible)**** Use ketamine +/- atropine IV/IO/IM to gain central access and airway if needed
Fluid and Catecholamine-resistant shock?	
PICU Team	Further management as per Paediatric Intensive Care/ retrieval service advice.

*lactate measurements are useful if available as they have prognostic ability if measured serially.

**Other bloods that may be indicated: coagulation studies, liver function tests, magnesium levels or any others indicated by the child's clinical picture.

***Balanced (buffered) fluids are used in preference to 0.9% sodium chloride, but if not available, 0.9% sodium chloride should be used.

**** These are starting dose ranges for these inotropes, and increases may be necessary but should be guided by PICU retrieval team/senior clinicians. Choice of inotropes is dictated by clinician preference, response to treatment and monitored parameters, and again decisions should be made in conjunction with PICU teams.

Warm shock – high cardiac output with low systemic vascular resistance.

Cold shock – low cardiac output with high systemic vascular resistance.

Fluid in mL kg^{-1} should be dosed for ideal body weight (max bolus 500 mL)

Illnesses affecting the central nervous system

Coma – the child with a diminished level of consciousness

A child's conscious level may be altered by illness, injury or intoxication. The level of consciousness may be assessed using the AVPU or Glasgow Coma Score (GCS). The GCS assesses 3 categories of response: eye-opening, verbal response, and motor response and is commonly used to assess the level of consciousness after traumatic injury. For non-verbal children, there is a modified paediatric version (Chapter 12).

AVPU is an easily performed assessment:

A	Alert
V	responsive to Voice
P	responsive only to Pain
U	Unresponsive

Recognition of coma in children

A Airway
As the child's level of consciousness diminishes, the likelihood of obstruction of the airway increases following the progressive loss of tone of surrounding soft tissue and supporting musculature. When the child becomes reactive only to pain, there may be loss of protective cough and gag reflexes leading to an increased risk of aspiration of stomach contents.

B Breathing
Coma may lead to slow respiratory rate and/or inadequate respiratory effort.

C Circulation
Depending upon the cause of the coma, circulation can be affected (e.g. hypovolaemic shock in septic shock or trauma) and should be managed accordingly.

D Disability
The assessment is based on AVPU (or GCS), posture and pupil reaction. Recording these values is essential and form part of the ongoing assessment and management of the child. Both pupils should be the same shape, size and react equally to light. If any pupil abnormalities are seen, this may indicate raised intracranial pressure or brain injury and should prompt further investigation (some drugs can cause pupil abnormalities, so check

this first (e.g. atropine, ipratropium bromide). After the initial ABCDE assessment, a more detailed neurological assessment is required to determine the cause of the change in the level of consciousness.

E Exposure
Causes such as meningococcaemia or other infective causes (e.g. vasculitis, SLE) may cause a decreased conscious level. The associated skin manifestations can help make the diagnosis (e.g. petechiae or purpura in meningococcal disease).

The management of coma in children

Open the airway and maintain its patency by appropriate means (e.g. airway opening manoeuvres, nasopharyngeal or oropharyngeal airway adjuncts, or tracheal intubation).

If protection against aspiration is required because of the loss of the protective upper airway reflexes, intubation must be performed by experienced personnel. Ventilatory support will then be required.

In children with a reduced level of consciousness, consider:

- Raised intracranial pressure (confusion leading to coma, falling heart rate and rising systemic blood pressure, abnormal pupils, posturing).
- Neuroimaging will likely be indicated either CT or MRI brain.
- If toxins/drugs/medication causes are suspected, then urine and blood samples should be collected early and sent for toxicology.
- In unexplained coma suspect metabolic causes and measure blood ammonia levels.
- If fits are prolonged despite anticonvulsant therapy, consider further investigations (e.g. electroencephalogram (EEG), metabolic tests). Don't forget any child or infant with seizures needs a blood glucose measurement.
- Involve PICU and/or neurosurgeons for advice early.
- Treatments are beyond the scope of this algorithm; refer to local protocols and RCPCH guidelines.

Seizures

Seizures are a common paediatric emergency. In the fitting child, an ABC approach to resuscitation still applies, but the child may only improve once the seizures have been controlled. There are many causes of seizures in children and infants (febrile seizures, genetic epilepsy, structural brain abnormalities, metabolic disturbance, meningoencephalitis, traumatic injury). Always exclude major metabolic disturbance as a cause (e.g. hypoglycaemia, hypocalcaemia, hyponatraemia, hyperammonaemia). A generalised seizure that has been ongoing for 5 min is unlikely to terminate without active management, and this is now the definition of convulsive status epilepticus (CSE).

Recognition of seizures

A Airway

There is a significant risk of upper airway obstruction during a seizure. This may be due to secretions or tongue/soft tissue hypotonia or, with loss of the protective upper airway reflexes with aspiration.

B Breathing

Respiratory failure is due to airway obstruction or a decreased level of consciousness, slowing the respiratory rate. Treatment of seizures can cause central nervous system depression, including respiratory arrest.

C Circulation

This is generally normal until decompensated respiratory failure. However, if the aetiology of the seizure is associated with other diseases (e.g. meningococcal disease or head trauma), circulatory failure may present earlier.

D Disability

Seizures should be controlled by antiepileptic drugs according to national guidelines. The first-line therapy is a benzodiazepine (diazepam, midazolam or lorazepam). However, a maximum of two doses (if required) should be administered because of the risk of respiratory depression.

E Exposure

As with coma, the skin may reveal the cause for the seizure, such as suspected infection or neurocutaneous disorders.

Management of seizures

Open the airway and maintain patency by appropriate means. Treat seizures according to national, local or the child's own seizure management plan (e.g. some children may not be able to tolerate benzodiazepines). Alternatively, a suggested guideline is given (Table 10.4), based on several recent international guidelines (i.e. Australia, US, New Zealand), which have been updated with evidence from recent randomised control trials studying the efficacy of levetiracetam, a second-line agent used in CSE.

Respiratory depression after benzodiazepine administration is common, and the child or infant may require respiratory support for a period of time after cessation of status epilepticus; this should be anticipated, and senior help sought. The blood glucose level should always be measured as hypoglycaemia is a treatable cause. Blood glucose levels < 3 mmol L^{-1} should be treated with 2 mL kg^{-1} 10% dextrose bolus.

Table 10.4 Management of seizures

Time	Management	
Seizure starts 0 min	Confirm clinically	Check ABC, high-flow O$_2$, attach monitoring Check blood glucose, treat < 3 mmol L^{-1}
5 min	1st line agent	**Midazolam** 0.3 mg kg^{-1} buccal* or intranasal* (max 10 mg) or **Lorazepam** 0.1 mg kg^{-1} IV/IO (max 4 mg) or **Midazolam** 0.15 mg kg^{-1} IV/IO (max 10 mg)
10–15 min	1st line agent	**Lorazepam** 0.1 mg kg^{-1} IV/IO (max 4 mg) or **Midazolam** 0.15 mg kg^{-1} IV/IO (max 10 mg) (Reconfirm epileptic seizure and prepare second-line agent of choice for next step.)
15–35 min	2nd line agent	**Levetiracam** 40 mg kg^{-1} IV (over 5 min, max 3 g) or **Phenytoin** 20 mg kg^{-1} IV (over 20 min with ECG monitoring) or **Phenobarbital** 20 mg kg^{-1} IV (over 5 min)
20–40 min	2nd or 3rd line agent	If preparation for deeper anaesthesia with intubation and ventilation complete, proceed to the next step. or Administer further alternative second-line drug **(levetiracetam, phenytoin, phenobarbital).**
20–40 min	3rd line agent	Rapid sequence induction of anaesthesia using **thiopental** sodium 4 mg kg^{-1} IV or **propofol** 1–1.5 mg kg^{-1} IV (with single-dose **rocuronium** if using NMB); **ketamine** and **midazolam** are alternatives. Intubation and ventilation; monitoring of neurological signs. Ongoing seizures are not always easy to identify; EEG monitoring.

*See BNFc for exact age-related doses

*ESETT/**ECLIPSE/***ConSEPT trials showed equal potency for phenytoin, levetiracetam, valproate (see further reading)

Levetiracetam has a good safety profile and is easy to administer

Children who frequently have seizures or CSE usually have an individually tailored guideline.

Do not give phenytoin too rapidly as it will cause bradycardia and or asystole.

Measure serum sodium and treat if < 125 mmol L^{-1} (3 mL kg^{-1} 3% sodium chloride)

Consider temperature control measures if hyperthermic

Consider meningitis, encephalitis and Raised ICP

Consider CNS haemorrhage if signs of trauma

There is no evidence for the ideal third-line agent: thiopentone, propofol, ketamine and midazolam may all be used.

Illnesses affecting metabolic and electrolyte balance

Diabetic ketoacidosis

Diabetic ketoacidosis (DKA) is caused by low insulin levels in the blood and may be seen in a child not known to have diabetes (i.e. as a newly presenting case). The following are key features of DKA:

- metabolic acidosis with bicarbonate < 15 mmol L^{-1} or pH < 7.3, AND blood ketones of > 3 mmol L^{-1}
- blood glucose levels are generally high > 11 mmol L^{-1} (note: children and young people with diabetes may develop DKA with normal blood glucose levels)
- hyperosmolality with resulting polyuria and dehydration.

Clinical features become more evident with worsening metabolic disturbance. They include dehydration, abnormal deep sighing respiration (Kussmaul breaths), vomiting, acetone smelling breath and drowsiness. The history may include increased urine output, increased thirst, weight loss, abdominal pain and confusion.

Careful fluid management is important in the treatment of DKA because of the risk of cerebral oedema. However, for the small number of children who initially present with circulatory failure (shock), recent guidelines have placed greater emphasis on adequate fluid resuscitation and treatment of shock as this can be fatal in DKA. Careful monitoring of fluid and insulin administration is needed, and expert advice is essential in managing such patients. Factors associated with an increased mortality include:

A) Cerebral oedema: occurs more frequently in younger children and newly diagnosed diabetes and has a mortality of around 25%. The cause of cerebral oedema is unknown, and evolution can be unpredictable.

B) Hypokalaemia: is preventable with careful monitoring and management.

C) Aspiration pneumonia: use a nasogastric tube in semiconscious or unconscious children.

D) Inadequate resuscitation: it is important to provide adequate resuscitation for children with DKA presenting with shock to prevent brain injury. Cerebral perfusion is influenced both by the circulatory perfusion pressure (blood pressure) and the intracranial pressure in incipient cerebral oedema.

Recognition of DKA

A Airway

This is safe if consciousness is not compromised, but careful and repeated assessment is required in the presence of an altered level of consciousness.

B Breathing

Children are often breathing quickly to compensate for their metabolic acidosis. If the child is shocked, give 100% oxygen by face mask. Avoid intubation if at all possible.

C Circulation

Assess for signs of circulatory failure. Signs of shock are very rare but can occur and include tachycardia, poor peripheral pulses, prolonged CRT and hypotension.

D Disability

Assess the level of consciousness using the Glasgow Coma Score (GCS score) or AVPU. Continue hourly neurological observations looking for signs or symptoms of raised intracranial pressure (e.g. headache, irritability, posturing, falling GCS score, rising BP with bradycardia, unequal or poorly reactive pupils). Monitor blood glucose, blood ketones, sodium and potassium. In reduced levels of consciousness, there is the risk of aspiration owing to the loss of protective airway reflexes.

E Exposure

Fever is not a feature of DKA, but infection may have a role in precipitating a crisis. Consider infection when any of the following are present: fever, hypothermia, raised blood lactate, hypotension, refractory acidosis.

Management of the child presenting with DKA

The following describes the early management of children with DKA, and this is based on guidelines from the National Institute of Clinical Excellence (NICE NG18, 2020 update) and BSPED Guideline for the Management of Children and Young People under the age of 18 years with Diabetic Ketoacidosis (2021), which should be referred to for ongoing management (Table 10.6).

Request assistance from a senior decision-maker and:
- admit to a paediatric ward or high dependency bed (whichever can provide one-to-one nursing care and the appropriate monitoring) if there is severe DKA (pH < 7.1) and/or child < 2 years
- admit to paediatric intensive care if blood glucose > 50 mmol L^{-1} and/or persistent shock and/or signs raised ICP.

A Airway

Ensure the airway is patent.

Table 10.5 Severity of DKA and degree of dehydration

Severity	Degree of dehydration	
Mild	5% dehydration	Venous pH 7.2–7.29 or, serum Bicarbonate < 15 mmol L^{-1}
Moderate	5% dehydration	Venous pH 7.1–7.19 or, Bicarbonate < 10 mmol L^{-1}
Severe	10% dehydration	Venous pH < 7.1 or, Bicarbonate < 5 mmol L^{-1}

Table 10.6 Early management of DKA in children; adapted from NICE guidelines August 2015 (updated December 2020) NG18

Identify DKA	History of polyuria, polydipsia and weight loss. May have confusion, abdominal pain and hyperventilation. • Blood glucose > 11 mmol L^{-1} • pH < 7.3 • Blood bicarbonate < 15 mmol L^{-1} • Ketones: blood beta-hydroxybutyrate > 3 mmol L^{-1} or urine ketonuria ++ and above Note: Usually not vomiting, acidotic or drowsy unless more than 5% dehydrated
Resuscitation	**A** ensure airway patency, insert NG tube if reduced conscious level or vomiting to decrease gastric distension **B** 100% oxygen via a face mask with reservoir bag + titrate to oxygen saturations 94-98%; avoid intubation unless respiratory arrest or respiratory failure when anaesthetic assistance urgently required **C** establish IV access, take venous bloods (pH, PaCO$_2$, bicarbonate, sodium, potassium, urea, creatinine, beta-hydroxybutyrate levels, glucose), monitor ECG, identify shock • Give a fluid bolus 10 mL kg^{-1} of balanced isotonic crystalloid or 0.9% sodium chloride over 30 min to children with NO shock • Give a fluid bolus 10 mL kg^{-1} of balanced isotonic crystalloid or 0.9% sodium chloride over 5-10 min and re-assess; repeat to a maximum of 40 mL kg^{-1}; inform PICU if shock is persists **D** seek and identify signs and symptoms of raised intracranial pressure – headache, confusion, irritability, posturing, falling GCS, rising BP with bradycardia. Treat with 3% sodium chloride or mannitol, seek PICU advice and call an anaesthetist. Consider CT brain to determine the cause. **E** Consider sepsis if fever, hypothermia, hypotension, lactic acidosis, refractory acidosis
Intravenous therapy: fluids and insulin	For children with dehydration, nausea and vomiting: Calculate fluid requirements (FR) for each child Aim: to correct fluid deficit over 48 h FR = Maintenance fluids for 48 h + fluid deficit Subtract 10 mL kg^{-1} from fluid requirement for children who did not present with shock Do not subtract resuscitation fluid volumes from fluid requirements for children who presented in shock Isotonic balanced crystalloids or 0.9% sodium chloride initial fluid of choice – add potassium once passing urine and serum potassium is in normal range (usually < 5.5 mmol L^{-1}); add 5% dextrose to fluid when glucose less than 14 mmol L^{-1} 1–2 h after intravenous fluids commenced, start insulin infusion at 0.05–0.1 units kg^{-1} h^{-1} (0.05 units kg^{-1} h^{-1} for children < 5 years old recommended) Monitor serum potassium and treat hypokalaemia Do not give intravenous bicarbonate to correct acidosis
Observations	Strict fluid balance Hourly capillary blood gas and blood glucose measurements Capillary blood ketone levels 1–2 h (ideally point of care testing) Initially two-hourly U+E's Hourly BP, HR, RR, temperature Hourly assessment of level of consciousness Half hourly neuro observations including level of consciousness in children with severe DKA and children < 2 years old. Urgently escalate symptoms of headache, bradycardia, changes in level of consciousness or changes in ECG (ST and T wave changes may indicate hypokalaemia)

Maintenance fluids calculation	Fluid deficit (mL) = % dehydration x weight (kg) x 10
4 mL kg^{-1} h^{-1} for first 10 kg of body weight	Fluid requirement (FR) over 48 h for a 10 kg child = maintenance requirement for 48 h + (fluid deficit – initial fluid given) (if no shock) (Note: max FR allowance for 5% dehydration = 3750 mL, 10% dehydration = 7500 mL)
2 mL kg^{-1} h^{-1} for second 10 kg of body weight (11–20 kg)	Example: 5% dehydrated, no shock at presentation, given 10 mL kg^{-1} 0.9% saline = (4 x 10 x 48) + (5 x 10 x 10) – (10 x 10) = 1920 + 500 – 100 = 2320 mL over 48 h = 48 mL h^{-1}
1 mL kg^{-1} h^{-1} for each kg of body weight above 20 kg (up to max of 75 kg)	

Diabetic ketoacidosis

B Breathing

Intubation should be avoided unless the patient has a GCS < 8, has a respiratory arrest or has poor respiratory effort. Intubation and ventilation are potentially dangerous as the children often have a low pH due to metabolic acidosis, which they are compensating for by hyperventilating (to reduce $PaCO_2$). Insert a nasogastric tube to prevent aspiration of vomit.

C Circulation

Obtain vascular access and check venous blood gases (pH, $PaCO_2$, bicarbonate, lactate), blood sugar, urea and electrolytes, including serum potassium and serum ketones (beta-hydroxybutyrate). Attach a cardiac monitor and monitor BP and HR as part of the assessment and re-assessment for the presence of shock.

- If no signs of shock, give 10 mL kg^{-1} of 0.9% sodium chloride or balanced isotonic crystalloid solution over 60 min (subtract this fluid volume from the calculated deficit).
- If signs of shock present (tachycardia, poor peripheral pulses, prolonged CRT, hypotension), give a 10 mL kg^{-1} fluid bolus of isotonic balanced crystalloid fluid or 0.9% sodium chloride over 5–10 min and re-assess. If signs of shock persist, fluid boluses may be repeated up to a total maximum of 40 mL kg^{-1}. If shock persists after this, inotropes should be considered (in shock, the volume of resuscitation fluid is not subtracted from the calculated deficit).

Treat DKA with intravenous fluids if the child or young person is not alert, is nauseated or vomiting, or is clinically dehydrated but with caution and re-assess as per guidelines in Table 10.5.

Do not give intravenous/intraosseous bicarbonate as its use is associated with an increased risk of cerebral oedema.

Assess the degree of dehydration. The aim is to correct the extent of dehydration slowly over 48 h. This is by administering maintenance fluids plus the fluid deficit calculated from the assessed degree of dehydration. Commence IV fluids for maintenance and rehydration initially with balanced isotonic crystalloid solutions or 0.9% sodium chloride; add potassium once renal failure excluded.

If there are any signs of reduced conscious level or raised intracranial pressure, consider cerebral oedema.

Start IV insulin infusion at 0.05–0.1 units kg^{-1} h^{-1}, approximately 1–2 h after starting IV maintenance fluids and replacement fluids. Lower dose insulin infusion is advised for younger children (< 5 years old) at 0.05 units kg^{-1} h^{-1}. If serum potassium is low < 3 mmol L^{-1}, then give potassium and delay starting insulin until the serum potassium is within normal range.

Sodium (Na$^+$)

Sodium is the major cation (positive ion) in the extracellular, and hence intravascular, fluid compartment. Hence the sodium concentration in the blood largely determines plasma tonicity (osmolality). Disturbances in sodium levels can cause, or occur due to fluid shifts between the different fluid compartments in the body, disrupting homeostasis and disturbing cellular function.

Hyponatraemia

The normal range of sodium in the blood is 135–145 mmol L^{-1}, and hyponatraemia is defined as serum sodium < 135 mmol L^{-1}. Hyponatraemia can develop because of excess free water intake, excessive loss of sodium from the kidney or gastrointestinal tract, retention of free water by the kidney, but rarely from deficient intake of sodium.

Plasma tonicity is fiercely defended by the body because of its importance in maintaining homeostasis. Usually, the body can maintain serum sodium in the normal range despite wide variations in fluid ingestion. This is achieved by the kidney's ability to generate dilute urine and excrete free water in response to changes in serum osmolality and intravascular volume status. A hormone called anti-diuretic hormone (ADH) is secreted from the pituitary when the body detects a high blood tonicity or low blood volume. This hormone acts on the kidney, making it conserve water, so increasing intravascular volume.

In most children, hyponatraemia is acquired during hospitalisation. The reasons for this are two-fold: firstly, particularly sick children, are unable to handle water normally, and they can develop the syndrome of inappropriate anti-diuretic hormone (SIADH). In this scenario, ADH is secreted even though plasma tonicity and or blood volume are normal or high, and this can result in hyponatraemia. This may be further exacerbated if hypotonic fluids are used as intravenous fluid therapy. Triggers for SIADH include morphine administration, artificial ventilation, intracranial conditions, pneumonia, asthma and barbiturates. This is why sick children in PICU are often fluid restricted and not given full maintenance fluids.

Other conditions that can lead to hyponatraemia include heart failure and nephrotic syndrome (where there is increased total body water); diuretic use and reduced sodium intake; loss of sodium via the gastrointestinal or urinary tract (e.g. cerebral salt wasting, gastroenteritis, fistulas).

Most of the signs and symptoms of hyponatraemia occur because of its effects on the central nervous system. When serum sodium and hence blood osmolality falls, water enters the brain, causing cerebral oedema. Cerebral oedema causes symptoms such as headache, nausea, vomiting, irritability and seizures. The manifestations of these symptoms can vary depending upon how quickly hyponatraemia develops, the level of sodium reached and the duration of the hyponatraemia. Seizures are very unusual at sodium levels > 125 mmol L^{-1} but become increasingly common at levels below 120 mmol L^{-1}. Other signs and symptoms include tachycardia, muscle cramps, hypotension and muscle weakness.

Management of the child with hyponatraemia

A Airway
Not usually compromised unless a reduced level of consciousness or seizures.

B Breathing
May have a reduced respiratory rate if a reduced level of consciousness.

C Circulation
Obtain vascular access and measure blood electrolytes. In hypovolaemic hyponatraemia states, there may be a need to give fluid resuscitation to restore haemodynamic stability; thereafter sodium should be corrected slowly at a rate of increase of not more than 0.5 mmol L^{-1} h^{-1}.

D Disability
If sodium level is < 125 mmol L^{-1} and the patient is seizing, then the sodium level should be corrected to 125 mmol L^{-1} as this would treat any seizures related to hyponatraemia. If the seizures continue after correction, then other causes should be sought. Treatment is with 3 mL kg^{-1} of 3% sodium chloride given over 20 min with repeated blood testing to ascertain the rate of change in measured serum sodium levels.

For hyponatraemia associated with euvolaemia or hypervolaemia fluid restriction and or diuretics may be useful. Again, the serum sodium should be corrected at a rate of change of no more than 0.5 mmol L^{-1} h^{-1}. This becomes increasingly important the longer the duration of hyponatraemia. This is because when hyponatraemia develops slowly, there is a slow cerebral adaptation to protect the brain from the injurious effects of hypo-osmolality. This protective mechanism leaves the brain susceptible to demyelination syndrome during

treatment if the correction is rapid, as there are significant fluid shifts between the different fluid compartments of the brain. Further management is directed at finding and correcting the underlying cause.

Hypernatraemia

Hypernatraemia is defined as serum sodium > 145 mmol L^{-1}. It represents a deficit of total body water relative to total body sodium. It is commonly caused by the loss of free water but can also be caused by excessive salt intake.

Plasma tonicity is increased in hypernatraemia, which causes cellular dehydration.

The brain is particularly vulnerable to these effects; cell shrinkage can result in seizures and encephalopathy. Shrinkage of brain tissues can lead to tearing of cerebral blood vessels, causing intracranial haemorrhage (i.e. a subdural haemorrhage as the dural veins become disrupted and blood accumulates in the subdural space).

Most at risk are critically ill children, those who are neurologically impaired and infants who are unable to respond to their thirst trigger.

Causes include:
- water depletion (e.g. diabetes insipidus)
- water depletion exceeding sodium depletion (e.g. gastroenteritis and diarrhoea, breastfeeding failure)
- sodium excess (e.g. administration of hypertonic solutions, infant formula made up incorrectly)

Signs and symptoms start to become more common at serum sodium levels of > 160 mmol L^{-1} and are more common when hypernatraemia develops acutely.

The signs and symptoms of severe hypernatraemia (usually > 170 mmol L^{-1}) include: irritability, lethargy, altered level of consciousness, seizures, ataxia, tremor, hyperreflexia, increased muscle tone and fever.

Management of the child with hypernatraemia

A Airway
Not usually compromised unless a reduced level of consciousness or seizures.

B Breathing
May have reduced respiratory rate if a reduced level of consciousness.

Sodium

C Circulation

Obtain vascular access and measure blood electrolytes.

Initially, in hypovolaemic hypernatraemia states, fluid resuscitation may be needed to restore haemodynamic stability.

Rehydration should then be over 48 to 72 h because rapid rehydration of prolonged hypernatraemia states (with rapid decreases in serum sodium levels) will result in cerebral oedema. Blood sodium level should be corrected slowly at a rate of decrease of not more than 0.5 mmol L^{-1} h^{-1}.

In severe hypernatraemia with levels in excess 170 mmol L^{-1}, 0.9% sodium chloride should be used to rehydrate, and potassium added once the patient is passing urine. Further management should be directed at finding and correcting any cause.

Potassium (K⁺)

The causes of hyperkalaemia and hypokalaemia are given in Table 10.7.

The normal range for serum potassium is 3.5–5.0 mmol L^{-1}

The K⁺ gradient, from the intracellular to extracellular space, determines the electrical conduction of certain cells; this is particularly important for myocardial cells as it will affect their contractility. Even limited increases in serum K⁺ can be responsible for decreased conduction and diminished cardiac contractility. Blood pH has a direct effect on K⁺; acidosis increases serum K⁺ (by 0.5–1.1 mmol L^{-1} for each 0.1 decrease in pH).

Table 10.7 Causes of potassium disturbance

Hyperkalaemia	Hypokalaemia
Renal failure (acute/chronic)	Gastrointestinal losses (e.g. diarrhoea, vomiting)
Acidosis Adrenal insufficiency Addison's disease Secondary	Alkalosis
Excessive potassium intake	Volume depletion
Intake of K⁺ sparing medication	Diuretics
Cell lysis (e.g. in tumour treatment, tissue infarction, trauma, rhabdomyolysis)	Insufficient potassium intake
Haemolysis	Malnutrition
Massive blood transfusions	Insufficient K⁺ intake
K⁺ supplements, certain drugs	

Hyperkalaemia

Hyperkalaemia is characterised by muscular weakness, paralytic ileus, respiratory arrest and heart conduction disturbances leading to arrhythmias and eventually to cardiac arrest.

Typical ECG changes seen in hyperkalaemia are dependent on both the K⁺ level and the associated rate of increase in K⁺ level.

Initially, there may be T wave elevation (peaked T waves), but as K⁺ levels rise, a prolonged PR interval is seen with flattening of the P wave, then widening of the QRS. Eventually, the child may develop an idioventricular rhythm and ventricular fibrillation as serum K⁺ rises. A normal ECG, however, does not exclude the risk of the child developing a life-threatening arrhythmia.

False hyperkalaemia values can result from haemolysis of the blood due to difficult capillary blood sampling, so unexpected high levels in an otherwise asymptomatic child should be rechecked. In children who are symptomatic or for whom hyperkalaemia is not unexpected, levels should still be rechecked, but this should not delay management.

Management of hyperkalaemia

The treatment of hyperkalaemia (Figure 10.3) is dependent on the speed of occurrence of the symptoms (acute rises are more often symptomatic) and the clinical state of the child, or if they show toxic ECG changes. It includes:

- intravenous calcium gluconate OR calcium chloride to antagonise the toxic effects of hyperkalaemia at the myocardial cell membrane
- sodium bicarbonate IV (if acidosis or renal failure is present)

- insulin-glucose IV infusion. This will facilitate potassium uptake into cells. Treatment can lower serum potassium by 0.6-1 mmol L^{-1}. Check blood glucose at 15 min and then every 30 min thereafter.
- salbutamol administration either via a nebuliser or intravenously. Salbutamol should be given alongside insulin-glucose in severe hyperkalaemia as there is a synergistic effect.
- haemodialysis/peritoneal dialysis
- hydrocortisone in cases of suspected adrenal insufficiency.

If the child has an elevation of the serum K^+ levels without symptoms, excess K^+ may be removed from the body by the use of:

- diuretics (e.g. furosemide)
- ion exchange resins (calcium resonium given orally or rectally). The onset of the effect of these resins is slow, but this treatment can be started early (as soon as the K^+ level is increased).

Figure 10.3 Management of hyperkalaemia

Mild hyperkalaemia > 5.5 mmol L^{-1} + asymptomatic +normal ECG	**Moderate hyperkalaemia** 6–7 mmol L^{-1} + asymptomatic + normal ECG	**Severe hyperkalaemia** > 7 mmol L^{-1} + symptomatic + ECG abnormalities
• Stop any K^+ supplements • recheck K^+ result • consider no treatment • +/- salbutamol nebuliser • +/- furosemide • +/- calcium resonium PO/PR	• Stop any K^+ supplements • salbutamol nebuliser • insulin/dextrose IV infusion • furosemide • +/- calcium resonium PO/PR • +/- bicarbonate if metabolic acidosis	• Stop any K^+ supplements • calcium gluconate/calcium chloride IV • salbutamol nebuliser/IV+ insulin/dextrose IV infusion • bicarbonate IV if metabolic acidosis • CVVH/dialysis • +/- calcium resonium • +/- hydrocortisone (if adrenal insufficiency suspected)

1. Calcium gluconate IV 10% 0.5 mL kg^{-1} slow IV (max 20 mL) OR calcium chloride IV 10% 0.1–0.2 mL kg^{-1} slow IV (max 10 mL). Onset < 3 min; lasts 30 min

2. Insulin/dextrose IV bolus: 10% dextrose 10 mL kg^{-1} (or 5 mL kg^{-1} 20% dextrose via a central line only) + short acting insulin 0.1 units kg^{-1} IV (max 10 units), give over 5 min. Onset 15 min; peak 30 min; duration 2–3 h. Check blood glucose at 15 min and then every 30 min thereafter. May need to add dextrose to maintenance fluid subsequently to keep blood glucose 6–10 mmol L^{-1}

3. Salbutamol nebuliser: patient < 10 kg, 2.5 mg 1–2 h; patient > 10 kg, 5 mg 1–2 h (max dose 10 mg)

4. Salbutamol IV (severe and symptomatic): 4 mcg kg^{-1} bolus IV. Onset 30 min; duration 2–3 h

5. Sodium bicarbonate IV 1–2 mmol L^{-1} in patients with metabolic acidosis (avoid giving in IV line with calcium)

6. Furosemide 1 mg kg^{-1} IV (max 20 mg)

Potassium

Hypokalaemia

Hypokalaemia (K^+ < 3.5 mmol L^{-1}) is characterised by muscular weakness, constipation, paraesthesia and tetany.

Severe hypokalaemia (< 2.5 mmol L^{-1}) can cause life-threatening arrhythmias (VF, pVT, PEA or asystole), paralysis, rhabdomyolysis, paralytic ileus and metabolic alkalosis.

Management of hypokalaemia in a child

Treatment of hypokalaemia (2.5–3.5 mmol L^{-1}) includes the early recognition of the cause. Patients treated with digitalis are at special risk of developing arrhythmias.

Treatment of severe hypokalaemia (< 2.5 mmol L^{-1}) or hypokalaemia associated with arrhythmias consists of careful intravenous K^+ infusion (preferably via central access) with ECG monitoring. Close attention to the site of infusion is required if administered peripherally.

This is best performed in a high dependency or PICU setting as life-threatening arrhythmias can occur. An infusion of 0.5 mmol L^{-1} h^{-1} of KCl is given until the arrhythmia resolves and/or the K^+ level is > 3.5 mmol L^{-1}. A total dose of 2–3 mmol kg^{-1} KCl may be required; administration of K^+ should be reduced as soon as the child is clinically stable.

Calcium

Hypercalcaemia

Hypercalcaemia usually presents with long-standing anorexia, malaise, weight loss, failure to thrive and vomiting. Other symptoms are convulsions, coma, polyuria, dehydration, hypokalaemia, bradycardia, arterial hypertension and ECG changes (e.g. short QT, widening of QRS complexes, AV block).

Causes include:
* hyperparathyroidism, hypervitaminosis A or D
* idiopathic hypercalcaemia of infancy
* malignancy
* thiazide diuretic abuse
* skeletal disorders.

Management of hypercalcaemia in children

Symptomatic hypercalcaemia requires urgent treatment; an underlying reason for hypercalcaemia presenting acutely or found incidentally must be determined.

Initial treatment consists of fluid resuscitation with 0.9% sodium chloride. Infusion of twice the calculated basic daily fluid requirement is delivered, providing the degree of dehydration, cardiac function and blood pressure permits significant fluid administration.

Levels of both serum K^+ and magnesium (Mg^{2+}) should be monitored. Furosemide can be useful in patients with fluid overload; however, in children with renal insufficiency and oliguria, dialysis may be necessary.

Hypocalcaemia

Causes include:
* vitamin D deficiency
* hypoparathyroidism (di George syndrome, magnesium deficiency, familial)
* renal failure.

Specific symptoms are:
* signs of neuronal irritation or convulsions
* laryngeal stridor
* muscle weakness and bone pain
* ECG changes: QT prolongation, AV block, VF.

Management of hypocalcaemia in children

The treatment of severe hypocalcaemia (without hypomagnesaemia) includes intravenous or intraosseous administration of calcium gluconate. Oral supplements of calcium may be needed. Vitamin D administration is often needed owing to clinical and biochemical levels of insufficiency.

If hypocalcaemia is associated with hypomagnaesemia, Mg^{2+} replacement will also be necessary.

Highly infectious diseases and patients in isolation

Resuscitation where there is high risk of infection:

- Assuring the safety of the rescuer has always been a priority in resuscitation guidelines; therefore, resuscitation events will require healthcare workers to take extra precautions in cases where there is a high infection risk.

- In such situations, staff should always be aware of and follow national guidance on the use of personal protective equipment (PPE). An example of such guidance for the COVID-19 pandemic can be found at www.resus.org.uk/COVID-19-resources.

- Procedures and techniques that limit the risk of disease transmission (for instance, by aerosol spread) are to be preferred.

- For resuscitation service planning, it is recommended that local decision-makers decide the level of risk within each clinical area and follow contemporary national guidelines to ensure appropriate and optimal treatment.

10: Summary learning

The conditions described in this chapter are common causes of paediatric illness and potential causes of cardiorespiratory arrest in children.

Use the ABCDE approach for early recognition and treatment to prevent cardiorespiratory arrest.

Call for expert help early when specialist procedures are needed.

10

My key take-home messages from this chapter are:

Further reading

ILCOR Worksheets on therapeutic hypothermia. www.americanheart.org

Alberta Medical Association; Alberta Clinical Practice Guideline Working Group. Guideline for the diagnosis and management of croup, 2008.

Resuscitation Council UK guidance on the management of anaphylaxis http://www.resus.org.uk/pages/faqAna.htm

NICE guidelines NG 18 August 2015 (updated November 2016). Bronchiolitis in Children. NICE Guideline (NG9). June 2015.

British Thoracic Society, Scottish Intercollegiate Guidelines Network

British guideline on the management of asthma in Children 2019.

https://pathways.nice.org.uk/pathways/sepsis)

Weiss S, et al. Surviving Sepsis Campaign International Guidelines for the Management of Septic Shock and Sepsis-Associated Organ Dysfunction in Children. Pediatr Crit Care Med. 2020;21(2);e52-e106

RCPCH decreased conscious levels www.rcpch.ac.uk/sites/default/files/201803/2015_decreased_conscious_level_-_full_clinical_guideline_0.pdf

Hoffman JIE, Kaplan S. The incidence of congenital heart disease. Journal of the American College of Cardiology. 2002; 12 (39). 1890-1900.

https://www.nice.org.uk/guidance/ng217 Epilepsies in children, young people and adults. NICE guidelines NG217 (updated April 2022).

Trinka, E, Cock, H, Hesdorffer, D, Rossetti, A, Scheffer, I, Shinnar, S, Shorvon, S & Lowenstein, D. A definition and classification of status epilepticus--Report of the ILAE Task Force on Classification of Status Epilepticus. Epilepsia. 2015. 56: 1515-23

Kapur et al. Randomised Trial of Three Anticonvulsant Medications for Status Epilepticus. N Engl J Med 2019;381:2103-2113.doi:10.1056/NEJMoa1905795

Lyttle M, Rainford NE et al. levetiracetam versus phenytoin for second-line treatment of paediatric convulsive status epilepticus (EcLiPSE): a multicentre, open-label, randomised trial. Lancet, Volume 393, Issue 10186, 2125 – 2134

Dalziel SR, Borland ML et al; PREDICT research network. Levetiracetam versus phenytoin for second-line treatment of convulsive status epilepticus in children (Concept):an open-label, multicentre, randomised controlled trial. Lancet. 2019 May 25;393(10186):2135-2145

Early management of DKA in children; adapted from NICE guidelines August 2015 (updated December 2020) NG18.

P. Van de Voorde, et al., European Resuscitation Council
Guidelines 2021: Paediatric Life Support,

Resuscitation (2021), https://doi.org/10.1016/j.
resuscitation.2021.02.015

RCUK anaphylaxis guidelines 2021. www.resus.org.uk/library/
additional-guidance/guidance-anaphylaxis/emergency-treatment

Mahoney BA, Smith WA, Lo DS et al. Emergency interventions
for hyperkalaemia. Cochrane Database Syst Rev. 2005 Apr
18(2):CD003235

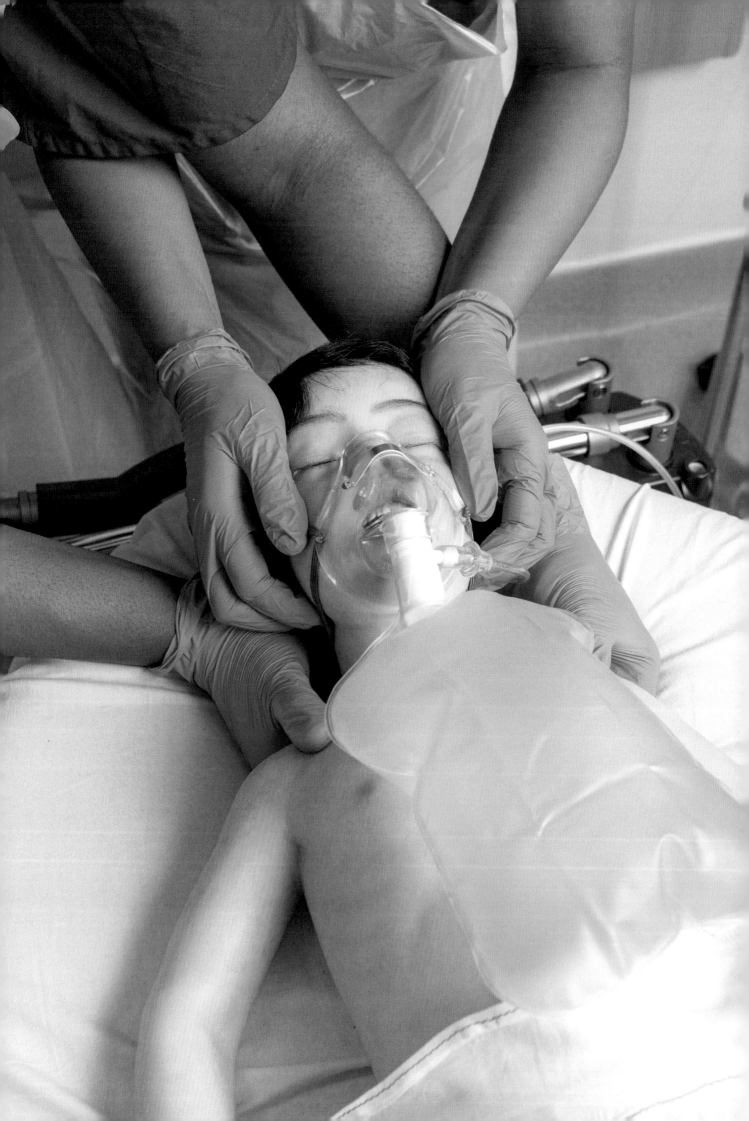

The injured child

Introduction

Blunt trauma is seen in 80% of paediatric cases in the UK; of these, two-thirds of life-threatening paediatric trauma is related to brain injury. Mortality from trauma is significantly increased if the triad of acidosis, hypothermia and coagulopathy are present.

Injury patterns in children vary from those seen in adults, owing to the different physiological and anatomical responses to trauma. In children, there is a relatively smaller muscle mass, less subcutaneous tissue and increased elasticity of ribs and other bones. This means that, in the child, more of the impacting energy is transmitted to underlying organs such as the lungs (often without rib fractures) or abdomen (with damage to visceral organs). Internal injury must, therefore, always be considered as there may have been significant force involved without external signs being present. The history of the mechanism of injury must always be sought, and the clinical consequences of how the impacting energy has been dispersed through the child's body must be considered.

Blunt trauma is seen in 80% of paediatric cases in the UK

The <C>AcBCDE approach in trauma

When dealing with an injured child, appropriate resuscitative measures must be carried out as soon as problems are identified. These measures must be applied by an effective team using a structured approach to ensure maximum benefit.

This structured approach involves every team member coordinating their activity via a trauma team leader (TTL) who has oversight of their actions. This means that the primary survey (<C>AcBCDE) and resuscitation are being performed simultaneously. This is followed by:

- X-ray series: chest and pelvis. Note that the cervical spine X-ray may be deferred as part of the secondary survey. Some centres may choose to perform a trauma CT scan (head, neck, chest and abdomen including pelvis) instead, but this is not universal.
- secondary survey
- emergency treatment
- definitive care.

The general principles of resuscitation for the injured child are similar to those of the critically ill child. However, there are a few important differences described in this chapter, particularly regarding the coagulopathy of trauma, the principles of damage control resuscitation and surgery. As in all resuscitations, there is an emphasis on team-working.

Table 11.1 The <C>AcBCDE approach

Treat first what kills first	
<C>	Catastrophic external haemorrhage control
Ac	Airway and cervical spine stabilisation
B	Breathing
C	Circulation
D	Disability neurological status (AVPU, pupils, posture)
E	Exposure (and Environment) undress the child, keep them warm and understand the history and consequences of the traumatic event

The team approach in trauma

Treatment of trauma in children demands a skilled team that is able to work in parallel while performing dedicated tasks. The TTL, who coordinates the management of the child, should allocate and coordinate the tasks, focusing on the <C>AcBCDE approach in that order. Ideally, team members should have their roles easily identified (e.g. labels on their tops, names on their scrubs etc.).

The major trauma units (MTU) are designated district general hospitals which have the capacity to manage certain levels of injured patients as determined by pre-hospital triage. This triage system will allocate more severely injured patients to the regional major trauma centres (MTC), which will have extensive facilities for dealing with immediate and shorter-term care of patients up to discharge back to the district general hospital and/or other rehabilitation services. This system allows patients to bypass the nearest hospital in favour of the MTC and has led to a recorded improvement in mortality figures for trauma patients in the UK.

The optimal trauma team comprises:

- paediatric emergency medicine specialist
- paediatric trauma nurses/ paediatric emergency nurses
- radiographer
- paediatric anaesthetist
- paediatric intensivist
- paediatric surgeon/ General surgeon/trauma surgeon
- other specialists may be involved, particularly after the secondary survey (e.g. paediatric radiologist, neurosurgical opinion, orthopaedic surgeon, plastic surgeon, cardiothoracics, interventional radiologist).

Whilst this is an optimal major trauma team, it is not always possible. However, experienced senior help must be sought urgently, ideally before the child arrives, by pre-alert. Following the alert, the team should be assembled and the available details made known so that roles can be allocated and consideration of the history allows for preparation ahead of the child arriving, e.g. for organising a CT of the head and neck in advance, or the instigation of a major haemorrhage policy. Other teams who may be required can also be called to attend as it is easier to stand down teams after the initial assessment is conducted than to wait for their arrival.

Primary survey

Catastrophic external haemorrhage, airway compromise, respiratory failure, circulatory failure and brain injury can co-exist following trauma. The primary survey is a rapid systematic evaluation, which identifies life-threatening problems using the <C>AcBCDE approach. It is completed in the first minutes of the initial assessment of the child.

Resuscitation occurs throughout the primary survey, with problems being treated as soon as they are found: 'treat first what kills first'.

The TTL will decide on the need for analgesia during the primary survey so that either IV/IO (or, if indicated, intranasal) pain relief can be given. There should be an emphasis on maintaining a calm and controlled environment and that any parents/carers are looked after by a designated member of staff. The child should be spoken to throughout in a reassuring manner, even if pre-verbal.

Adhere to the structured process of <C>AcBCDE. Some children may have 'distracting' injuries, the presence of which must not interrupt the primary and secondary surveys, or otherwise life-threatening injuries may be missed. Distracting injuries are usually very painful injuries or injuries, the appearance of which may divert attention from the structured approach of the primary survey (e.g. degloving injuries, severe burns, severe extremity fractures). For painful injuries, strong analgesia should be administered as soon as possible; if there is a significant anatomical disruption (e.g. amputation), this should be covered to prevent infection following the primary survey after documentation (and preferably having been photographed).

Monitoring should be attached as soon as possible (SpO$_2$, ECG, respiratory rate, BP) during the primary survey. Measurement of the body temperature is also important as warming devices may be required if the child has been exposed to a cold environment for a period of time (body heat loss can occur quickly in the pre-hospital setting).

<C> Catastrophic external haemorrhage

This is external bleeding that will be un-survivable unless an intervention is promptly made. This is usually due to penetrating trauma, (e.g. knife injury, blast injury) or other invasive mechanisms and is, therefore, less commonly seen in children.

If identified, the area of bleeding should have direct pressure applied, preferably with a haemostatic dressing. Haemorrhage from a limb is managed with a tourniquet being applied to a long bone above the injury.

Ac Airway and in-line cervical spine immobilisation

Airway

If cervical spine (C-spine) injury is suspected, try to open the airway using the jaw thrust manoeuvre while manually immobilising the cervical spine (Figure 11.1). However, opening the airway takes priority, and therefore, some slight head extension may be necessary; very gently increase the amount of extension until the airway is just open. Clear the oropharynx of debris, blood, vomit and other secretions by gentle suction under direct vision. The neck is inspected for distended veins, wounds, subcutaneous emphysema or tracheal deviation. It may be necessary to assist the airway by using an oropharyngeal airway, remembering that this will not protect the airway in the event of vomiting, as vomit can be inhaled. If the child tolerates an oropharyngeal airway, this indicates loss of the gag reflex and intubation should be considered. In severe trauma, a tracheal tube is used to secure the airway, or when intubation is not possible, a surgical airway or needle cricothyroidotomy (Chapter 3) is performed (this may be required when there has been severe facial trauma).

In-line cervical spine immobilisation

Immobilisation is indicated in high-energy trauma, signs of potential spinal injury and decreased consciousness. If a child is resisting immobilisation, this should be discontinued as a distressed and immobilised child is more likely to worsen existing cervical damage rather than be protected from it. If a child is ambulant, they should be helped to lie on a trolley whilst being spoken to in a calm and reassuring manner.

A quick examination of the child's back using a minimum of lateral elevation (approximately 45 degrees) whilst maintaining spinal immobilisation can be made when the child is placed on the scoop stretcher by paramedics. A formal log roll for a fuller assessment can be made later when pelvic stability has been established; this avoids destabilising any clots that may have formed. As part of pre-hospital management, the child may then be transferred to a vacuum-mattress from a scoop stretcher before transfer to hospital, depending on urgency. Ideally, children should remain on a scoop stretcher for less than 30 min due to the risk of pressures sores.

Regardless of being on a scoop stretcher or a vacuum-mattress, specific attention must be paid to in-line C-spine immobilisation. Compared to an adult, a child has a relatively large head, immature vertebral bodies (with less tensile strength) through which the spinal cord travels, strong elastic intervertebral ligaments, flexile joints capsules, and easily compressible

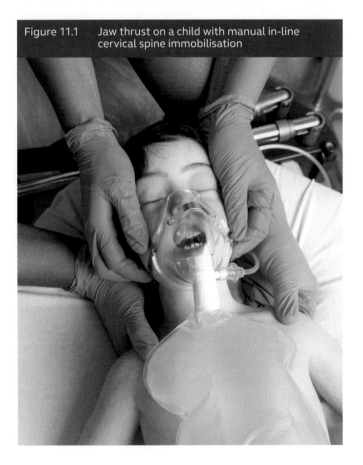

Figure 11.1   Jaw thrust on a child with manual in-line cervical spine immobilisation

soft tissue in the neck. As these structures are pliable, injury to the cervical spinal cord, although uncommon, may occur even without radiographic abnormality being seen on either X-ray or CT scan. This is known as spinal cord injury without radiological abnormalities (SCIWORA).

In-line immobilisation of the c-spine can be maintained manually by a single rescuer throughout the ongoing resuscitation, although this prevents one rescuer from doing other tasks. As an alternative, to immobilise the c-spine, the use of head blocks (or equivalent) is advocated. These head blocks can be either positioned within the vacuum-mattress, strapped to the scoop stretcher or taped to the fixed parts of the trolley.

There is much controversy concerning the use of cervical collars, especially in children. Cervical collars might induce problems in airway management (collars make mouth opening difficult and can cause respiratory constriction) or cerebral perfusion (compression of the veins in the neck can cause venous congestion and a rise in intracranial pressure). There is also no proof of their added value in terms of preventing further c-spine injury, especially if the collar does not fit well, as is often the case in children. Therefore, the standard use of collars is no longer advised. Collars might still have a place during the extraction of a severely injured child or later on in the definitive care of a child with a proven c-spine injury (for instance, post-surgery). If a collar is used, it should be a good fit (size, adequate positioning) and regularly checked to see that it is not causing any of the problems noted above.

B Breathing and ventilation

Evaluate the effectiveness of breathing and ventilation after the airway is opened, and high-flow oxygen commenced.

If breathing is ineffective, ventilation must be assisted by BMV with 100% oxygen and tracheal intubation if indicated (Table 11.2).

If tracheal intubation is required, any cervical spine stabilisation devices must be removed and manual in-line stabilisation maintained during the intubation; a skilled operator is required for the process of intubation. The oral route is preferred for tracheal intubation as the nasotracheal route can lead to neck extension (worsening cervical spine injury), damage to adenoid tissue (with associated haemorrhage), and in the case of basilar skull fracture, direct damage to the brain.

Emergency anaesthesia for tracheal intubation with cricoid pressure should be considered as the stomach may be full. If cricoid pressure impedes ventilation or intubation, however, it should be removed (Chapter 3). Correct tube placement must be confirmed with end-tidal CO_2 and a chest X-ray (the tip of the tracheal tube should lie between vertebral bodies T2 and T3).

Table 11.2 Considerations for intubation and assisted ventilation

Inadequate oxygenation by bag-mask ventilation
Prolonged or controlled ventilation required
Glasgow coma score < 8, Glasgow motor score < 4 or 'P' or 'U' on AVPU score
Respiratory failure (hypoventilation and/or hypoxia despite 100% oxygen)
Flail chest, severe facial injuries, or head injury with seizures, severe facial fractures
Inhalation injury with burns around the mouth or rest of the face, carboneous sputum or a hoarse voice
Respiratory arrest

Hyperventilation

This should not be performed in children with head injuries as cerebral vasoconstriction induced by hypocapnia aggravates ischaemic brain injuries. The $PaCO_2$ in children with traumatic brain injury (TBI) should be maintained in the lower normal range (4.5–5 kPa).

Gastric distension

Significant gastric distension can occur with swallowed air and BMV. This impairs diaphragmatic movements and affects ventilation. Gastric distension increases the risk of vomiting and aspiration of the stomach contents. A gastric tube should be inserted following intubation. The oral route is preferred in cases of craniofacial trauma (owing to the risk of maxillofacial or basilar skull fractures). The position of the gastric tube must be checked after insertion.

C Circulation and haemorrhage control

The assessment of cardiovascular status and the restoration of normal circulating volume and haemostasis are key elements of managing a child with haemorrhagic shock; hence, two routes of vascular access must be secured in children who have suffered severe trauma. At the same time, blood samples for cross-match, blood gas analysis (haemoglobin and lactate levels) and laboratory studies must be taken (Table 11.3). Some centres also have access to near-patient haemostatic testing, which can aid in the management of any coagulopathy (e.g. thromboelastogram).

Staff should wear personal protective equipment (e.g. gloves, protective clothing, visor/goggles), and ideally, this should be donned as part of the pre-alert preparedness.

Blood loss can be visible (i.e. external) or hidden (i.e. internal). Trauma induced coagulopathy is the single highest predictor of death, and prevention of coagulopathy is essential. Remember, mortality is further increased with the triad of coagulopathy, hypothermia and metabolic acidosis. Most MTCs and MTUs will have major haemorrhage protocols in place for the treatment of these patients outlining the use of blood products.

Tranexamic acid has been shown to reduce mortality in adult trauma patients, and early use is vital for efficacy. Whilst there is less evidence in children, current recommendations for children who have suffered major trauma with severe blood loss are to give tranexamic acid within 3–4 hours of injury.

Children with burns lose fluids from the burned surface, and specific formulas are available to aid with ongoing fluid management after initial resuscitation (see burns section).

Traumatic haemorrhage

Open fractures can cause large quantities of blood to be lost. Splinting of limb fractures (re-establishing normal anatomical position) reduces blood loss, pain and tissue damage (remembering to give analgesia first). Pelvic fractures or major long bone closed fractures may also be associated with soft tissue damage and the extravasation of blood. Such injuries, when isolated, do not generally lead to hypovolaemic shock in children. In adolescents, when a significant bleeding is suspected from a pelvic fracture with pelvic ring disruption, a pelvic binder should be applied. Such fractures require urgent consultation with orthopaedic colleagues and potentially the use of interventional radiology.

Internal haemorrhage:

If hypovolaemia persists despite control of external haemorrhage and the need for fluid resuscitation persists, internal haemorrhage must be excluded. Intra-thoracic, intra-abdominal, retroperitoneal and pelvic bleeding are the main causes of life-threatening internal haemorrhage in trauma patients. Intra-abdominal haemorrhage (e.g. rupture of an organ such as the spleen, liver, major blood vessels) may present with peritonism, abdominal distension (which does not decompress with a gastric tube) and signs of circulatory failure. However, on occasions, there may be very few signs, and hence there must be a high index of suspicion, especially if there is a history of abdominal trauma.

An early focused thoracic and abdominal ultrasound scan may detect free fluid. However, a negative ultrasound examination does not rule out severe internal bleeding in children. Children with significant free fluid and continuing haemodynamic instability might need immediate surgical intervention. The gold standard to detect internal bleeding remains contrast-enhanced CT scan (although this has to be balanced against the risk of radiation exposure and the risk of removal to an area with limited resuscitative capabilities).

Closed head trauma is not associated with hypovolaemia, and another source of bleeding must be sought if hypovolaemic shock is present in a child with head injuries. The exception to this is an acute extradural haemorrhage in the newborn.

Evaluation of blood loss

The total circulating blood volume in children is around 70 mL kg^{-1} (depending on age).

A decrease in blood pressure is a late sign (often > 40% of total blood volume is already lost), and therefore not very useful to initiate or guide treatment.

Evaluation of blood loss (and category of hypovolaemic shock) depends on the assessment of heart rate, the volume of the peripheral pulses, peripheral perfusion (capillary refill time and skin temperature), level of consciousness and BP. The child should be repeatedly reassessed as there may be rapid alterations in the circulatory status, such as the development of internal haemorrhage (e.g. intra-abdominal bleeding). Response to treatment must also be assessed to see if further interventions are required.

Vascular access

The mainstay of treatment for hypovolaemic shock is intravascular fluid replacement. Circulatory access is usually gained most quickly by inserting either two peripheral, short, wide-bore cannulae or two IO needles (ensuring no IO lines are placed distally to fracture sites (Chapter 5)). When access is obtained, blood should be taken and sent for blood typing and cross-match, baseline biochemistry, coagulation and full blood cell count, blood gas analysis and lactate.

Treatment of hypovolaemic shock

The patient is initially given a 10 mL kg^{-1} bolus of balanced isotonic crystalloid fluid or 0.9% sodium chloride, which should preferably be warmed to prevent the worsening of hypothermia. Monitoring of the clinical response to each fluid bolus is essential to guide therapy. A further 10 mL kg^{-1} of balanced isotonic crystalloid or 0.9% sodium chloride may be administered if there is an inadequate or no response to the initial fluid bolus. If there is an inadequate response, crystalloid should be replaced with blood products to prevent a dilutional coagulopathy. Local protocols will dictate the early use of blood products, and protocols for massive transfusion will clarify the ratio of packed red blood cells (PRBC) to fresh frozen plasma (FFP), cryoprecipitate and platelets (e.g. The Association of Anaesthetists of Great Britain and Ireland (AAGBI) guideline recommends 1:1 PRBC and FFP with cryoprecipitate and platelets adjusted according to blood results). In all children with massive haemorrhage, tranexamic acid should be started within 3–4 h of injury and administered at a dose of 15 mg kg^{-1} (loading dose over 10 min) followed by an infusion of 2 mg kg h^{-1} for at least 8 h, or until the bleeding has stopped.

Table 11.3   Laboratory parameters to aim for

Normal base deficit and lactate level – a trend in base deficit and lactate help monitor the progress of the patient.
Haemoglobin level 70–90 g L^{-1} Platelet count > 100 x 10^9 L^{-1}
Normal coagulation testing, including fibringogen 1.5 g L^{-1}
Normal ionised calcium
Thromboelastography/thromboelastometry (if available, this is a point of care test looking at clot formation in the blood)

Intra-abdominal bleeding may be managed conservatively or by angiographic embolisation. Surgery is usually avoided if at all possible but monitoring is key to picking up any children who may be deteriorating from such a bleed. The TTL will need to discuss the clinical condition with an experienced surgeon to determine whether operative intervention is necessary to stop internal bleeding. Damage control surgery should focus on bleeding control and brain protection. The duration of surgery is kept to a minimum, with subsequent definitive surgery being undertaken when the child has recovered from the physiological disruption of the traumatic event.

D Disability

The child's disability is determined from their level of consciousness according to the AVPU or Glasgow Coma Scale (GCS), posture and examination of the pupils for size, symmetry and response to light. Beware of hypoxia, hypovolaemia or hypoglycaemia, which can cause symptoms such as aggression or altered level of consciousness.

Level of consciousness

The Glasgow Coma Scale (GCS) was designed for adult traumatic head injuries and has been modified for use in children (Table 11.4). It allows a more accurate assessment of the head injury and is, therefore, better when reassessing the progress of management interventions, particularly in the trauma setting. It is more complicated than AVPU to use, especially in the initial assessment of the sick child. Another challenge is using GCS in the non-verbal child (either because that milestone hasn't been reached yet, or the child has a developmental delay or has complex needs). Therefore, AVPU can be used in the initial assessment of the child, and when more time allows, a GCS can be calculated using a chart for reference. An AVPU score of P (i.e. response to pain), Glasgow motor score of 4 or less, and a total GCS score of 8 or less defines a level of consciousness where protective

Table 11.4   Paediatric Glasgow Coma Scale (GSC)

	> 5 years	< 5 years	Pre-verbal children	Score
Eye opening	Spontaneously	Spontaneously	Spontaneously	4
	To verbal command/sound	To verbal command/sound	To verbal command/sound	3
	To pain	To pain	To pain	2
	No response	No response	No response	1
Verbal response	Orientated	Alert, babbles, coos, words or sentences to usual ability	Smiles/coos appropriately	5
	Disorientated/confused	Inappropriate words	Cries but consolable	4
	Inappropriate words	Persistent cries & screaming	Persistent inappropriate crying and/screaming	3
	Incomprehensible sounds	Grunts	Grunts, agitated and restless	2
	No sound	No sound	No response to pain	1
Motor response	Obeys commands	Normal spontaneous movements	Normal spontaneous movements	6
	Localises to pain	Localises to pain or withdraws to touch	Localises to pain or withdraws to touch	5
	Flexion withdrawal from pain	Flexion withdrawal from pain	Flexion withdrawal from pain	4
	Flexion abnormal withdrawal to pain	Flexion abnormal withdrawal to pain	Flexion abnormal withdrawal to pain	3
	Extension to pain	Extension to pain	Extension to pain	2
	No response	No response	No response	1

airway reflexes are unlikely to be present. There is, therefore, a risk of aspiration of the stomach contents at this level of consciousness, and tracheal intubation must be considered to protect the airway.

Pupils

The pupils must be examined for size and direct response to light. A unilateral dilated pupil in association with head injury may indicate an intracranial bleed on the same side or raised intracranial pressure. This is a neurosurgical emergency and requires urgent neurosurgical opinion, emergency CT head and consideration for measures to reduce intracranial pressures (ICP) such as 3% sodium chloride, analgesia, sedation, controlled oxygenation and ventilation. The child should be accompanied to CT by a team that is able to instigate resuscitation if required.

Posture

Any focal/lateralising signs should be recorded together with the child's posture. Arms flexed towards the trunk represents decorticate abnormality, whereas if the child's arms are extended, this may indicate decerebrate pathology. Both of these postures are worrying and may indicate raised-intracranial pressure; the underlying cause must be sought and treated.

Figure 11.2   Decerebrate and Decorticate posturing

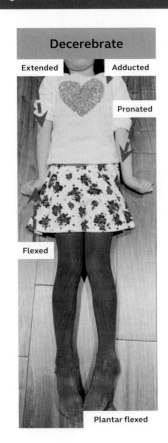

Decerebrate

Extended   Adducted

Pronated

Flexed

Plantar flexed

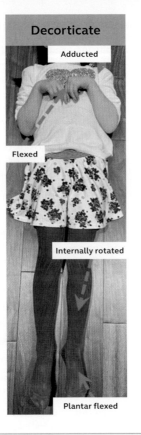

Decorticate

Adducted

Flexed

Internally rotated

Plantar flexed

For all trauma patients, the child's vital signs and neurological status must be recorded regularly and the results interpreted in the context of the child's clinical state. A change in 'Disability' should prompt a full reassessment of the patient.

E Exposure

The child's clothes should be removed appropriately so that any injuries can be seen in the secondary survey.

As the child has a large body surface to weight ratio, heat loss occurs relatively quickly, and they should be covered between examinations and interventions. Warming devices (e.g. overhead radiant heaters, warming blankets, and fluid warmers) should be used to keep the child warm. Marked hypothermia can be deleterious, especially in hypovolaemic shock.

Radiology

1. X-rays

Routine radiological investigations are carried out at the end of the primary survey, namely: chest, pelvis and cervical spine. X-rays of any limb injury must wait until the child is stable and the secondary survey has been completed. The X-rays of the limbs should have an anterior-posterior view and lateral view so as not to miss any fractures.

2. CT

Many centres offer swift access to trauma CT scanning (head, neck, chest, abdomen and pelvis with contrast) for severely injured children instead, and this will be the radiological investigation of choice for children with traumatic brain injury. A decision to take the child to CT must always consider the risks of radiation exposure and the requirement for safe transportation to the CT with a team able to resuscitate the child should deterioration occur.

3. Point of Care Ultrasound (POCUS)

Portable ultrasound machines are increasingly utilised to identify underlying injuries. An ultrasound is a fast and non-invasive investigation performed by a trained clinician at the patient's bedside. The chest can be scanned at certain points with the ultrasound probe, looking for a pneumothorax, haemothorax or cardiac tamponade. The abdomen is also scanned to look for free peritoneal fluid, which may indicate bleeding. Remember, a normal ultrasound scan does not rule out any injuries, and further investigations may be required (e.g. CT scan). Life-threatening abnormalities identified clinically should be managed urgently and appropriately. Therefore, treatment should not be delayed by performing POCUS.

Secondary survey

The secondary survey is a full examination to detect any occult injury. The child should be told what is happening even if they appear to be unconscious. The need for full exposure should be made clear, but the child's dignity must be maintained. Further information about the mechanism of injury and forces impacted should be sought.

The secondary survey should only start when all immediate life-threatening injuries have been treated. The vital signs relating to <C>AcBCDE should be regularly assessed during and after the secondary survey; deterioration in the child's clinical signs requires the primary and then the secondary survey to be repeated, stopping to deal with any abnormal clinical features as they are found. Emergency treatments for abnormalities found in the secondary survey must be identified and managed as soon as possible after life-threatening injuries are treated.

History

A short history informs the management of the child and can be remembered by the acronym AMPLE (Table 11.5).

- **Allergy:** Allergies must be recorded especially to drugs that may be used (e.g. penicillin).
- **Medications:** Details of current medications (e.g. if the child has a chronic illness such as epilepsy, diabetes or asthma) are important because the drugs used in these conditions may impact the child's management.
- **Past medical history:** The child's past medical history may explain some of the physical signs, such as cerebral palsy, although injury must still be excluded.
- **Last meal:** The closer the injury to the time of the last meal, the greater the risk of vomiting and potential aspiration; cricoid pressure may be required to protect the airway during intubation (Chapter 3).
- **Environment:** Asking about the environment/events gives information about the energy involved in the injury and potential clinical consequences.

Table 11.5 AMPLE for history taking in secondary survey

Treat first what kills first	
A	Allergy
M	Medication
P	Past medical history
L	Last meal
E	Environment (history of the accident, mechanism of injury

Definitive care

Definitive care is the final part of the structured approach to trauma.

Good note taking and appropriate referral are essential in providing optimum treatment. A paediatric MTC is able to provide damage control surgery, interventional radiology, paediatric critical care, delayed definitive surgery and complex rehabilitation coordination.

Types of Injury

The following types of injury will now be considered:

- traumatic brain injury and raised intracranial pressure, cerebral lesions, extradural haematoma
- chest trauma (e.g. pneumothorax, haemothorax, flail chest, cardiac tamponade, rib fractures, pulmonary contusions, tracheobronchial tree injuries, great vessel injuries, traumatic diaphragmatic hernia, use of chest drains)
- abdominal trauma
- skeletal trauma, crush injuries of the abdomen and pelvis, traumatic amputation, open long bone fractures, compartment syndrome, cervical spine injury
- button and coin battery ingestion
- burns
- non-accidental injury.

Traumatic brain injury (TBI)

Brain injuries are responsible for 70% of deaths in the first 48 h following paediatric trauma.

Assessment
- history of injury (mechanism of injury, loss of consciousness, headache, vomiting, amnesia, seizures)
- general assessment (<C>AcBCDE), bruises, lacerations, fractures, bleeding from ears and nose or focal neurological pathology
- <C>AcBCDE reassessment should be carried out on a regular basis
- CT head (when the child can be safely transported to and managed in CT).

Treatment
- Primary brain damage occurs at the time of the trauma and is generally irreversible. Aggressive treatment must be given to prevent secondary brain damage, which may be due to:
  - hypoxia from hypoventilation, airway obstruction, pulmonary contusion, aspiration or seizures (with or without hypoglycaemia)
  - ischaemia, which is associated with hypotension, focal/generalised cerebral oedema, extradural/subdural haematoma.

- Hypoxia should be ameliorated by administration of 100% oxygen and, if indicated, BMV. Tracheal intubation may be necessary. The underlying cause of hypoxia must also be treated (e.g. pneumothorax).

- Secondary brain damage can also be minimised by avoiding systemic hypotension and by treating raised intracranial pressure. Both hypoglycaemia and hyperglycaemia can also worsen the outcome, therefore, ensure careful bedside blood glucose monitoring.

Avoid hypotension and hypoxia in the management of patients with TBI.

Raised intracranial pressure:

Raised intracranial pressure (RICP) (e.g. from cerebral oedema) can lead to herniation of the brain, at first of supra-tentorial contents (cerebral hemispheres) through the cerebellar tentorium and if swelling continues (or there is a posterior fossa bleed) through the foramen magnum causing brain death as the skull has limited ability to expand. In infants, prior to fusion of the skull sutures, a raised, tense anterior fontanelle may be found.

RICP should be identified (ideally prevented) and treated rapidly. It is clinically indicated by depression of conscious level, abnormal pupil size and reactivity and Cushing's triad of elevated systemic BP, bradycardia and 'sighing' respirations. Later signs may include decerebrate and or decorticate posturing.

Steps to diminish the likelihood of RICP are in Table 11.6.

Hypovolaemic shock in brain injuries

Isolated closed head injuries do not usually cause hypovolaemic shock, and internal haemorrhage must be considered as a cause. Other causes such as intrathoracic or intra-abdominal trauma, pelvic and long bone fractures must be ruled out. Scalp lacerations, and in certain cases, acute extradural haemorrhage in the newborn, can lead to a significant blood loss, so the scalp must be carefully inspected.

The most common immediate cause of death in trauma is hypovolaemic shock. Fluid and blood transfusions, when indicated, are essential to maintain adequate cerebral blood flow to prevent worsening of any co-existing brain injury.

Cerebral lesions

A CT scan may demonstrate treatable conditions such as:

- skull fractures (compound and depressed, including basilar skull fractures associated with 0.4–5% risk infection)

- intracranial haemorrhages (extradural haematoma, subdural haematoma, cerebral contusions and subarachnoid haemorrhage)

Table 11.6   Steps to diminish the likelihood of RICP

1.	The femoral veins are preferred for central line insertion, as canulating the internal jugular veins can reduce venous drainage from the brain.
2.	The head should be maintained in the neutral position, and the head and chest should be elevated to 30°, once systemic hypotension has been treated to aid venous drainage. Flexion of the body when achieving elevation should be avoided to protect the spinal cord.
3.	Mean arterial pressure (MAP) must be maintained as below to preserve cerebral perfusion pressure (with vasopressors if necessary): 60 mmHg (0–2 Years) 70 mmHg (2–6 Years) 80 mmHg (> 6 Years)
4.	Maintain normoxaemia (PaO$_2$ 10–13 kPa). Hypoxia, especially when combined with hypoperfusion, will induce secondary brain injury. The impact of hyperoxia is unclear at present, and you should aim for normal PaO$_2$ or SpO$_2$ between 94–98%.
5.	The PaCO$_2$ should be kept between 4.5–5.0 kPa (i.e. within the low-normal range). Hyperventilation should only be carried out under careful supervision if there is an acute rise in ICP.
6.	Hypertonic sodium chloride or mannitol must be given if there is evidence of RICP. Monitoring of serum osmolality and urine output via urinary catheterisation (via the suprapubic route if there is urethral trauma) is essential. In unilateral lesions without evidence of RICP consult a neurosurgical specialist before administering.
7.	Hyperglycaemia and hypoglycaemia must be avoided.
8.	Seizures should be treated with benzodiazepines and antiepileptic medication as required.
9.	Provide adequate analgesia and sedation. Pain and stress increase cerebral metabolic demands, leading to increased cerebral blood flow and ultimately a further increase in ICP.

- midline shift of white and grey matter
- signs of cerebral oedema and RICP (absent sulci, slit-like cerebral ventricles).

Extradural haematoma

Extradural haematomas are life-threatening emergencies requiring extremely urgent drainage by a neurosurgeon. A rapidly expanding extradural haematoma can cause cerebral herniation, so time is of the essence even if the child is clinically unstable.

Systemic arterial hypertension

Systemic hypertension associated with bradycardia and irregular respiration (Cushing's triad) suggests RICP. The systemic hypertension should not be treated with antihypertensive agents, but RICP should be managed appropriately.

Hyperglycaemia, hypoglycaemia and seizures

Hyperglycaemia, hypoglycaemia and seizures may aggravate ischaemic cerebral lesions and worsen cerebral oedema. Administration of glucose-containing solutions must be avoided during resuscitation unless given to treat documented hypoglycaemia. Blood sugar levels must be monitored, and seizures treated promptly.

Chest trauma (primary survey)

Life-threatening conditions such as tension pneumothorax, massive haemothorax, flail chest and cardiac tamponade can be identified and treated during the primary survey. If the child deteriorates during the secondary survey or later due to one of these conditions, the primary survey must be repeated.

Pneumothorax

Pneumothorax means that there is air in the pleural space, between the lung and the internal thoracic wall, which compresses the lung and impedes ventilation. There are three main types – simple, tension and open. Respiratory failure can be caused by all three.

All forms of pneumothorax can be diagnosed clinically.

Simple pneumothorax

This represents a limited air leak into the pleural space, which causes the lung to collapse without there being significant haemodynamic signs.

A small simple pneumothorax may only be identified on the secondary survey and chest X-ray.

It may be managed conservatively provided there is continuous monitoring of the child's physiological parameters to ensure there is no deterioration in the clinical condition.

Immediate chest drainage is required if the child requires ventilation. This is because if a simple pneumothorax is not discovered prior to intubation, the pressures involved in ventilation can convert a simple pneumothorax to a tension pneumothorax.

Tension pneumothorax

When air is forced into the pleural cavity (a limited space) without means of escape, it accumulates and comes under pressure. This pressure can displace the mediastinum to the opposite side of the chest, causing compression of the great vessels interfering with venous return, causing obstructive shock with a concomitant fall in systemic BP. The jugular venous pressure is raised if there is no associated hypovolaemia.

Signs
- hypoxia
- absent/decreased breath sounds on the affected side
- affected side resonant on percussion
- neck vein distension
- tracheal deviation away from the side of the tension pneumothorax; this is usually a late, pre-terminal sign.

Treatment
- airway opening
- oxygen (100%) by a non-rebreathe mask with reservoir or BMV.
- needle thoracocentesis (the insertion of a cannula into the second intercostal space in the mid-clavicular line on the side of the tension pneumothorax (Figure 11.3)). When the needle of the cannula is removed, a hiss of escaping air may be heard as the pressure within the pleural space is released. The cannula is left to vent the air if the patient is ventilated, but if spontaneously breathing, it will need to be capped and be aspirated intermittently until a chest drain is placed.
- In experienced and trained hands, an alternative is to perform a needle thoracocentesis or finger thoracostomy in the 5th intercostal space mid-axillary line. (This will likely be out of the scope of practice for many EPALS providers, but this may occur pre-hospital by a critical care team).

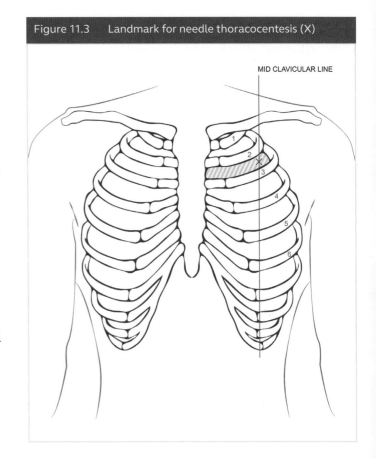

Figure 11.3   Landmark for needle thoracocentesis (X)

Chest drain insertion should be undertaken as soon as possible, provided it doesn't delay progressing the assessment and management of the patient.

If the child deteriorates at any stage following the needle thoracocentesis, air may have reaccumulated, reforming the tension pneumothorax. This may be due to the cannula kinking. Needle thoracocentesis must be repeated, and a chest drain inserted as soon as possible.

Open pneumothorax

Open pneumothorax results from a penetrating chest wound and makes a sucking noise.

When the child breathes in, negative intrathoracic pressure is generated (which normally draws air into the lungs with each inspiration), and air rushes in through the wound into the pleural space. This then leads to inefficient ventilation and displacement of the mediastinum with each breath causing cardiovascular instability.

If the open chest wound is obstructed, causing a one-way valve effect, a tension pneumothorax can also develop.

Signs
- penetrating chest wound (examine front and back)
- audible air passage through the wound
- decreased chest wall movement on the affected side
- decreased breath sounds on the affected side
- increased percussion noted on the affected side
- a tension pneumothorax can develop from an open pneumothorax.

Treatment
1. airway opening.
2. oxygen (100%) by face mask or BMV
3. close the defect with a chest seal dressing (e.g. Russel or Asherman), which will seal the wound and allow entrapped air to escape through a valve. These are more effective than the previously used occlusive dressing taped down on three sides.
4. chest drain insertion on the same side as the pneumothorax but in an area away from the wound.

If a tension pneumothorax is present, treat accordingly. If positive pressure ventilation is required, a chest drain must be sited as soon as possible.

Massive haemothorax

This is due to blood accumulating in the thoracic cavity as a result of a pulmonary parenchymal injury associated with pulmonary vessel or chest wall injuries. A haemothorax may contain a significant proportion of a child's total circulatory blood volume.

Signs
- hypoxia
- hypovolaemic shock
- decreased chest wall movements on the affected side
- decreased breath sounds on the affected side
- decreased percussion noted on the affected side
- neck veins may be flat, not full or distended.

Treatment
1. airway opening
2. oxygen (100%) by a non-rebreathe mask with reservoir or BMV.
3. vascular access with two large-bore intravenous cannulae or intraosseous needles
4. fluid infusion (10 mL kg^{-1}) bolus(es); blood should be used as soon as it is available
5. insertion of a chest drain.

As blood loss can be rapid via the chest drain, fluid replacement must be available and circulatory access secured before its insertion. Temporary clamping of the chest drain and an urgent thoracotomy may be required if the initial blood drainage is > 20 mL kg^{-1}, with persistent loss requiring continuing blood transfusion.

Flail chest

Flail chest is where two or more ribs are broken in two or more places so that they are not connected to the rest of the rib cage and do not move in conjunction with it on expiration and inspiration.

Hypoventilation may occur, and respiratory failure can develop as a result of pain and severe pulmonary contusions that usually accompany a flail chest. This is very uncommon in childhood, owing to the child's increased chest wall elasticity.

Cardiac tamponade

Cardiac tamponade generally results from penetrating rather than blunt injuries. Therefore, cardiac tamponade is not often seen in paediatric trauma. The heart is pierced, and blood fills the pericardial sac. This limits the space for cardiac contraction, causing obstructive shock. Cardiac tamponade requires emergency thoracotomy.

Chest trauma (secondary survey)

Rib fractures

Rib injuries are always significant as they suggest considerable trauma in children. Underlying chest and abdominal injuries must be suspected.

Upper rib (1–3) and clavicle fractures suggest injury to the major vessels, the mediastinum, and the bronchus.

Fractures of the middle ribs (4–9) are associated with pulmonary contusion and haemothorax, while the lower ribs (10–12) are linked to liver and splenic injuries.

Ensure analgesia and examination for underlying damage, such as thoracic or abdominal injury.

Pulmonary contusion

Pulmonary contusion is common in childhood, even in the absence of fractures.

It results from the disruption of pulmonary capillaries and the filling of the alveoli with blood, thus leading to hypoxia.

Treatment is based on oxygenation, and mechanical ventilation may be required. Analgesia and respiratory physiotherapy are essential components of the management of pulmonary contusion.

Tracheobronchial tree injuries

Tracheobronchial tree ruptures are associated with a pneumothorax or haemothorax with subcutaneous emphysema.

They should be considered in the presence of a persistent large air leak after insertion of a chest drain.

Great vessel injuries

Great vessel injuries are rapidly fatal, except when the leak is contained within the vessel wall.

The child may present with shock, and a high index of suspicion should be triggered by a widened mediastinum on the chest X-ray.

Diagnosis is confirmed by CT-angiography, and urgent surgical treatment is required.

Traumatic diaphragmatic hernia

A traumatic diaphragmatic hernia occurs more often following abdominal trauma (both blunt and penetrating) and is more common on the left side.

Diagnosis can be made from hearing bowel sounds on chest auscultation and seeing bowel within the chest cavity on chest X-ray. Often the child will refuse to lie down.

These injuries may occur with lap seat belts, and treatment is surgical repair.

Chest drains

Chest drains are flexible plastic tubes with one or more side ports inserted to drain the pleural space when air and/or fluid have collected within this space, causing pressure on the lungs (Figure 11.4).

Conditions requiring chest drain Insertion

- pneumothorax – air
- haemothorax – blood
- pleural effusion – fluid
- chylothorax – chyle
- empyema – pus
- post-op (cardiac or thoracic surgery).

Two techniques may be used to insert chest drains:

For small and medium bore chest drains, a Seldinger technique using a guidewire and dilator can be used.

For larger bore chest drains, a blunt dissection technique is recommended.

All procedures must be done with aseptic precautions. Chest drain insertion is painful, so adequate analgesia and sedation or anaesthesia should be used.

Landmarks for insertion

4th or 5th intercostal space between the anterior axillary line and mid-axillary line. Insert just above the rib at the lower border of the chosen intercostal space to avoid the neurovascular bundle that runs below the ribs. Insertion should be performed by those with expertise in the procedure.

Once the chest drain has been inserted into the pleural space, it is sutured to the chest wall, and the entry point covered with a sterile transparent dressing. A chest X-ray is performed to confirm the position of the chest drain. The child will require ongoing analgesia as the pleural surface is well innervated, so chest drains are uncomfortable.

The chest drain is then connected to an underwater seal drain (UWSD) system; this creates a one-way system allowing air and fluid to leave the pleural space without allowing air or fluid to enter the pleural space.

When moving a child with a chest drain from a trolley to a bed, the chest drain will need to be briefly clamped near the proximal (chest) end. This is a safety precaution to prevent accidental entrainment of fluid or air.

If a child with a chest drain needs to be transferred to radiology or another facility, the chest drain can temporarily be attached to a one-way flutter valve (e.g. Heimlich valve, Pneomostat).

Most UWSD systems have three chambers:

- One chamber provides the underwater seal; this has a set volume of water in the chamber, with the distal end of the chest drain tubing below the water level. This prevents air and fluid from re-entering the pleural space.

- The second chamber to allow the measurement of any fluids drained from the pleural space.

- The third chamber allows the application of negative suction pressure to the system.

The UWSD system must be kept below the level of the patient to allow proper functioning of the system and allowing gravity to aid with drainage of the pleural space. Providers looking after children with a chest drain should familiarise themselves with the equipment, which requires regular checking to ensure ongoing safety.

Abdominal trauma

The clinical ability to determine the presence of intra-abdominal bleeding is poor without accompanying investigation; note that abdominal haemorrhage is often associated with blunt trauma. If there is any suggestive history or sign, such as distension or contusions on the abdominal wall, surgical opinion and investigations are urgently required. Abdominal ultrasound (which can be rapidly obtained at the bedside) may be helpful in detecting free fluid, which suggests free blood in the abdominal cavity; however, remember a negative scan does not rule out intra-abdominal injury. An abdominal CT scan with contrast will be diagnostic.

Signs
- abdominal wall contusion
- abdominal wall bruising, lacerations or penetrating wounds
- abdominal distension
- abdominal or shoulder tip pain
- peritoneal irritation or peritonitis
- hypovolaemic shock unresponsive to fluid resuscitation.

Gentle examination of the abdomen should be carried out as it may reveal an area of tenderness and rigidity suggestive of intra-abdominal haemorrhage. Gastric and urinary bladder drainage may help in the assessment by decompressing the abdomen. A vaginal examination should only be performed by a clinician with expertise in gynaecological trauma and only if indicated. The external urethral meatus of the penis should be examined for blood as well as the scrotum for any collection of blood. The rectal examination should only be carried out once during the secondary survey, ideally by the surgeon responsible for deciding if operative treatment is required.

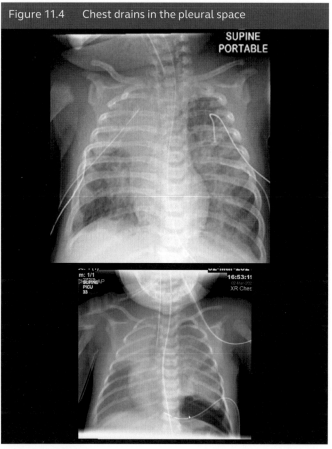

Figure 11.4   Chest drains in the pleural space

Investigations
- Blood tests: full blood count, cross-match, urea, electrolytes, amylase, bedside estimation of blood glucose, and clotting profiles.

- X-rays: of the three secondary survey X-rays, the chest and pelvic bones may suggest intra-abdominal injury (e.g. free gas under the diaphragm), soft tissue swelling and incorrect location of the gastric tube (as in traumatic diaphragmatic hernia).

- Ultrasound may show the presence of free fluid within the abdominal cavity; laceration of intra-abdominal organs such as the liver or spleen.

- Diagnostic peritoneal lavage should not be performed.

- CT scan of the abdomen is the imaging investigation of choice for every severely injured child. Any child with significant injury going to the CT scan must be escorted by a competent team. In children with less severe presumed injuries (less severe trauma mechanism), the decision to do an abdominal CT scan must be balanced against the risks of radiation exposure.

Treatment
Most children with visceral injury are managed non-surgically but on a site where there is a supervising experienced surgeon and team on-site, ready to operate should the child deteriorate. Indications for operative intervention include penetrating injury, perforated bowel, refractory hypovolaemic shock (i.e. unresponsive to fluid resuscitation).

Skeletal trauma

Skeletal trauma is rarely life-threatening; its appearance, however, must not detract from adherence to <C>AcBCDE steps of managing an injured child.

The few life-threatening conditions in skeletal trauma which are treated in the primary and secondary survey include:

- crush injury of the abdomen and pelvis
- traumatic amputation of an extremity, either partial or complete.
- massive long bone open fracture.

Additionally, neurovascular injuries and compartment syndrome should be identified early as they can become limb-threatening.

Crush injury of the abdomen and pelvis

Crush injury of the abdomen and pelvis is associated with hypovolaemic shock, which remains resistant to fluid resuscitation until the pelvic disruption is stabilised and injured vessels are occluded.

Stabilisation is initially achieved with a pelvic binder and then by using an external pelvic fixator, radiological intervention or by operative means.

Urgent surgical consultation together with an interventional radiologist and TTL is required. Limit the number of examinations of pelvic stability as this may increase bleeding.

Never insert a urinary catheter unless a urethral injury has been ruled out.

Traumatic amputation

In complete amputation, blood loss is usually limited owing to the transected blood vessels going into spasm for a limited time. In partial amputation, there may be considerable blood loss as blood vessel spasm may not occur; urgent management is needed. The child may need to be treated for hypovolaemic shock.

Direct pressure should be applied to the bleeding vessels with a haemostatic dressing or gauze. A tourniquet should be placed proximally on a limb to help stop torrential bleeding – this is only a short-term measure to provide time to definitive surgical management to stop the bleeding.

An amputated limb should be isolated in a sterile bag and then kept cool (avoiding direct contact with any ice being used as a coolant) until a surgical opinion about the feasibility of surgical re-attachment is obtained.

Open long bone fractures

This is usually obvious and needs immediate treatment. If there is an associated exsanguinating haemorrhage; direct pressure should be applied to the bleeding vessels with a haemostatic dressing or gauze.

Splinting the limb so that the correct anatomical position is achieved will help to reduce blood loss, pain, tissue damage and the risk of compartment syndrome.

Antibiotics should be administered during the secondary survey.

Expert orthopaedic help is needed to manage this condition, ideally, conjointly with expert plastic surgical opinion.

Limbs

The extremities should be inspected for bruising, swelling, deformity, laceration, and any evidence of open fractures.

Gentle palpation should be undertaken to establish any areas of tenderness and to evaluate the surface temperature and capillary refill time.

Ask the child to move as much as they are able to (this does require comprehension on the part of the child about what is being asked of them) and to demonstrate what functionality of the limb is like.

The neurovascular status of the limb, especially distal to the injury, must be recorded and acted upon (e.g. the absence of pulses distal to a supracondylar fracture can be limb-threatening unless managed urgently).

Table 11.7   Vascular limb injury

Assessment of the vascular status of the limb relies on determining:
The presence and quality of peripheral pulses distal to the injury.
Capillary refill time and skin temperature gradient compared with the rest of the body.
Sensory and motor function (i.e. neurological status of the limb).
A large bruise or haematoma is suggestive of vascular injury, particularly if it continues to increase in size.
Emergency treatment of vascular limb injury:
1. Fluid resuscitation with 10 mL kg^{-1} bolus(es) with haemostasis of obvious bleeding. Consider administering blood products early to prevent a dilutional anaemia.
2. Pain relief.
3. Alignment and immobilisation by splintage (if pain increases after immobilisation, then ischaemic injury and/or compartment syndrome must be excluded).

Compartment syndrome

This occurs when the interstitial pressure is higher than the capillary tissue pressure in the fascial compartment, resulting in local muscle ischaemia. It may occur, for example, in a circumferential burn of the upper arm or a fracture of the limb (e.g. tibia, fibula fracture).

In the case of a burn that impedes venous blood drainage out of the limb (which has a maximum venous BP of 10–15 mmHg), compartment syndrome can be seen when the systemic arterial flow into the arm continues as the systemic BP is much higher than the venous BP. There is a 'damming up' of blood within the muscle of the limb, and the increasing pressure is transmitted to the tissues via the capillary bed, leading to muscle ischaemia and cellular necrosis.

Signs
- pain accentuated by passive muscle stretch
- decreased sensation
- swelling
- muscle weakness.

Distal pulses only disappear when the intra-compartmental pressure rises above arterial BP. Initial treatment is the releasing of any constrictions. Surgical intervention may be required (i.e. fasciotomies to try to save the limb).

Cervical spine injury

Compared to an adult, a child has a relatively large head, immature vertebral bodies (with less tensile strength) through which the spinal cord travels, strong elastic intervertebral ligaments, flexible joint capsules and easily compressible soft tissue in the neck.

As these structures are pliable, injury to the cervical spinal cord may occur without radiographic abnormality being seen (SCIWORA). This holds true for the rest of the spine.

Although spinal cord injury is uncommon, the cervical spine must be immobilised along with the rest of the spine until spinal cord injury can be clinically excluded by neurological examination.

Signs
- severe multiple injuries
- significant trauma to the head, neck and back
- any trauma associated with high deceleration forces such as high-velocity traffic accidents
- falls from heights.

Conscious children may complain of pain in the affected vertebra(e).

In the assessment, the six 'Ps' should be evaluated:
- pain
- position
- paralysis
- paraesthesia
- priapism
- ptosis (for upper cervical lesions).

If pain, tenderness or swelling located to the spinal area are present, even in the absence of neurological signs, a spinal injury must be ruled out. Magnetic resonance imaging should be considered, especially if SCIWORA is suspected (this may involve a general anaesthesia to obtain definitive images).

Treatment
- Treatment is based on the <C>AcBCDE process. Airway obstruction is common in such patients, and a jaw thrust manoeuvre should be carried out, avoiding movement of the cervical spine.
- Cervical immobilisation using manual in-line stabilisation or head blocks with two points of attachment to prevent neck movement must be employed.
- Ventilation should be assisted if there is respiratory failure or risk to the airway. Tracheal intubation is a skilled technique and should be carried out by an experienced intubator. It requires in-line cervical spine immobilisation by an assistant.

Button and coin battery ingestion

Button and coin batteries are used in numerous household items and can be accidentally ingested by children. Often, they are swallowed unwitnessed, and there aren't always immediate clinical consequences. They can sometimes cause immediate difficulties with swallowing, vomiting and retching (with or without an adult witnessing the ingestion). This will depend on the size of the battery and the diameter of the child's oesophagus (which is related to their age).

A delayed presentation will include the following symptoms:
- airway obstruction
- wheezing
- vomiting
- chest discomfort
- difficulty swallowing, decreased appetite, refusal to eat
- coughing, choking or gagging when eating or drinking.

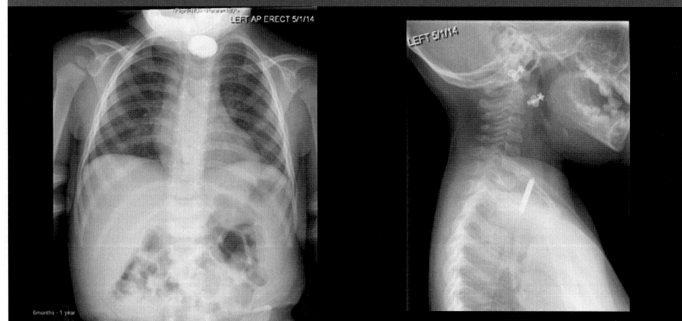

Figure 11.5   X-rays showing coin battery ingestion

Fully charged batteries will cause more damage; however, used batteries will have sufficient electrical charge to cause significant liquefaction necrosis to tissues. The electrical charge causes tissue damage within hours, which can lead to early oesophageal perforation, and the erosive process can continue once the battery has been removed. If there is a delay in removing this foreign body, it can lead to life-threatening complications from tracheal and major blood vessel (e.g. aorta) fistulas. The latter can lead to major haemorrhage or death.

A suspicion of a button/coin battery ingestion should lead to a chest X-ray to show where it is lodged (Figure 11.5). Specialist management will be urgently required to remove the battery, and this may require a time-critical transfer to a children's hospital with ENT, thoracic and cardiac surgery. Ongoing follow-up will be required following the removal of the battery, because of the potential of long-term complications.

Magnets being ingested can cause bowel obstruction by compressing loops of bowel together, and in some cases, cause a volvulus. Multiple magnets will join together and may not be passed through the digestive system. Surgical removal will, therefore, likely be needed as soon as possible.

Thermal Burns

Burns (thermal injuries) are described by depth:

- **Epidermal burns** are injury to the epidermal layer only, causes erythema and pain, the skin remains intact and appears dry (no blisters) and typically heals within seven days without treatment. This is commonly seen with sunburn. This area should be omitted from any burns surface area calculations (otherwise, the fluid resuscitation amount will be too high and result in fluid overload with poorer outcomes).

- **Superficial partial-thickness burns** involves the superficial layers of the skin (epidermis and superficial dermis). The skin will look blistered and pale pink as blood supply to the area is maintained (blisters may not be apparent immediately). Superficial partial-thickness burns are very painful as sensory nerve endings are exposed. These typically heal in 2–3 weeks without scarring. It is included in the burns surface area calculation.

- **Deep partial-thickness burns** involves the superficial and deeper layers of skin (epidermis and majority of the dermis). The examination may find areas of dry/moist skin, blotchiness, erythema and blisters. Capillary refill time may be decreased as blood supply to the area is affected. It may or may not be painful, as the burn may not be the same depth in different areas. Healing typically takes three or more weeks; surgery may be required to aid healing and prevent scarring.

- **Full-thickness burns** involves the epidermis, full-thickness of the dermis, and may involve subcutaneous tissue and deeper structures (muscle, bone). This affected area will appear white (waxy initially before becoming leathery/firm in texture) or charred, absent capillary refill as surface blood vessels coagulated. Traditionally this was described as painless due to loss of pain receptors in the deep dermis; however, the sensation of pain may occur from inflammatory mediators and areas of mixed depth. Full-thickness burns require surgical debridement and grafting in order to heal and minimise scarring/contracture formation.

Burns to the face, hands, feet and perineum are always considered serious; they have specific management considerations regardless of their depth.

The total body surface area (TBSA) percentage of the areas involved should be calculated from a paediatric burns chart. These charts show the age-related percentage BSA of the head, limbs, trunk and body. A useful method of quickly determining TBSA is to estimate the area of the burn from the size of the child's palm with their fingers spread out as this is approximately 1% TBSA (this works well for small burns or very large burns in which the area of unburnt skin is estimated). The 'rule of nines' cannot be applied to a child younger than 14 years. For any child with significant burns, including burns to the face, hands, feet and perineum, discussion with the regional burns unit should occur for both advice and ongoing management.

A Airway

The upper airway may be compromised owing to injury from burns or chemical irritants from noxious agents (present in smoke). As oedema quickly follows, the airway may deteriorate rapidly, and even the suspicion of potential airway compromise should prompt immediate consideration of tracheal intubation; delay may make intubation impossible. Worrying features include facial burns, singed eyebrows or carbon stained sputum, hoarse voice, stridor or decreased level of consciousness. The use of low pressure cuffed tubes is preferable in view of expected problems with mechanical ventilation. Ongoing facial swelling should be anticipated, and therefore, the TT should not be cut short.

B Breathing

In severe cases, there may be circumferential burns to the thorax, which limits its movement and hence respiratory effort. Surgical incisions to release these tissues may be required to reduce the constricting effect of the burns (escharotomies). Particles inhaled during fire may contribute to respiratory distress and must be removed by suction after intubation or bronchoscopy. Oxygen 100% should be administered to all cases of severe burns/suspected inhalation injury as there may be carbon monoxide poisoning (irrespective of the oxygen saturation level). If possible, measure the carbon monoxide level and continue 100% oxygen until carbon monoxide < 10%.

C Circulation

Significant burn injuries are associated with increased fluid losses (evaporative) and the redistribution of fluid from intravascular to extravascular spaces. Burns of 10% TBSA or more require fluid replacement as calculated by the Parkland formula:

(TBSA % x Bodyweight (kg) x 4 mL day^{-1})

Half of this total is given in the first 8 h from the time of the burn and the second half in the next 16 h. Maintenance fluids should be given in addition for all children less than 30 kg.

Fluid resuscitation (10 mL kg^{-1} of isotonic fluid) is necessary if there are signs of shock with careful reassessment after each bolus. The quantity of fluid given as fluid boluses should subsequently be subtracted from the total fluid as calculated by the Parkland formula. Careful fluid-balance monitoring is necessary in the management of burned children. Whilst the Parkland formula is used to calculate initial fluid requirements, ongoing fluid requirements should be titrated to maintain a urine output of approximately 1 mL kg^{-1} h^{-1}, so that fluid overload does not occur. This can cause additional complications, such as abdominal compartment syndrome and is associated with worse outcomes.

If metabolic acidosis, coma or cardiovascular instability with no clear cause, consider the possibility of cyanide poisoning (inhaled as a component of smoke). Treat based on the clinical picture and surrogate markers (e.g. lactate > 7, reduced arteriovenous oxygen gradient < 10%, elevated anion gap acidosis) with hydroxocobalamin (cyanokit).

Pain relief

Any child with anything other than a minor burn should be given morphine, IV or IO (0.1 mg kg^{-1}) titrated to their needs. Initial routes of administration of opioids such as diamorphine or fentanyl can be given via the intranasal route until an intravascular route is secured. If necessary, intravascular access (IV or IO) can be placed through areas of burnt skin using an aseptic technique.

Wound care

Wound care should be started as soon as possible to avoid infection and reduce pain. Hypothermia should be avoided. The child's tetanus status should be determined to identify if a tetanus booster is required.

Non-accidental injury

Non-accidental injury may present as a physical injury. This is only one form of child abuse; others include nutritional deprivation, neglect, emotional or sexual abuse and deliberate poisoning. There may be a history of domestic violence. Non-accidental injury needs to be considered in all presentations of the critically unwell child where there are symptoms and signs that are consistent with known patterns of inflicted injury or when there is no clear mechanism or pathology accounting for the clinical presentation.

The decision about whether an injury could be intentionally inflicted relies on a detailed clinical assessment and medical history. Consider whether the injuries sustained could be the result of an accident, or if the injuries could be the result of the reasonable activities of daily living for a child of that age and development and whether the mechanism of injury is unexplained or reported as inflicted. In addition, there may be features of potential neglect (e.g. inadequate supervision and/or delayed presentation) that will need to be addressed.

As with all critically unwell children, the priority is to first assess and treat with the ABCDE approach. Once the child is stable, if there is a suspicion of child abuse, then the child protection experts should be involved immediately (usually this is the general paediatric team or dedicated safeguarding team). If there are any concerns surrounding the immediate safety of the child, or their siblings, the parent/carer or the healthcare staff, then this should be referred at the time to the senior clinician who will inform the police.

There are certain signs that may alert a healthcare professional to potential child protection concerns and the possibility of non-accidental injury:

- The general condition and appearance of the child: is the child dressed in appropriate clothes, at an expected level of cleanliness, free from infestations? If inserting an airway adjunct or intubating, is the child's dental hygiene satisfactory? When determining the child's weight for resuscitation purposes, take note of the child's appearance to see if this is grossly compatible – does the child appear notably thin or overweight or malnourished?

- Delayed presentation to seek medical assistance: if there was a delay in presenting to hospital, is there a suitable reason?

- Unexplained or unusual patterns of injury: during the ABCDE assessment, injuries may be seen that are not readily explained by the presenting medical history or are deemed unlikely to have been caused by the proposed mechanism of trauma (e.g. injuries found in locations not affected by the presenting trauma, unrelated fractures found incidentally on radiology assessment or bruising with unusual patterning). A body map should be created with all injuries clearly indicated.

- Accidental v non-accidental injuries: consider whether the injuries are compatible with the child's level of development or motor function (particularly relevant in children with motor development delay).

- Inconsistent histories: once the child has been stabilised, consider if there are varying versions of the history provided. These could come from the child, parent, staff member or accompanying person. Accurate and contemporaneous documentation is essential.

Remember, you are not being asked to determine whether the child you are resuscitating has been subject to child abuse. This is the role of safeguarding experts. However, safeguarding of all children is the responsibility of all healthcare professionals, and you are expected to raise any concerns you may have with a senior clinician and then with those colleagues who can then investigate further.

11: Summary learning

Trauma is the second highest cause of death in children over 10 years old.

Treat first what kills first – deal with life-threatening problems as they are found (<C>AcBCDE).

Trauma management requires surgical expertise and a team approach.

Secondary survey is a thorough head-to-toe examination, front and back.

If the child deteriorates, repeat the primary survey.

Airway patency can be rapidly lost in upper airway burns.

Non-accidental injury must be considered in injured children.

My key take-home messages from this chapter are:

Further reading

Pang D, Pollack IF. Spinal cord injury without radiographic abnormalities in children: the SCIWORA syndrome. J Trauma. 1989; 29: 654-664.

Faculty of Clinical Radiology. Paediatric trauma protocols. The Royal College of Radiologists, 2014.

Association of Anaesthetists of Great Britain and Ireland. https://anaesthetists.org/Portals/0/PDFs/Guidelines%20PDFs/Guideline_blood_components_alternatives_2016_final.pdf?ver=2018-07-11-163753-007&ver=2018-07-11-163753-007

https://www.rcpch.ac.uk/resources/guidance-resources-child-protection-evidence

https://www.rcemlearning.co.uk/reference/major-trauma-burns/

Pre-hospital care

12

For the purposes of the chapter, the term 'child' will include neonate and infant.

Team approach and safety in the pre-hospital environment

Assessing and managing children out of the hospital environment brings a different set of challenges. The team is smaller, specialist help is not immediately available, safety is crucial, and the environment can be difficult to operate in.

Safety has been discussed in previous chapters, and this has further emphasis when working in an unfamiliar environment. The emergency services have had training and have experience in working in these situations. They will assess safety by specifically assessing the scene for any hazards, assessing any potential danger to themselves (so that they don't become a further casualty) and assessing the situation of the patient(s). Scene safety could include stopping the traffic before approaching the casualty, and therefore it is recommended to take a short pause beforehand to assess safety.

Environmental factors such as temperature extremes, adverse weather, noise, and movement can affect the child's condition and make a clinical assessment more difficult. Sometimes it will be necessary to move a child to an area where 360° access to the child is possible to allow a more thorough assessment. This could be another room in a house or in the back of an ambulance.

Depending on the number and composition of the team, the team members may not be known to each other prior to arriving at the scene. Bystanders may know the casualty (such as family members), or they may be a trained first aider who was nearby. It is imperative to quickly work out who is present and what skills they have so that that team members can take up the most appropriate roles. Family members can help console an unwell child and give you essential information to help diagnose the problem and present a timeline of events.

The ambulances services in the UK use a publication called JRCALC (Joint Royal Colleges Ambulance Liaison Committee), which standardises the management of patients. This includes an 'age per page' section which, depending on the child's age, gives a weight with corresponding drug doses. If you are first on scene and the child is unresponsive and unknown to bystanders, it may be possible to ascertain the child's approximate age by checking the label on their clothes.

Depending on the situation described to the ambulance call handler, the speed and composition of the team members involved in the ambulance response will vary. In seriously unwell children and those in cardiorespiratory arrest, an immediate response will be activated. This may occur while the call handler is taking further information or giving life-saving advice over the telephone. Multiple ambulance personnel, including paramedics, will be dispatched. Additionally, a pre-hospital critical care team may be sent to provide specialist skills at the scene (e.g. major trauma, cardiorespiratory arrest) via road or helicopter. These specialist teams, which have doctors with pre-hospital training, are able to supplement the management provided by paramedics (e.g. advanced analgesia, emergency anaesthesia, red cell administration and surgical procedures).

Initial assessment of the unwell or injured child in the pre-hospital environment

In Chapter 2 (Recognition and initial management of the seriously ill child), the ABCDE assessment was discussed. This was supplemented by the <C>AcBCDE approach in the injured child chapter to take into account the possibility of catastrophic haemorrhage (<C>) and cervical spine injury.

Depending on the situation, during the safety assessment, and before approaching the child, gain any history of what has happened; the trained responder should decide on the best assessment approach. If there is a history of trauma or obvious injuries, the <C>AcBCDE is the most suitable approach. If the child is seriously unwell due to a medical complaint, then the ABCDE is appropriate. If there is any doubt or if both a serious illness and injury are present, then the <C>AcBCDE approach should be used.

Table 12.1   The <C>AcBCDE approach

Treat first what kills first	
<C>	Catastrophic external haemorrhage control
Ac	Airway and cervical spine stabilisation
B	Breathing
C	Circulation
D	Disability neurological status (AVPU, pupils, posture)
E	Exposure (and Environment) undress the child, keep them warm and understand the history and consequences of the traumatic event

<C> Catastrophic external haemorrhage

If catastrophic external haemorrhage is present, for example, an amputated limb, injured femoral artery or open long bone fracture, this needs to be managed first. This is because the continued bleeding will lead to the child dying of hypovolaemic shock from exsanguination, despite any ABC interventions. Therefore, if large amounts of external bleeding are present, direct pressure with a dressing should be applied.

The ambulance service will carry haemostatic dressings that help the blood clot and further reduce blood loss. Continuously pressing with your fingers will provide more direct pressure than your palm. Releasing the pressure will likely restart the bleeding, and therefore removing the pressure to reassess the injury is not advised.

Haemorrhage from a limb is managed with a tourniquet being applied to a long bone above the injury. These can be improvised using a belt or scarf by wrapping it around the limb once and then twisting the ends until it tightens. Clinically designed tourniquets are carried by the emergency ambulance crews and may be used if they are immediately available. If the child is conscious, the amount of compression caused by the tourniquet will likely be painful; strong analgesia will be required.

The child should be transported to hospital as a priority, and if a tourniquet is applied, the time it was first applied must be passed on to the ambulance service ready to handover to the hospital trauma team.

Ac Airway with in-line cervical spine immobilisation

The airway should be managed as discussed in previous chapters, and a stepwise approach may be required if the clinical situation is dynamically changing.

If there is potential for a cervical spinal injury, cervical immobilisation management will also need to be performed. Additionally, if there is concern about a spinal injury, the jaw thrust technique should be used and not a head tilt chin lift.

When assessing the airway outside, it may be more difficult to hear breath sounds with or without a stethoscope. You may need to reassess this again when the child has been moved to somewhere quieter. Looking and feeling may need to be relied upon more than usual initially.

B Breathing

Assessment of breathing should be performed as you would usually do during an ABCDE assessment. As above, if the ambient noise is loud, certain aspects of the examination may not be successfully performed. They can be done once the noise has dissipated. If the child is cold, the saturation probe may not be accurate, and it may also be affected by movement artefact in a moving ambulance.

In critically ill children, those presenting with acute hypoxaemia or in the peri-arrest situation give high-concentration oxygen immediately via a non-rebreathe mask with reservoir.

For children who demonstrate absent or inadequate breathing, assisted ventilation may be required. BMV with or without airway adjuncts is the simplest and safest method of providing this in children. Use of advanced airways (SGA, TT) should only be inserted by those experienced in their use and if BMV is ineffective. Whilst tracheal intubation provides a definitive airway, it is more challenging in the pre-hospital environment, and it can be more difficult to detect complications (e.g. prolonged desaturation, unrecognised oesophageal intubation, bronchial intubation); additionally, for most children, there have been no demonstrated advantages of early intubation. If an advanced airway is used, capnography should be used to confirm the airway's placement and monitor for complications.

C Circulation

The assessment of circulation should follow the same process as described earlier. It may not be possible to measure a non-invasive blood pressure, depending on the availability of appropriately sized blood pressure cuffs. Establishing vascular access may be more difficult compared to a healthcare environment. The positioning of the child, expertise in cannulating neonates/infants, acute stress/pain and a cold environment can add to an already challenging situation. In some circumstances, intraosseous access will be required in seriously unwell children.

D Disability

Frequently assess and reassess AVPU. This is a good marker of improvement or deterioration in a seriously unwell child. The pupillary response, posture and tone of the child should be assessed. Glucose can easily be measured and is often low in an unwell child. Oral glucose or IM glucagon can be administered if IV is difficult. Glucagon is used to release glucose into the bloodstream from the body's glycogen stores. Paramedics can administer it to children who have a reduced conscious level due to hypoglycaemia when IV access is difficult.

If the expertise is available and time allows, a detailed GCS can be performed in addition to AVPU. This allows a more detailed assessment of a neurological injury, especially in drowsy or responsive children. More information about the use of GCS is described in Chapter 11.

E Exposure

Examination of other areas needs to be weighed against exposure to the cold, wind or rain. The child's and family's privacy needs need to be respected too. So, if possible, exposure should be limited and brief if required. Otherwise, it should be completed once in a warm and sheltered environment, such as indoors or in an ambulance.

Drowning

Drowning causes respiratory impairment from immersion (at least face and upper airway covered) or submersion (all the body) in water or another fluid. The most common and detrimental consequence of drowning is hypoxia. The duration of hypoxia is the critical factor in determining the outcome.

Terms such as dry or wet drowning, near-drowning or silent drowning should not be used.

Safety

Personal safety is always a priority. Attempt to save the child without entry into the water. Try to reach the child with a rescue aid (e.g. stick, clothing), throwing a rope or a buoyant rescue aid or using a boat. If entry into the water is essential, a floating device (e.g. buoyant rescue aid) should be used.

The child should be removed from the water by the fastest and safest means available. Remove the individual from the water in a horizontal position to avoid post-drowning hypotension and cardiovascular collapse if possible.

A Airway

Cervical spine injury is rare, and c-spine immobilisation is difficult to perform in the water. Therefore, cervical spine immobilisation is not indicated unless a severe injury is likely (e.g. diving, waterslide use). Open the airway by jaw thrust if possible.

B Breathing

In-water rescue breathing should be performed only if the rescuer is trained to do so. Otherwise, rescue breathing must be started when out of the water (or in shallow water) if there is no spontaneous breathing after opening the airway.

C Circulation

If there are no signs of life start chest compressions.

Table 12.2   Modifications to ALS in drowning

Advanced life support in drowning	
Ac	Open and maintain airway, consider cervical spine immobilisation.
B	High-flow oxygen should be given during the initial assessment of the spontaneously breathing child.
	Non-invasive ventilation or CPAP may also be applied if hypoxia persists.
	Early tracheal intubation and ventilation should be considered in children who are not responding to these measures or have a reduced level of consciousness.
C	Assess circulation for hypovolaemic shock and give a bolus of fluid as indicated but avoid fluid overload.
	If the patient is hypothermic, warm to 32–34°C then allow passive rewarming.

D Disability

A blood glucose should be measured as this can often be low in a drowned child. Seizures should be managed as usual but these should be differentiated from shivering, which is a normal response when cold following drowning. Abnormal pupil responses would suggest a concomitant head injury and this should be managed at the same time.

E Exposure

Look for any other injuries that may have occurred at the same at the drowning, such as trauma. The child is likely to be cold, so wet clothing should be removed, blankets should be used to reduce further heat loss and they should be moved to a warm environment. The receiving hospital should be advised of any hypothermia so that they can have additional warming equipment immediately available on arrival at hospital.

Hypothermia

Hypothermia is diagnosed when the body's core temperature falls below 35°C; a higher threshold may be considered in infants (Table 12.3). Young children are at risk because they have a high body surface area to weight ratio, resulting in a faster rate of heat loss. It is usually a consequence of environmental causes such as drowning and exposure (worse when both wet and windy). However, in teenagers, consider drug and alcohol ingestion as complicating factors; note that sepsis can present with mild hypothermia.

The body regulates falling core temperature by generating heat (e.g. shivering, increasing levels of thyroxine and adrenaline) and by heat conservation (e.g. peripheral vasoconstriction). Early signs and symptoms in children will be cold extremities and shivering (note - infants less than 6 months old do not shiver).

Core temperature is best measured using an oesophageal or rectal thermometer where possible, as tympanic thermometer measurements may be unreliable. Low reading thermometers may be needed in hypothermia.

Hypothermia can be mild, moderate, or severe. The risk of death increases as the core temperature drops below 32°C and temperatures below 28°C are immediately life-threatening.

Assessment

ABCDE approach, unless suspicion of traumatic injury where an <C>AcBCDE approach may be more appropriate.

- Airway: ensure open and safe.
- Breathing: assess ventilation rate, chest movement and monitor SpO_2 if able to obtain saturation trace.
- Circulation: assess heart rate, rhythm, pulses and monitor blood pressure and ECG for moderate and severe cases.
- Disability: assess level of consciousness, posture, responsiveness, pupil response and blood glucose.
- Environment: accurate assessment of core temperature is very important.

Table 12.3   Classification, signs and symptoms of hypothermia

Classification	Temperature	Signs and symptoms	
Mild hypothermia	32–35°C	34–35°C	Shivering +++; pale, cold to touch, quiet and sleepy
		< 34°C	Increasing confusion, altered judgement, fatigue, nausea
		32–33°C	Shivering stops, apathy, ataxia, usually stable haemodynamically but may have atrial arrhythmias
		Tachycardia, tachypnoea, cold diuresis (as kidney loses concentrating ability) – may present as incontinence; may develop red, cold skin and/or hypoglycaemia	
Moderate hypothermia	28–32°C	Bradycardia, hypotension, hypoventilation, hyporeflexia, further reduction LOC	
		Slurred speech, inability to complete simple tasks	
		Atrial arrhythmias	
		28–30°C	Pupils dilated and minimally responsive to light
		28°C	Ventricular arrhythmias (including VF), fixed dilated pupils
Severe hypothermia	< 28°C	Unconscious, unresponsive, fixed pupils, rigid muscles, areflexia, slow shallow breathing (may be just 1 breath per min) or apnoeic	
		VF and further myocardial depression – pulses hard to detect	
		'appears dead'	
		20°C	Asystole

Management

Conscious individuals with mild hypothermia (temperature > 32°C) are usually successfully treated with simple external rewarming measures: remove wet clothes, dry patient, warm blankets, cover with a 'space blanket' and transfer to a warm environment. For infants and small children, cover the head with a hat where possible as the surface area of the head is a large proportion of overall body surface areas. Warm 41°C packs may be used over the chest, abdomen and groins.

For children with a core temperature below 32°C

- Children with moderate and severe hypothermia should be transferred to hospital for active rewarming.

- Remove wet clothing and cover with dry warm coverings; careful handling is required to prevent precipitating arrhythmias.

- Monitor core temperature, HR and rhythm, check glucose (and electrolytes if possible).

- An echocardiogram may be helpful in the assessment of hypothermic patients when signs of life are absent, pulses are difficult to detect, and the ECG is very slow.

- Open airway, give warmed and humified oxygen.

  - if not breathing, ventilate with high-concentrations of warm, humidified oxygen. The chest wall can be stiff in hypothermia due to muscle rigidity which can make ventilation more difficult.

  - intubation and other interventions may precipitate VF, so this should be done with care by experts.

- If the child is pulseless, start BLS and assess the heart rhythm; muscle rigidity will make chest compressions more difficult to perform.

  - Hypothermia substantially reduces the effectiveness of defibrillation and resuscitation drugs. It is reasonable to attempt defibrillation, but if this is unsuccessful, continue chest compressions until core temperature > 30°C, when drugs and defibrillation are more likely to be effective. Only give drugs when the core temperature is > 30°C as earlier administration may result in accumulation whilst cold with resultant toxicity when rewarmed. Once 30°C core temperature is reached, give drugs but double the drug dose intervals until 35°C.

  - Never diagnose death and stop resuscitation until the patient has been rewarmed to at least 32°C or cannot be rewarmed despite active measures. In some cases, hypothermia can exert a protective effect on the brain, and vital organs and intact neurological recovery can occur even after prolonged cardiorespiratory arrest if deep hypothermia develops before asphyxia.

  - Consider Extracorporeal CPR where facilities are available to support this.

- Rewarming

  - For patients with altered consciousness, both active external and internal rewarming is required.

  - Active rewarming is best performed in hospital. Methods employed include:

    - Warmed IV fluids: start with pre-warmed 0.9% sodium chloride at 40°C if there is no evidence of hypoglycaemia. Hypokalaemia is common, and electrolytes should be regularly monitored. Patients may require large volumes of fluid during rewarming as vasodilation causes expansion of the intravascular space. Continuous haemodynamic monitoring essential.

    - Gastric or bladder lavage using 0.9% sodium chloride warmed to 40°C.

    - Peritoneal lavage with potassium free dialysate or 0.9% sodium chloride at 40°C; use 20 mL kg^{-1} cycled every 15 min.

    - Ventilation with humified gas heated to 42°C.

    - Pleural lavage/haemodialysis/extracorporeal life support.

    - Active external rewarming: overhead warmers and/or warm air system (e.g. Bair hugger, thermal mattress).

  - Check blood gases, potassium, glucose and blood haematocrit with every few degrees of warming.

  - Actively rewarm to 32°C, then allow passive rewarming. Once the patient's core temperature is above the fibrillation threshold of 32°C, there is less urgency in rewarming.

  - Monitor the heart rhythm being aware that peripheral rewarming and vasodilatation can result in cold, acidotic blood being shunted to the core with a drop in temperature, hypotension and again, an increased risk of arrhythmias.

  - Avoid subsequent hyperthermia; keep < 36.5°C.

Pre-hospital management of paediatric illnesses

Once any life-threatening conditions have been identified and managed, more information can be gathered by paramedics or other pre-hospital clinicians. If a child requires an immediate transfer to hospital for further management, this additional information gathering may need to be curtailed or even omitted.

However, if able, a detailed history should be taken from any caregivers present, including the presenting complaint, social and family history, past medical history, previous hospital admissions or recent contact with primary care clinicians. In addition, the history of the child's oral/feeding intake, activity levels, wet nappies, sleeping patterns, immunisation, developmental milestones and any complications during pregnancy or delivery can help formulate a diagnosis. Clues from the environment and interaction with caregivers will also provide valuable information.

The ABCDE assessment approach and treatment of specific illnesses are managed similarly by critical care practitioners to those in hospital guidelines. Some treatments are not available out of hospital (unless an advanced practice paramedic or pre-hospital critical care team are in attendance), and these are listed in Table 12.4. Therefore, the initial treatment of acute illness will be delivered before and during a transfer to hospital. It is often difficult to know if a compensated state will lead to decompensation, especially in children with complex needs or in the very young, and therefore there is a low threshold for further assessment in hospital. Remember that a tiring or exhausted child is an ominous sign, as is a decreasing level of consciousness or responsiveness towards the caregiver.

Table 12.4   Treatments unavailable pre-hospital

Paediatric illness	Treatments unavailable pre-hospital*
Asthma	Intravenous medications – magnesium infusion, aminophylline infusion, salbutamol infusion
Sepsis	Vasoactive infusions (inotropes or vasopressors)
Status epilepticus	3rd line treatment – rapid sequence induction
Hypoglycaemia	Continuous glucose infusion
Ingestion of toxins	Specific antidotes (naloxone available)
*Unless a pre-hospital critical care team is in attendance. Some of these treatments may then be available.	

Out-of-hospital cardiorespiratory arrest in infants and children

Outcomes for children after out-of-hospital cardiorespiratory arrest (OHCA) are poor. Data on cardiorespiratory arrest in children under 18 years of age from an OHCA audit in England between January 2014 and December 2018 indicated that there were on average 570 paediatric OHCA per year, with an incidence of cardiorespiratory arrest of 5 per 100 000 children under 18 years of age. The median age of the children was 3.3 years old, and 58% were male. A bystander, family member or EMS crew witnessed the OHCA in one-third of cases; however, only 60% received bystander CPR. A medical cause for OHCA was given for two-thirds of patients, with 7% asphyxiation, 6% trauma, 2% drowning and 1% toxic ingestion (remaining aetiologies unknown). The presenting cardiac rhythm was asystole in 66%, with only 6% in a shockable rhythm; an AED was used in just 1.2% of cases.

Overall outcome for ROSC at hospital handover by emergency medical services teams was 18% and survival to hospital discharge of 9%.

Survival after OHCA relies on early recognition and CPR from bystanders. When an ambulance is called, ambulance service telephone dispatchers will assist bystanders in identifying cardiorespiratory arrest and starting CPR before the ambulance arrives. Most paediatric cardiorespiratory arrests are not caused by primary cardiac problems but are secondary to other causes, usually hypoxia. However, in cases where the likelihood of a primary shockable rhythm is extremely high, such as in sudden witnessed collapse, if easily accessible, the bystander/rescuer should apply an automated external defibrillator (AED) at the time of calling EMS. When there is more than one bystander/rescuer, a second bystander/rescuer should immediately call for help and then collect and apply an AED (if feasible).

AEDs are available in many public places (e.g. train stations, shopping centres), and in many areas, the ambulance dispatcher will be able to tell bystanders the location of the nearest AED. There have been continuing reports of safe and successful use of AEDs in children less than 8 years, demonstrating that AEDs can identify arrhythmias accurately in children and are extremely unlikely to advise a shock inappropriately.

A bystander being willing and able to perform timely BLS before the ambulance arrives is crucial in improving outcomes for both children and adults who have an OHCA. This highlights the importance of the Restart a Heart initiative and the inclusion of CPR within the national school curriculums; both initiatives aim to

Table 12.5   Type of responder/level of training

Type of responder/level of training	BLS sequence for cardiorespiratory arrest	
Bystander with no CPR training	EMS dispatcher directed CPR – Adult sequence with paediatric modifications	– 5 rescue breaths – 30 chest compression : 2 breaths
	Chest compressions only	Chest compressions only No mouth-to-mouth breaths
Healthcare provider and lay rescuers trained in 'adult' BLS e.g. first aider or adult based healthcare worker in the vicinity	BLS with paediatric modifications	– 5 rescue breaths – 30 chest compression : 2 breaths
Healthcare professionals with a duty to respond to paediatric emergencies e.g. paramedic	Paediatric BLS	– 5 initial rescue breaths – 15 chest compression : 2 breaths

improve the knowledge and skills of a larger number of laypeople who can then deliver bystander CPR. Early BLS, rapid activation of the Emergency Medical Service and prompt, effective advanced life support is crucial in improving mortality and morbidity. Once cardiorespiratory arrest has been confirmed, the sequence of actions in paediatric BLS will depend upon the level of training of the rescuer attending (Chapter 4). These are summarised in Table 12.5.

As can be seen from the table above, it is possible for the different ratios of CPR to be delivered to a child in cardiorespiratory arrest. It may mean that as the training of responder increases, there may be a change in compressions: breaths ratio during the early stages of cardiopulmonary resuscitation. The paramedics will then add advanced resuscitation management to the ongoing BLS.

BLS is more effective when the rescuer is proficient in its delivery, but even suboptimal CPR gives a better result than no CPR at all. Hence rescuers unable or unwilling to provide mouth-to-mouth ventilation should be encouraged to perform at least compression-only CPR. A child or infant is far more likely to be harmed if the bystander does nothing.

Debriefing

Following an out-of-hospital resuscitation attempt, an immediate debrief with the attending EMS team can provide both a learning opportunity and support for the team. Debriefing in a structured manner allows a review of the non-technical elements of resuscitation such as communication, leadership and team working. Ideally, the debrief is led by a person trained and capable of leading the session in a constructive manner.

If a defibrillator with the capability to monitor CPR quality has been used, this data can be used to inform the debrief and drive quality improvements.

Out-of-hospital cardiac arrest outcomes (OHCAO) database

Ongoing, systematic collection and analysis of data about out-of-hospital cardiorespiratory arrest and bystander CPR is essential to the planning, implementation, and evaluation of effective CPR programs. The British Heart Foundation and Resuscitation Council UK established a national OHCAO registry in partnership with the National Association of Ambulance Medical Directors and the University of Warwick. The OHCAO registry collects process and outcome information about patients treated by ambulance services for cardiorespiratory arrest and is based on the international Utstein template. The registry will provide a tool to support local quality improvement initiatives and will facilitate measuring the impact of resuscitation interventions.

Recognition of life extinct

The pre-hospital care teams will follow protocols when life extinct is ultimately recognised and discuss with local organisations for transfer to hospital for post bereavement care.

Resuscitation of the newborn out-of-hospital

The process of resuscitating a newborn is discussed in detail in Chapter 13. However, some babies are born in unexpected places (e.g. in the back of cars or at home.) Babies born unexpectedly outside the hospital are likely to involve the emergency services and the community midwives.

The principles of resuscitation are identical to the hospital setting. Whenever a baby is born unexpectedly, there is often great difficulty in keeping them warm, but it is particularly important to avoid hypothermia as it causes an increase in both morbidity and mortality. Drying and wrapping the newborn, turning up the heating in the home or ambulance and closing windows and doors are all important in maintaining the body temperature. Pre-term babies will be at greater risk of getting cold. Alternatively, newborns > 30 weeks gestation maintaining adequate spontaneous respirations may be dried, kept warm, and nursed skin-to-skin. If care of both the mother and the newborn requires transportation to the hospital, this will need to be discussed according to local guidelines.

Packaging a patient prior to transfer

The paramedic team will package the patient appropriately depending on the child's condition and/or injuries. This will include lying on the transfer trolley with its standard straps, modified paediatric straps or on a caregivers lap with a restraint. Injured children may be transferred on a scoop stretcher if it is a short transfer time or in a vacuum mattress. The latter provides immobilisation and insulation.

Pre-alert and patient handover

The receiving emergency department should be alerted as soon as possible if a child is seriously unwell or in cardiorespiratory arrest. A structured method is used by the ambulance services to pass the important pieces of information in a short amount of time. Typically, this is done using 'ATMIST' along with an estimated time of arrival and if a specific hospital response is required (for example a resuscitation team or trauma team).

Table 12.6 A structured approach to providing key information – the ATMIST mnemonic

	Medical	Trauma
A	Age	Age
T	Time of onset	Time of incident
M	Medical complaint/history	Mechanism of injury
I	Investigations (brief examination of findings)	Injuries (top to toe)
S	Vital Signs (first set and significant changes)	Vital Signs (first set and significant changes)
T	Treatment, including ETA and any specialist resources needed on arrival	Treatment, including ETA and any specialist resources needed on arrival
ETA – expected time of arrival		

When the pre-hospital team arrive at hospital with the patient, an ATMIST handover is given to the receiving team. Unless CPR is ongoing, this is a hands-off handover so that all the team members can listen to the important information without distraction. Once the handover has been taken, the team leader will then lead the team in the assessment/management of the child.

12: Summary learning

Team approach and safety in the pre-hospital environment.

Initial assessment of the unwell or injured child in the pre-hospital environment.

Drowning children must be removed from water by the fastest and safest means.

Pre-hospital management of paediatric illnesses and cardiopulmonary resuscitation.

Out-of-hospital cardiorespiratory arrest.

Patient packaging, pre-alert and patient handover.

My key take-home messages from this chapter are:

Further reading

Association of Ambulance Chief Executives (Great Britain) & Joint Royal Colleges Ambulance Liaison Committee 2019, JRCALC clinical guidelines 2019, Class Professional Publishing, Bridgwater.

The Out of Hospital Cardiac Arrest Outcome registry warwick.ac.uk/fac/sci/med/research/ctu/trials/ohcao

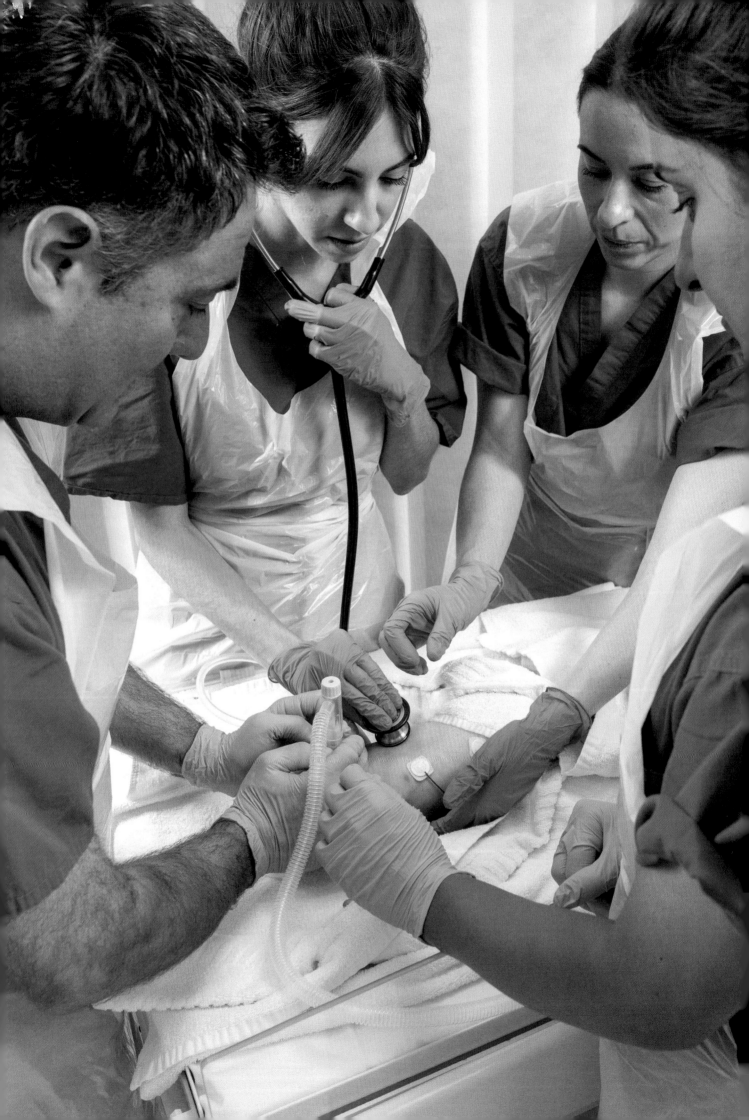

Babies born outside the delivery room

In this chapter

Principles of supporting transition and, when required, resuscitation of the newborn outside the delivery room.

Care of the umbilical cord

Algorithm for Newborn Life Support

Preterm newborns

Discontinuation of resuscitation

The learning outcomes will enable you to:

Identify the equipment required for newborn resuscitation

Formulate strategies for support and newborn resuscitation of the newborn infant

Undertake an assessment of the newborn infant and take appropriate actions

Identify differences in preterm babies

Think about when to consider discontinuation newborn resuscitation

---

The approach to newborn babies differs from that in all other age groups as the fetus, with its fluid-filled lungs and dependence on the placenta for respiratory function, transitions to a newborn infant whose air-filled lungs take over. The majority of newborns make this transition without any help; a few will need a bit of support, and a tiny minority will need resuscitation. In most cases, you will merely need to support that transition rather than resuscitate the baby.

Birth outside the delivery room

Ideally, someone trained in newborn resuscitation should be present at all deliveries. However, some babies can be born in unexpected places (e.g. emergency departments and pre-hospital settings). For these situations, it is important that clinicians have some understanding of the differences between the newborn baby and other age groups.

Whenever a baby is born unexpectedly, there is often great difficulty in keeping them warm, but this is very important to avoid both morbidity and mortality. Drying and wrapping, turning up the heating and closing windows and doors are all important in maintaining the body temperature.

Hospitals with emergency departments should have guidelines for resuscitation at birth, summoning help and post-resuscitation transfer of babies born within the department.

Babies born unexpectedly outside the hospital are likely to involve the emergency services. However, the principles of supporting the transition (and resuscitation if required) are identical to the hospital setting. Transport will need to be discussed according to local guidelines. These babies will be at greater risk of being both preterm and of getting cold.

> Whenever a baby is born unexpectedly, there is often great difficulty in keeping them warm, but this is very important to avoid both morbidity and mortality

Strategy for assessing and resuscitating a baby at birth

Resuscitation is likely to be rapidly successful if begun before the baby has become so anoxic that all potential for respiratory activity has vanished. The apnoeic baby may be in primary (seen before the onset of gasping) or terminal apnoea (which, as the name suggests, is a preterminal event after gasps have ceased); early intervention and support can prevent the baby in primary apnoea progressing to the more ominous gasping phase and on to terminal apnoea (Figure 13.1).

Equipment

Most newborn babies will not need any help to transition to breathing air. A few will need some support, but only a tiny minority will require resuscitation (i.e. A, B, C, D). Non-maternity settings should have contingency plans to cope with any newborn baby that may present. Equipment which may be required to resuscitate a newborn baby is listed in Table 13.1. This will vary between departments; however, most babies can be resuscitated with a flat surface, warmth, knowledge and a way to deliver air or oxygen at a controlled pressure.

Table 13.1   Equipment for newborn resuscitation

Equipment
A flat surface
Source of warmth, hat and dry towels
A plastic bag or wrap (for preterm babies)
A suction system with catheters size 6, 8, 10, 12 F
Stethoscope and or saturation monitor with appropriate probe type
Round (or anatomical) face masks sizes 00, 0, 1
Paediatric self-inflating bag or pressure-limiting device (T-piece)
Source of air and oxygen (preferably with blender)
Oropharyngeal airways size 000, 00, 0, 1
Laryngeal mask airway device size 1
Laryngoscopes with miller/macintosh blades size 0 and 1
Nasogastric tubes sizes 5, 8 F
Device to clamp cord
Scissors to cut cord
Tracheal tubes sizes 2.5, 3.0, 3.5, 4.0
Tracheal tube stylet size 2 mm
Umbilical catheters (artery forceps, tie, blade to cut the cord, 0.9% sodium chloride flush, 3-way tap, syringes 1 mL, 2 mL, 5 mL, 10 mL, 3.0 silk suture, sharps bin)
Adhesive tape
Colorimetric exhaled CO_2 detector (or suitable alternative)
Appropriate PPE

Call for help

Call for help if you expect or encounter any difficulty or if the delivery is outside a labour suite. In hospital, alert the paediatric or neonatal team. Outside a hospital setting, alert the community midwife or delivery suite and, if necessary, call 999 and request paramedic support.

Start clock

When the baby is delivered, start the clock (if available, otherwise note the time of birth).

At birth

- Unless the umbilical cord has snapped, do not rush to clamp or tie it. This can wait until after you have dried and assessed the baby.

- Dry the baby quickly and effectively. Remove the wet towel (or whatever you have used) and wrap in fresh dry, warm towels (or suitable alternatives). For very small or significantly preterm babies (i.e. those born before 32 weeks gestation), an alternative is to place the wet baby in a food-grade plastic bag and then under a radiant heater; the radiant heater is essential for this technique though.

- While you are addressing thermal control, assess the baby and decide whether any intervention is needed.

- Your assessment should also guide you when you clamp and cut the cord. Unless immediate resuscitation is required, delaying cord clamping for at least 60 s is recommended. Ideally, this should be after the lungs are aerated. When ready, the cord should be clamped or tied 4–5 cm from the skin.

- If the baby is thought to need assistance, then this becomes the priority, and the cord may need to be clamped in order to deliver that assistance. This is especially likely in deliveries occurring in unexpected areas. When cutting the cord, make sure it is securely clamped or tied to prevent blood loss.

- In babies > 28 weeks gestation, umbilical cord milking (from an intact or cut cord) may be an alternative to delayed cord clamping when resuscitation is required.

Keep the baby warm

The temperature of a newborn should be maintained between 36.5°C and 37.5°C. Studies of preterm babies show that for each 1°C below 36.5°C the baseline risk of mortality increases by over 25%. Ideally, delivery should take place in a warm room, and an overhead heater should be switched on. If possible, keep the environment warm at 23–25°C.

Dry the baby immediately and then wrap in a dry towel. If this is not addressed at the beginning of resuscitation, it is often forgotten. Most heat loss is caused by evaporation

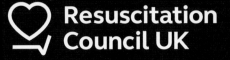

Newborn life support

(Antenatal counselling)
Team briefing and equipment check

Birth
Delay cord clamping if possible

Start clock / note time
Dry / wrap, stimulate, keep warm

Assess
Colour, tone, breathing, heart rate

Ensure an open airway
Preterm: consider CPAP

If gasping / not breathing
- Give 5 inflations (30 cm H_2O) – start in air
- Apply PEEP 5–6 cm H_2O, if possible
- Apply SpO_2 +/- ECG

Reassess
If no increase in heart rate, look for chest movement

If the chest is not moving
- Check mask, head and jaw position
- 2 person support
- Consider suction, laryngeal mask/tracheal tube
- Repeat inflation breaths
- Consider increasing the inflation pressure

Reassess
If no increase in heart rate, look for chest movement

Once chest is moving continue ventilation breaths

If heart rate is not detectable or < 60 min[-1] after 30 seconds of ventilation
- Synchronise 3 chest compressions to 1 ventilation
- Increase oxygen to 100%
- Consider intubation if not already done or laryngeal mask if not possible

Reassess heart rate and chest movement every 30 seconds

If the heart rate remains not detectable or < 60 min[-1]
- **Vascular access and drugs**
- Consider other factors e.g. pneumothorax, hypovolaemia, congenital abormality

Update parents and debrief team
Complete records

Preterm < 32 weeks

Place undried in plastic wrap + radiant heat

Inspired oxygen
28–31 weeks 21–30%
< 28 weeks 30%

If giving inflations, start with 25 cm H_2O

Acceptable pre-ductal SpO_2	
2 min	65%
5 min	85%
10 min	90%

TITRATE OXYGEN TO ACHIEVE TARGET SATURATIONS

APPROX 60 SECONDS

MAINTAIN TEMPERATURE

AT ALL TIMES ASK "IS HELP NEEDED"

Figure 13.1   Newborn life support algorithm   197

from the wet skin; babies have a large surface area to volume ratio; thus, heat can be lost very quickly. Drying effectively and wrapping the baby in a warm, dry towel (or equivalent) is the most important factor in avoiding hypothermia. Cover the baby's head with a hat as it represents a significant proportion of the baby's surface area. A naked wet baby will become hypothermic despite a warm room and a radiant heater, especially if there is a draught.

Thermal care in preterm babies is addressed slightly differently (see preterm babies).

Assessment of the newborn baby

While you dry and wrap the baby, make an initial assessment of their:

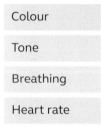

Colour

Tone

Breathing

Heart rate

Colour
Is the baby blue or are they pale? Note: even a healthy baby may remain blue until 5 min of age.

Tone
Is the baby vigorous and flexed or are they floppy?

Breathing
Is the baby crying? If not crying, are they breathing regularly, gasping or not breathing at all?

Heart rate
Use a stethoscope to assess the heart rate. Is it fast, slow, very slow or absent?

It is important to make an initial assessment and then to regularly re-assess the newborn at fairly short intervals of 30 s so that one can judge the impact of interventions. Heart rate and breathing are the main parameters that point to the need for resuscitation. However, a baby who is pale and peripherally shut down is more likely to be acidotic, and a baby who is floppy (atonic) is likely to be unconscious – if you see these, you should call for help as soon as possible. Subsequent assessments should focus on heart rate and breathing.

Respiration

Most babies will establish spontaneous regular breathing sufficient to maintain the heart rate > 100 min^{-1} within 3 min of birth. These babies will often cry. The non-crying baby deserves special attention as it often indicates a need for support or resuscitation. The non-crying but breathing baby should also be closely monitored. If apnoea or gasping persists after drying, intervention is required.

Heart rate

An initial assessment of heart rate is vital because its increase will be the first sign of success during resuscitation. The quickest and most effective way to assess heart rate early on is to listen to the cardiac apex using a stethoscope. Palpating peripheral pulses is not practical and not recommended, and palpation of the umbilical pulse is unreliable when this is < 100 min^{-1}.

Consider using an oxygen saturation monitor (one designed to pick up a trace on a baby and is resistant to movement artifact) in the baby requiring support or resuscitation. Apply the probe to the right hand or wrist (pre-ductal). This can give an accurate and continuous reading of heart rate and saturations within 90 s of application. ECG monitoring may also be used, but pulseless electrical activity (PEA) is a recognised phenomenon even in the newborn.

A heart rate below 100 min^{-1} in a baby without effective breathing requires immediate intervention. A heart rate below 100 min^{-1} in a baby with effective breathing requires reassessment every 30 s to ensure that it continues to rise; if it does not, intervention is required.

Colour

Attempting to judge oxygenation by assessing skin colour is unreliable, but it is still worth noting the baby's colour at birth and any changes thereafter. Very pale babies who remain pale after resuscitation may be hypovolaemic as well as acidotic.

Using an oxygen saturation monitor allows assessment of both heart rate and saturation within about 90 s of application. Oxygen saturations in healthy babies in the first few minutes of life can be considerably lower than at other times (Table 13.2).

This initial assessment will categorise the baby into one of the three following groups:

1. Regular respirations, heart rate fast (> 100 min^{-1}), blue but with a good tone. These are healthy babies. Avoid clamping and cutting the cord too early. They should be kept warm by drying and being placed skin-to-skin with their mothers under a cover when they may also be put to the breast.

2. Irregular or inadequate respirations, heart rate slow (< 100 min⁻¹), blue, normal or reduced tone. If gentle stimulation (such as drying) does not induce effective breathing, the airway should be opened. If the baby responds then no further resuscitation is needed. If there is no response, progress to lung inflation. This will, in most cases, necessitate clamping and cutting of the cord to move the baby to a resuscitaire (or similar).

3. Apnoeic, heart rate very slow (< 60 min⁻¹) or absent, blue or pale, floppy. This baby will require support and possible resuscitation. Clamp and cut the cord if you have to move the baby to a resuscitaire. Open the airway and then inflate the lungs. A reassessment of any heart rate response or confirmed chest wall movement then directs further resuscitation. Re-assess the heart rate and respiration at regular 30 s intervals throughout.

The combination of apnoea, low or absent heart rate, pallor and floppiness at the initial resuscitation suggest a significant hypoxic insult and possible need for prolonged resuscitation (in many cases requiring additional help). Nonetheless, the initial management of such babies remains the same by ensuring that the baby does not become hypothermic.

After the assessment, any supportive or resuscitative intervention should follow the sequence:

A	Airway

B	Breathing – initially inflating and then ventilating the lungs

C	Circulation

D	Drugs – with the use of drugs in a few selected cases

Table 13.2 Time from birth and acceptable preductal oxygen saturations

Time from birth	Acceptable (25th centile) preductal saturation (%)
2 min	65% SpO₂
5 min	85% SpO₂
10 min	90% SpO₂

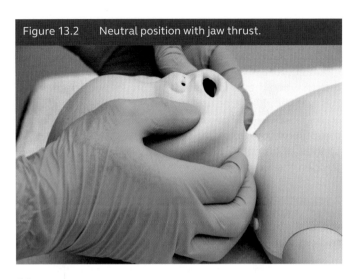

Figure 13.2 Neutral position with jaw thrust.

Airway

The baby should be positioned with the head in the neutral position (Figure 13.2). The newborn baby's head has a large, often moulded, occiput, which tends to cause the neck to flex when they are supine on a flat surface. However, overextension may also collapse the newborn baby's pharyngeal airway, leading to obstruction. A 2 cm thick folded towel placed under the neck and shoulders may help to maintain the airway in a neutral position.

In the very floppy baby, jaw thrust (using either a single-handed or a two-handed approach) may be needed to bring the tongue forward and open the airway (Figure 13.2).

Laryngeal mask airways

In infants > 34 weeks gestation and > 1500 g a laryngeal mask airway may be used as an alternative means of establishing an airway when basic airways manoeuvres and a two-person (two-handed) technique have been unsuccessful, and when tracheal intubation is either unsuccessful or not feasible. Using a laryngoscope during the insertion may also ensure that the oropharynx is clear of any particulate matter that could cause obstruction.

Suctioning

Routine oral and nasopharyngeal suctioning in newborns has not shown to improve respiratory function and may cause a delay in other necessary simple airway manoeuvres. Routine suctioning for both clear and meconium-stained fluid is therefore not recommended. Blind deep pharyngeal suction should not be performed as it may cause vagally induced bradycardia and laryngospasm.

If, despite all airway interventions, obstruction is suspected and suctioning is attempted, it should not exceed 150 mmHg (20 kPa) and be under direct vision using a laryngoscope.

Meconium-stained liquor is relatively common and occurs in up to 10% of births. Meconium aspiration with airways obstruction is a rare event, usually occurring in term infants before delivery. Suction of the baby's nose and mouth when the head is on the perineum will not prevent this and should not be undertaken. The crying baby has an open airway and does not need help. If the baby born through meconium-stained liquor is pale, floppy and apnoeic, the priority is to address thermal care and then to open the airway and begin inflation breaths. Only then, if the chest does not move despite airway interventions, it would be appropriate to inspect the oropharynx and suction any particulate meconium under direct vision.

Breathing (inflation breaths and ventilation)

Use a transparent face mask big enough to cover the nose and mouth of the baby. The first five breaths should be inflation breaths in order to expel the fetal lung fluid from the alveoli and aerate the small airways. Inflation breaths are sustained for 2–3 s beginning at a pressure of 30 cm H_2O in term babies (and a lower pressure of 25 cm H_2O in preterm babies < 32 weeks gestation) when using a continuous gas supply, a pressure-limiting device and a mask. If no such system is available, or you are not familiar with it, then a 500 mL self-inflating bag with a blow-off valve set at 30–40 cm H_2O can be used. This is especially useful if compressed air or oxygen is not available.

Where possible, start resuscitation of babies born at > 32 weeks gestation in air. Less than 32 weeks use 21–30% and less than 28 weeks use 30%. There is now good evidence for this in term babies, and oxygen toxicity is a real concern with premature babies. Use of supplemental oxygen should be guided by pulse oximetry with reasonable levels listed and on the algorithm (Table 13.2 and Figure 13.1).

The chest may not move during the first 3 inflation breaths as fluid is displaced. Successful inflation is usually indicated by either a rapidly increasing heart rate or a heart rate that is maintained at > 100 min⁻¹. Therefore, re-assess the heart rate after delivery of the first 5 breaths. If no chest rise is seen and there has been no increase in heart rate, re-assess your airway opening technique and repeat the inflation breaths. Consider other airway opening manoeuvres.

Once the chest is inflated, and the heart rate has increased, or the chest has been seen to move, ventilation should be continued at a rate of 30 min⁻¹. Continue ventilatory support until regular breathing is established.

If the heart rate remains slow after inflation breaths and you have seen the chest move, ventilate for 30 s then re-assess the heart rate. If you have not seen the chest move, recheck the airway and repeat the inflation breaths.

If the heart rate remains slow after the 30 s of ventilation, increase the inspired oxygen concentration to 100% and begin chest compressions. Consider pulse oximetry if not already being used.

Circulation

Chest compressions will help to move oxygenated blood from the lungs to the heart and coronary arteries. It should only be commenced once the lungs have been successfully inflated and when the heart rate has not responded after 30 s of ventilation breaths.

The most efficient way of delivering chest compressions in the newborn is to encircle the chest with both hands so that the fingers lie behind the baby and the thumbs overlap on the lower third of the sternum (Figure 13.3). If there is a single person present, the two-finger technique (using the index and middle finger together over the lower third of the sternum) will be required, whilst the other hand is maintaining the airway. Compress the chest briskly, by one-third of its depth. In newborn babies, perform three compressions for each ventilation breath (3:1 ratio).

The purpose of chest compressions is to move oxygenated blood or drugs to the coronary arteries in order to initiate cardiac recovery. There is no point in starting chest compressions before effective lung inflation has been established. Similarly, compressions are ineffective unless interposed by ventilation breaths of good quality; consequently, synchronised rather continuous chest compressions are used as simultaneous delivery of compressions and breaths reduce the effectiveness of the breaths. A 3:1 rather than 15:2 ratio is used as this allows for more breaths per minute.

Figure 13.3　Chest compressions on a newborn infant: two thumbs encircling technique

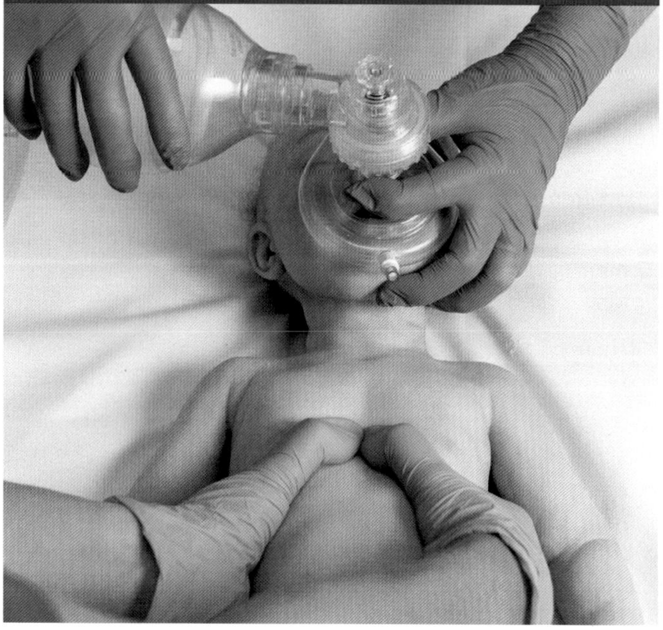

Re-assess the heart rate every 30 s (or continuously if a saturation monitor is used). Once the heart rate is > 60 min^{-1} and rising, chest compressions can be discontinued and the baby closely monitored. Maintain ventilations at 30 min^{-1} until effective breathing or mechanical ventilation is established.

Drugs

If, after adequate lung inflation and cardiac compressions, the heart rate has not responded, drug therapy should be considered. However, the most common reason for a lack of improvement in heart rate is a failure to achieve lung inflation; there is no point in giving drugs unless the airway is open, the lungs inflated and chest compressions are being given. Airway, breathing and circulation must be re-assessed as adequate before proceeding to drug therapy. Central venous access will be required via an umbilical venous line (or alternatively through an intraosseous needle). The outcome is poor if drugs are required.

Adrenaline

Adrenaline increases coronary artery perfusion during resuscitation, enhancing oxygen delivery to the heart.

Dosage
In the presence of profound unresponsive bradycardia or circulatory standstill, 20 microgram kg^{-1} (0.2 mL kg^{-1} 1:10 000) adrenaline may be given intravenously.

A dose range 10–30 micrograms kg^{-1} is acceptable which facilitates dosing based on estimated weight.

Subsequent doses may be administered every 3–5 mins if the heart rate remains < 60 min^{-1}.

Glucose

Hypoglycaemia is a potential problem for all stressed or asphyxiated babies.

Dosage
It is treated using a slow bolus of 2.5 mL kg^{-1} of 10% glucose intravenously. It may be necessary to follow this up with a secure intravenous infusion of 10% glucose. Hand-held glucometers are unreliable in neonates at glucose levels < 5 mmol L^{-1}.

Response to resuscitation

The first indication of success will be an increase in heart rate. Recovery of respiratory drive may be delayed. Babies who have been profoundly hypoxic for some time will tend to gasp first as they recover before starting normal respirations. These babies will have been in terminal apnoea. Those who respond by starting with normal breathing were less severely affected and will have been in primary apnoea. It is helpful to note the baby's respiratory recovery response during resuscitation.

Tracheal intubation

Most babies can be resuscitated using a mask system. However, tracheal intubation, if it is performed, is especially useful in prolonged resuscitations, preterm babies and meconium aspiration. It should be considered if mask ventilation has failed, although the most common reason for failure with mask ventilation is poor positioning of the head with consequent failure to open the airway or poor application of the mask resulting in a leak.

Fluid

Very occasionally, hypovolaemia may be present because of known or suspected blood loss (antepartum haemorrhage, placenta or vasa praevia, unclamped cord), or it may be secondary to loss of vascular tone following asphyxia.

Dosage
Volume expansion, initially with 10 mL kg^{-1}, may be appropriate. 0.9% sodium chloride can be used; if blood loss is acute and severe, non-cross-matched O-negative blood should be given immediately. However, most newborn or neonatal resuscitations do not require fluid unless there has been known blood loss or septicaemic shock.

Sodium bicarbonate

Any baby who is in terminal apnoea will have a significant metabolic acidosis. Acidosis depresses cardiac function.

Dosage
Sodium bicarbonate 1–2 mmol kg^{-1} (2–4 mL kg^{-1} of 4.2% solution) may be used to raise the pH and enhance the effects of oxygen and adrenaline.

Bicarbonate use remains controversial, and it should only be used in the absence of discernible cardiac output despite all resuscitative efforts or in profound and unresponsive bradycardia.

The technique of intubation is the same as for infants and is described in Chapter 3. A term newborn usually needs a 3.5 mm tracheal tube, but a range of sizes (2.5 mm to 4.0 mm) should be available.

Tracheal tube placement must be assessed visually during intubation and, in most cases, will be confirmed by a rapid response in heart rate on ventilating via the tracheal tube. End-tidal CO_2 detection will correctly identify most correctly sited tubes in the presence of any cardiac output. Detection of exhaled carbon dioxide should be used to confirm tracheal tube placement along with chest X-ray.

If you cannot intubate, or if it is difficult, then consider the use of a laryngeal mask airway.

Special cases

Preterm babies

Unexpected deliveries outside delivery suites are more likely to be premature. Premature babies are more likely to get cold (higher surface area to mass ratio) and more likely to become hypoglycaemic (fewer glycogen stores). There is good evidence to support the placing of babies of < 32 weeks gestation and/or < 1000 g up to their neck in a plastic bag. These babies are not dried but instead placed in the bag still wet and then nursed under a radiant heater.

Most preterm babies have not undergone the hypoxic insult seen in term babies who require assistance, and many breathe spontaneously. If possible, you should gently support this spontaneous breathing by using continuous positive airways pressure (CPAP) and avoid more aggressive respiratory support unless the baby is apnoeic.

The lungs of preterm babies are more fragile than those of term babies, but they have more compliant chest walls; thus, their lungs are more susceptible to damage from over-distension. You should start with a lower inflation pressure of 25 cm H_2O, but do not be afraid to increase this to 30 cm H2O if there is no heart rate response and no chest movement. Similarly, reduce the pressure if there is a good heart rate and chest movement seems excessive; very obvious chest wall movement, particularly in preterm babies of < 28 weeks gestation, may indicate excessive and potentially damaging tidal volumes. If you are using a pressure-limiting device (T-piece), you should ensure delivery of 5 cm H_2O of positive end-expiratory pressure.

Premature babies are more susceptible to the toxic effects of hyperoxia. For babies born > 32 weeks gestation, begin using air for resuscitation; if they are < 32 weeks, begin with 21–30% and < 28 weeks with 30%. Use a pulse oximeter early on to monitor both heart rate and oxygen saturations. If oxygen is being administered and oxygen saturations are above 95%, then begin to wean the oxygen. Table 13.2 shows acceptable (25th centile) preductal saturations at 2, 5 and 10 minutes.

Actions in the event of poor initial response to resuscitation

1. Check airway and breathing by asking:

    a) Is mask ventilation effective? Observe chest movement. Consider airway opening manoeuvres such as two-person jaw thrust.

    b) Do you need to intubate? If you cannot intubate or it is difficult, consider a laryngeal mask airway.

    c) Is the tracheal tube in the trachea? Auscultate both axillae, listen at the mouth for a large leak and observe movement. Use an end-tidal CO_2 detector to ensure tracheal tube position.

    d) Is the tracheal tube in the right bronchus? Auscultate both axillae and observe movement.

    e) Is the tracheal tube blocked? If there is doubt about the position or patency of the tracheal tube replace it. Use an end-tidal CO_2 detector.

    f) Is a longer inflation time or higher inflation pressure required?

2. If using air and oxygen saturations are slower than normal to increase despite chest movement, increase the oxygen concentration. It is reasonable to use 100% oxygen if chest compressions are being carried out. Does the baby have a pneumothorax? This occurs spontaneously in up to 1% of newborns at birth, but those needing action in the delivery unit are exceptionally rare. Auscultate the chest for asymmetry of breath sounds. A cold light source can be used to transilluminate the chest – a pneumothorax may show as a hyper-illuminating area.

3. Does the baby remain cyanosed despite breathing with a good heart rate? There may be a congenital heart malformation, which may be duct-dependent or a persistent pulmonary hypertension.

4. Is there severe anaemia or hypovolaemia? In cases of suspected blood loss (e.g. antepartum haemorrhage, placental abruption, etc.), 10 mL kg[-1] of O-negative blood or a volume expander should be given.

Discontinuation of resuscitation

The outcome for a baby with no detectable cardiac output for more than 20 min despite effective resuscitation is likely to be very poor. The decision to stop may depend on the circumstances of the delivery, the gestation of the baby and access to neonatal intensive care (including therapeutic hypothermia).

Stopping resuscitation early or not starting resuscitation at all may be appropriate in situations of extreme prematurity (< 23 weeks) or with birth weight of < 400 g. A best interest decision needs to be considered on a case-by-case basis for the infant.

13: Summary learning

Most babies need no more than drying, keeping warm and skin-to-skin with their mother. They also benefit from delayed cord clamping.

The key to successful resuscitation at birth is lung inflation.

Start resuscitation with air; only add oxygen if SpO_2 remains low despite good lung inflation and ventilation, or if you start chest compressions.

Drugs are rarely needed but, if they are, the prognosis is somewhat poorer.

My key take-home messages from this chapter are:

Further reading

Wyckoff MH, Wyllie J, Aziz K, et al; Neonatal Life Support Collaborators. Neonatal Life Support 2020 International Consensus on Cardiopulmonary Resuscitation and Emergency Cardiovascular Care Science With Treatment Recommendations. Resuscitation 2020;156:A156-A187.

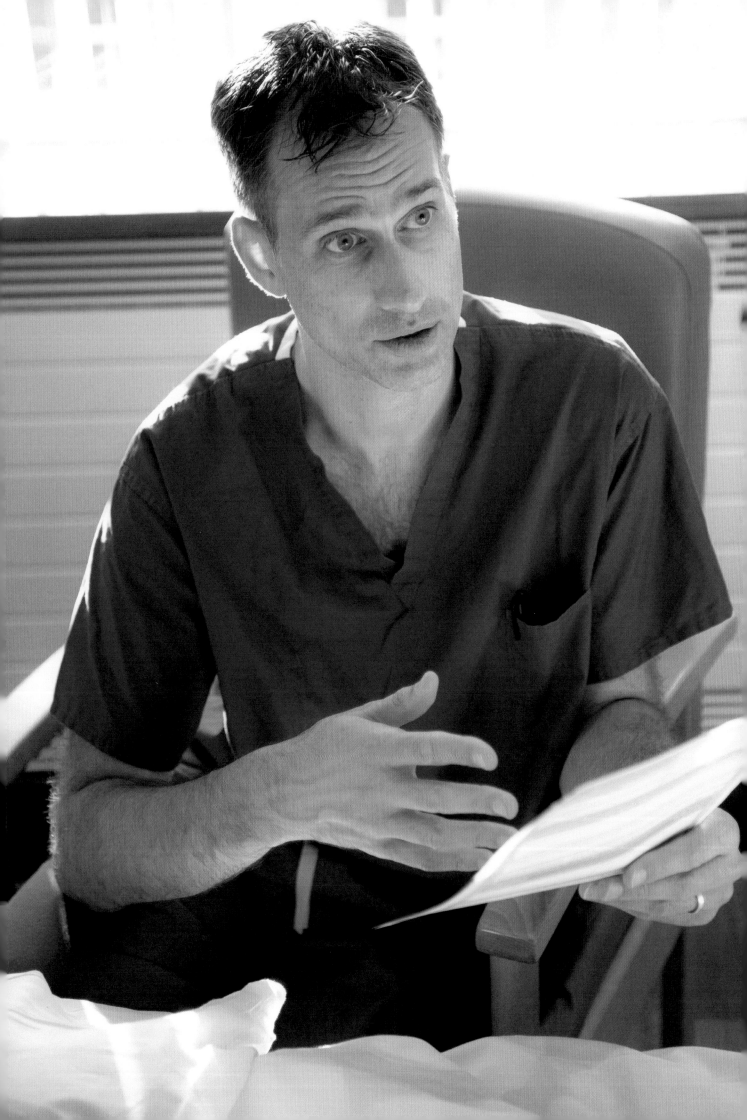

Ethical considerations in resuscitation

Ethical concepts and principles

Ethics is the field of study that attempts to understand human actions in a moral sense. Medical ethics is the study of the application of moral principles that guide the behaviour of healthcare professionals. Ethical principles are not immutable; they change over time and vary according to the social and cultural characteristics of the human populace.

Historically the ethics of medical practice was guided by the Hippocratic principle 'Do good and avoid harm' without any recognition of the patient's opinion. Now, the central role of the patient (or parents/guardians in the case of a child) in the decision-making process is recognised.

In the current approach to medical ethics, four guiding principles are considered:

- autonomy
- beneficence
- justice
- non-maleficence.

Dignity and honesty are frequently added as essential elements.

Autonomy

Autonomy requires people to be allowed and helped to make their own informed decisions, rather than having decisions made for them. A person with capacity must be adequately informed about the matter to be decided and free from undue pressure in making their decision. Autonomy allows an informed person to make a choice, even if that choice is considered illogical or incorrect by others, including health professionals. As a child's sense of autonomy evolves, children have a right to have their opinion taken into account when decisions are being made that affect them directly. An inclusive approach of both parents and guardians and the child is fundamental to ensure that the parents/guardians have been correctly informed and that they fully understand the clinical situation, the treatment plan, and alternatives before making a treatment decision. If the patient is not competent because of age or disturbance of mental capability, the parents/guardians must make the decision on their behalf. The patient has a right to confidentiality: the doctor must inform only the patient and those individuals they wish to be informed; this may cause conflict, particularly concerning sick adolescents.

There are only a few exceptions to this, for example, in the event of serious criminal actions or a notifiable disease, where not informing a relevant authority would seriously jeopardise public safety.

Competence

There may be occasions where a parent is absent and a condition is not life-threatening, so professionals feel they cannot treat a child without parental/guardian permission, but there is a degree of urgency. It may be a young person can give consent to treatment without the parent's consent, even if under 16 years. A framework can be used to determine if a young person under 16 years of age can give consent. The young person must understand the advice given and have sufficient maturity to consider the implications of what is involved. The child must be able to retain the information and comprehend the nature, purpose and consequences of the treatment (or lack of it), and be able to communicate their decision; this is known as 'Gillick competence'. There may be occasions where the clinician disagrees with the parents.

In a life-threatening situation, the clinician may act in the best interests of the child. If there is time, the case can go to court for a judicial decision.

If a competent child refuses treatment, then those with parental responsibility can consent to treatment if it is in the child's best interests despite their refusal. However, this should be limited to urgent situations where not treating might result in serious harm. In other situations, legal advice should be sought and referral to court considered.

Beneficence

All medical acts must be guided by the goal of achieving good for the patient whilst balancing benefit and risk. This principle requires that the patient is offered all available diagnostic procedures and potentially beneficial therapies.

Evidence-based clinical guidelines exist to assist decision-making. Increasingly, patients and guardians are involved as active partners in a personalised protocol or guideline development process, ensuring that patient's views and perspectives are captured in the guidance provided.

Justice

This requires spreading benefits and risks equally within a society to guarantee equal opportunities and rational distribution of resources. There should be no discrimination purely on the grounds of factors such as age, sex, race, religion, socioeconomics or disability. Justice does not imply an entitlement to expect or demand CPR for everyone. In addition, medical practice must conform to civilian and criminal law.

Non-maleficence

The actions of healthcare professionals must not cause harm. Treatments that are harmful must be avoided. The balance between risks and benefits of a proposed treatment for a patient must be evaluated carefully. Only treatments that have demonstrated efficacy should be used, but futility is difficult to define in a way that is precise, prospective and applies to the majority of cases.

Ethical aspects of paediatric life support

Cardiorespiratory arrest and other clinical emergencies can be unpredictable. There may not have been an opportunity to discuss treatment options with the child and/or parents/guardian before the event. In these circumstances, the principle of a child's autonomy is difficult to apply, and healthcare professionals must make the decisions about resuscitation. In these situations, consent for life-saving interventions is presumed.

For children, information must be given to the parents/guardians unless the nature of the emergency does not allow for this. If the parents/guardians are present, they can be given information as the resuscitation takes place; if they are not, the circumstances must be carefully documented in the child's medical records. In some cases, there may be conflicts of interest between parents, or they may refuse appropriate and effective treatment because of religious or other beliefs. If this occurs, the doctor must make a decision that protects the best interests of the child and should request both legal advice and advice of colleagues (Greif 2020). Carefully detailed documentation, including the reasons for the decision, is required.

Ethics and cardiorespiratory resuscitation

Various forms have been developed in different areas to record people's treatment decisions in advance. These might be referred to as a DNACPR plan or Advance Directive. RCUK favours the use of a standard process known as ReSPECT (Recommended Summary Plan for Emergency Care and Treatment).

When to start resuscitation

Life support should be started in the following circumstances:

- Sudden and unexpected cardiorespiratory arrest.
- Recent cardiorespiratory arrest. However, if there is a delay in initiating resuscitation following a cardiorespiratory arrest of more than 30 min, or if there are signs of established biological death, life support should not be started (with the exception of drowning and/or hypothermia).
- Potentially reversible causes precipitate cardiorespiratory arrest.
- Non-terminal illness. Resuscitation is not indicated if the cardiorespiratory arrest is the final natural end event in a process of dying after all available treatment options have been exhausted. The right to die with suitable dignity must be respected.
- There is no risk to the rescuer.

When to stop resuscitation

Resuscitation should be terminated when:

- There are signs of established biological death.
- The rescuer is too exhausted to continue or is in danger.
- Other individuals who have a greater chance of survival require simultaneous life support, but there are insufficient numbers of people to carry out resuscitation.
- A ReSPECT plan/anticipatory care decision exists, which indicates CPR attempts are not recommended.
- Newborn babies who fail to respond despite 20 min of intensive resuscitation are associated with a high risk of a poor outcome. It is appropriate to consider discussions with the team and family about the withdrawal of treatment if there has been no response despite the provision of all recommended steps of resuscitation and having excluded reversible causes.
- In children, consider and discuss the option of discontinuing resuscitation if life support has been continued for at least 30 min without evidence of a return of spontaneous circulation (other factors should also be considered such as cause, age, presenting rhythm).

However, resuscitation should be continued:

- in hypothermic children
- in cases of poisoning
- in persistent VF/pVT
- when a cardiorespiratory arrest occurs in children with invasive monitoring in place (whereby coronary perfusion pressure can be continuously assessed, ensuring that an adequate cardiac output can be generated to perfuse vital organs)
- when the team considers (based on specific circumstances) that resuscitation efforts must be maintained.

Organ donation

International consensus is that brain stem death is equivalent to the death of the person. This is recognised under UK law but not always in other countries. When brain stem death has occurred, the rationale for maintaining cardiorespiratory function is to allow further investigations, discussions and permissions for organ donation. In these circumstances, if cardiac activity stops, resuscitation would be inappropriate.

Organ donation should be requested in the event of brain stem death. The approach to the family of the potential organ donor must be sensitive and respectful. Frequently this request is accepted, usually 'to help other children'. Early referral to the 'Specialist Nurse for Organ Donation' team is advised to ensure expert family support is provided in this sensitive area and timely coordination is in place. Ideally, the donation should not impair the bereavement process of the child's family.

Sometimes parents change their mind many hours after a child's death when some organs may still be useful (e.g. corneas). Seek specialist advice as soon as possible.

Contraindications to organ donation are:

- cancers, except for certain non-metastatic brain tumours
- some metabolic diseases
- specific infections
- caution if history of intravenous drug addiction; further investigations may be indicated.

Making decisions about CPR

When someone is dying from an irreversible cause, CPR is unlikely to work but can subject them to an undignified death or even cause suffering and prolong the process of dying. Prolonging life at all costs is not an appropriate goal of medicine.

If a child is at risk of death or sudden cardiac arrest, consider in advance whether or not CPR could help them and whether they or their parents or guardians would want CPR. Whenever possible, make advance plans as shared decisions with parents, guardians and/or patients as part of a wider consideration of other care and realistic treatments that may or may not be appropriate for each child. Avoid focusing specifically on cardiac arrest, CPR or completing a form. Start by establishing a shared understanding of the patient's condition and likely future developments. Explore the child and parents' or guardians' priorities and preferences for their child's future care. Then discuss what types of care and realistic treatment will help them to achieve their goals of care, and whether or not they would want them, and explain relevant treatments that would not work or could do harm. Discuss CPR within this context of the broader treatment options, which might include, for example, emergency admission to hospital, various types of organ support such as ventilation, or antibiotics for life-threatening infection. Effective communication is essential to ensure that decisions about treatments such as CPR are made well and understood clearly by all those involved. The courts have made clear that there should be a presumption in favour of involving patients and/or parents and families in discussions about whether or not CPR will be attempted. This upholds the principle of autonomy and the provisions of the Human Rights Act (1998).

Recording parents', guardians' or a child's wishes about these other aspects of the child's care and treatment, alongside recommendations about CPR, can help to guide immediate decision-making by health or care professionals faced with helping that person (who they may not have met before) in an emergency. For example, this can be documented on the ReSPECT document.

Requirements for effective communication include providing information in a format that the parents, guardians and/or child can understand and checking that they have understood it. They may need time and more than one discussion before they can reach a shared decision that they are comfortable with. They should be offered opportunities for further discussion and be made aware that they may change their decision if they wish to. The use of structured communication tools or child and parent-focused leaflets may help.

Table 14.1 Examples of communication and preferred language when talking to the families for ReSPECT conversations (taken from ANZICS Statement on Care and Decision-Making at the End of Life for the Critically Ill)

Poor statements	Possible interpretation by families	Better statement
Do you want us to do everything	Do you care whether they live or die	We want to work out what is the right thing to do
The Medical team have decided	The family and their views do not matter at all	We are becoming concerned that the burden of continuing this sort of treatment outweighs the benefit

It is not necessary to discuss CPR with parents or guardians if there is no reason to expect the child to suffer a cardiorespiratory arrest or die. However, if any parent, guardian or child wants to discuss CPR, they must be given full opportunity to do so.

Make sure that you are familiar with the approach and policy that is used in your health and care community or organisation. Various forms have been developed in different places to record people's treatment decisions in advance. RCUK favours the use of a standard document that should be used and accepted by all health and care provider organisations, so that it is effective across geographical and organisational boundaries. It supports the use of the ReSPECT process (Table 14.1) and form: respectprocess.org.uk.

In addition, all health and care professionals must practise within the law. Laws relevant to CPR, including those on matters relating to capacity and consent, vary from nation to nation, both outside and within the UK. Detailed guidance, Decisions relating to cardiopulmonary resuscitation, has been published by the British Medical Association (BMA), Resuscitation Council UK and Royal College of Nursing (RCN). It includes guidance on ethical and legal aspects of decisions about CPR, but the ethical and legal principles that underpin this guidance apply equally to the broader planning approach taken by the ReSPECT process and other treatment escalation plans. As an EPALS provider, you should read and be familiar with that guidance and be familiar with relevant aspects of the law in the nation where you live and work.

Presence of parent/guardians during resuscitation

Parents/guardians of children suffering from chronic diseases may be used to witnessing medical procedures and are often present during the resuscitation of their children.

The majority of parents/guardians would like to witness their child's resuscitation; parents/guardians witnessing their child's resuscitation can see that everything possible has been attempted.

Families who are present at their child's death show less anxiety and depression, better adjustment and an improved grieving process when assessed several months later.

The opportunity to be present during resuscitation should be offered. If they decide to stay, a dedicated member of the team must be assigned to support the family with information in an empathetic manner. This also ensures safety is maintained during an emergency situation. When appropriate, physical contact with the child should be allowed, and wherever possible, they should be permitted to be with their dying child in the final moments. Many hospitals will have a procedure on how to perform this role and include training for the clinician.

The resuscitation team leader will decide when to stop resuscitation. This must be expressed with sensitivity and understanding.

Informing parent/guardians

When a child dies, it is the resuscitation team leader's duty to inform the parents/guardians. This is always a difficult task, particularly if the parents were not present at the resuscitation, and the suddenness of an event may make it difficult for the team leader to understand family dynamics and predict a response to bad news.

The following four principles may ease the process, preparation, communication, planning and follow-up:

- Select an appropriate environment (with assured privacy).
- The medical attitude must be professional, with a simple and clear explanation of the facts, but at the same time, it should be compassionate, and their emotional needs must be recognised. It is important to take a few moments to prepare what the team leader will say.
- Establish with certainty who the family members are and their relationship to the child.
- Explain with clarity that their child is dead (use the word "dead" specifically). Information should be given with empathy, compassion and sympathy. The details of the circumstances should be given clearly.

Use the child's first name and avoid 'empty introductory sentences' (he came in with.. and we tried.. but eventually failed) that postpone saying the only thing they are waiting to hear ('alive or dead').

- Encourage the parents/guardians to see and stay with their child. They should be encouraged to touch and hold their child.
- Explain the necessity of a post-mortem examination (if applicable), particularly in cases of sudden, unexplained or accidental death. Inform the parents/guardians that the police and the coroner are routinely informed if the child's death fits these circumstances and consider other safeguarding issues.
- Permission for post-mortem studies may be discussed, which may help better understand aspects of the child's condition or mode of death.
- Ask the parents/guardians about any religious requirements.
- Do not guess at the diagnosis but explain that the pathologist will try to ascertain the cause of death. Explain that all children's deaths are reviewed by an appropriate reviewing body, and it is normal in unexpected deaths that a rapid response team is convened to coordination investigations.
- Make an appointment for further discussion and information.

Verify
- name and address of parents
- date of birth of the deceased child
- arrival time in the emergency department (if relevant)
- time of death.

Inform
- paediatrician or general practitioner, giving the address where the parents are going and their contact details
- health visitor for children < 5 years or school nurse for children > 5 years
- social worker
- persons that the parents wish to be informed.

Document this information in the child's notes and ensure their safekeeping.

14: Summary learning

Ethics attempts to understand human actions in a moral sense.

In current medical ethics, the four guiding principles are: autonomy, beneficence, non-maleficence and justice.

Commencing the difficult conversation early between the patient family and medical team when end-of-life care or ReSPECT decisions have to be considered will support better communication between the patient/family and medical teams

Information must be given to the child as appropriate and to the parents/guardians.

The majority of parents would like to be present during resuscitation.

If the child dies, parents/guardians being present during resuscitation helps their grieving process.

My key take-home messages from this chapter are:

Further reading

Australian and New Zealand Intensive Care Society. ANZICS Statement on Care and Decision-Making at the End of Life for the Critically Ill. 1st edition. 2014 Melbourne,

Beckman AW, Sloan BK, Moore GP et al. Should parents be present during emergency department procedures on children, and who should make that decision? A survey of emergency physician and nurse attitudes. Acad Emerg Med 2002; 9: 154-8.

British Medical Association, Resuscitation Council UK and Royal College of Nursing. Decisions relating to cardiopulmonary resuscitation. 2007. www.resus.org.uk

Boie ET, Moore GP, Brummett C, Nelson DR. Do parents want to be present during invasive procedures performed on their children in the emergency department? A survey of 400 parents. Ann Emerg Med 1999; 34: 70-4.

Horisberger T, Fischer JE, Fanconi S. One-year survival and neurological outcome after pediatric cardiopulmonary resuscitation. Int Care Med 2002; 28: 365-8.

Powers KS, Rubenstein JS. Family presence during invasive procedures in the pediatric intensive care unit: a prospective study. Arch Pediatr Adoles Med 1999; 153: 955-8.

Meyers TA, Eichhorn DJ, Guzzetta CE et al. Family presence during invasive procedures and resuscitation. Am J Nurs 2000; 100: 32-42.

Robinson SM, Mackenzie-Ross S, Campbell Hewson GL, Egleston CV, Prevost AT. Psychological effect of witnessed resuscitation on bereaved relatives (comment). Lancet 1998; 352: 614-7.

Sharp MC, Strauss RP, Lorch RC. Communicating medical bad news: parents' experiences and preferences. J Pediatric 1992; 121: 539-46.

Taylor N, Bonilla L, Silver P, Sagy M. Pediatric procedure: do parents want to be present? Crit Care Med 1996; 24: A131.

Tsai E. Should family members be present during cardiopulmonary resuscitation? N Engl J Med 2002; 346: 1019-21.

Woolley H, Stein A, Forest GC et al. Imparting the diagnosis of life threatening illness in children. BMJ 1989; 298: 1623-6.

Youngblut JM, Shiao SYP. Child and family reactions during and after pediatric ICU hospitalisation: a pilot study. Heart Lung 1993; 22: 46-54.

I. Barata, J. LaMantia, D. Riccardi, et al: A Prospective Study of Emergency Medicine Residents' Attitudes toward Family Presence during Pediatric Procedures. The Internet Journal of Emergency Medicine. 2007; 3:number 2.

L.Nibert, D.Ondrejka Family presence during pediatric resuscitation: An integrative review for evidence-based practice Journal of Pediatric Nursing 2005; Volume 20: Issue 2,145-147.

http://www.rcn.org.uk/ data/assets/pdf_file/0006/545289/004471.pdf. accessed 23 Sept2015

Working together to safeguard children. http://www.workingtogetheronline.co.uk/chapters/chapter_five.html accessed 23 Sept 2015

Organ donation information for UK, Scotland, Wales, Northern Ireland https://www.organdonation.nhs.uk/about-donation/what-can-i-donate/ https://www.organdonationscotland.org/ http://organdonationwales.org/?skip=1&lang=en https://www.organdonationni.info/

www.respectprocess.org.uk

TIMMIS, V. 2020. Should family members be present at resuscitation? Arch Dis Child, 105, 506-508.

Oczkowski SJ, Mazzetti, I, Cupido C, Fox-Robichaud AE; 2015. Canadian Critical care Society. Family presence during resuscitation. A Canadian Critical Care Society. position paper. Can Respir J, 4: 201 – 5

MARK, K. 2020. Family presence during paediatric resuscitation and invasive procedures: the parental experience: An integrative review: Scand J Caring Sci.

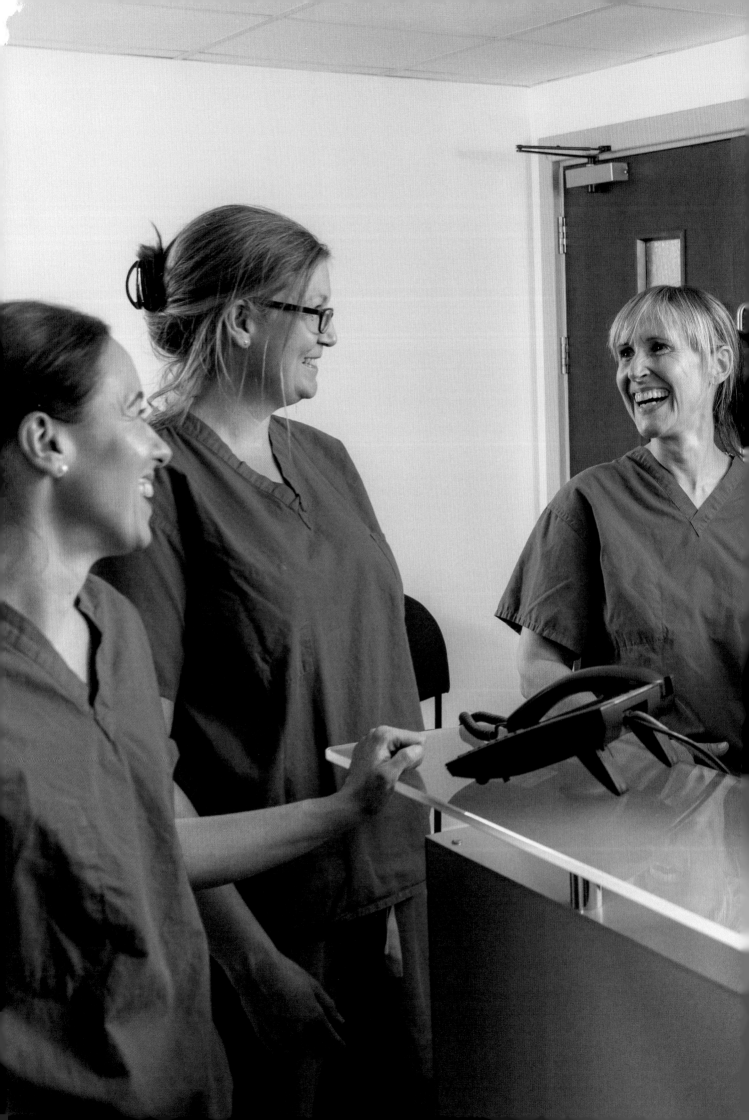

Non-technical skills in resuscitation

In this chapter

2

Non-technical skills

Situational awareness

Decision making

Team working

Team leadership

Task management and the importance of communication

Resuscitation teams and preparation

Quality and audit

The learning outcomes will enable you to:

Be an effective team member and team member

Consider the role of non-technical skills during resuscitation

Effectively use structured communication tools such as SBAR and RSVP

Introduction

Non-technical skills can be defined as the cognitive, social and personal resource skills that complement technical skills and contribute to safe and efficient task performance. More simply, they are the things that affect our personal performance. Non-technical skills of leadership and teamwork have been identified as important contributory factors to technical skill performance in both simulated settings and poor clinical outcomes in acute medical settings.

Paediatric resuscitation is particularly emotive, stressful and often time-critical. The skills of chest compressions, vascular access, defibrillation, and rhythm recognition are considered typically to be important aspects of paediatric resuscitation management. These are all technical skills that are learnt from books, lectures, courses and peers. Although they are important for the successful resuscitation of a child, there is another group of skills that is becoming increasingly recognised in medicine as equally important.

The importance of non-technical skills in emergencies is now widely accepted across many acute medical specialities, including surgery, anaesthesia, critical care and acute medicine. Examples of poor non-technical skills include poor communication, poor leadership, poor decision making, and absence of clarity in role allocation, all of which can lead to system errors. Episodes of resuscitation with documented system errors are associated with poor clinical outcomes. In the context of advanced life support, which is fundamentally a team effort, the contribution of teamwork and leadership is therefore expected to make a significant contribution to patient outcome. Understanding and improving non-technical skills may help to reduce human errors, creating more effective teams and improve patient safety. An effective team leader can help focus the team members, improve team commitment and act as the role model for others.

The key non-technical skills are:

- situational awareness
- decision making
- team working
- leadership
- task management.

Situational awareness

This can be described as an individual's awareness of the environment at the moment of an event and the analysis of this to understand how individual actions may impact on future events. This becomes particularly important when many events are happening simultaneously, for example, at a resuscitation attempt. High information input with poor situational awareness may lead to poor decision making with serious consequences. At a resuscitation, all those participating will have varying degrees of situational awareness.

In a well-functioning team, all members will have a common understanding of current events or shared situational awareness. It is important that only the relevant information is shared; otherwise, there is too much distraction or noise.

Situational awareness in resuscitation will include perception of environment and events taking place, comprehension of their meaning, and future projection.

Information gathering
What are the potential causes of cardiac arrest?
- location of arrest
- information from staff about events leading up to the arrest
- note the actions already initiated
- confirm who is present; names, skills, roles and who is leading.

Interpretation
What immediate steps are needed?
- confirm diagnosis
- check that a monitor has been attached and interpreting what it shows
- determine immediate needs and necessary actions.

Future planning
What are the next steps?
- consider the impact of interventions
- plan for next steps.

Decision making

This is defined as the cognitive process of choosing a specific course of action from several alternatives. At a resuscitation, the many decisions to be made usually fall to the team leader. The leader will assimilate information from the team members and from personal observation and will use this to determine appropriate interventions and shares these with the team. Typical decisions made at a resuscitation may include:

- likely reversible causes of the arrest
- appropriate treatment such as drugs or airway management
- how long to continue resuscitation
- appropriate post-resuscitation care.

Once a decision has been made, clear unambiguous communication with the team members is essential to ensure that it is implemented.

Team working

This is one of the most important non-technical skills that contribute to the successful management of critical situations. A team is a group of individuals working together with a common goal or purpose. In a team, the members usually have complementary skills and, through coordination of effort, work synergistically. Teams work best when everyone knows each other's name, when they are doing something they perceive to be important, and when their role is within their experience and competence. Optimal team function mandates a team leader.

There are several characteristics of a good resuscitation team member:

- **Competence** – has the skills required at a resuscitation and performs them to the best of their ability.
- **Commitment** – strives to achieve the best outcome for the patient.
- **Communicates openly** – articulates their findings and actions taken, raising concerns about clinical or safety issues, and listening to briefings and instructions.
- **Supportive** – enables others to achieve their best.
- **Accountable** – for their own and the team's actions.
- **Prepared to admit when help is needed.**
- **Creative** – suggests different ways of interpreting the situation.
- **Participates in providing feedback.**

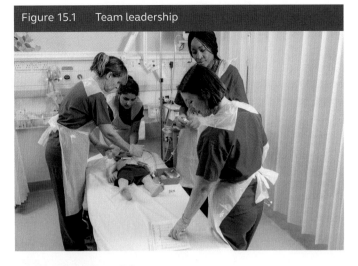

Figure 15.1 Team leadership

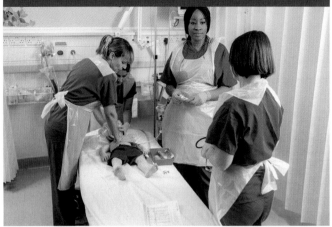

Figure 15.2 Team leader prioritising actions of the team

Team leadership

A team leader provides guidance, direction and instruction to the team members to enable successful completion of their stated objective (Figure 15.1). They lead by example and integrity. Team leaders need experience, not simply seniority. Team leadership can be considered a process; with training, it is available to everyone within the team and not restricted to those with leadership traits.

There are several attributes recognisable in a good team leader:

- knows everyone in the team by name and knows their capability
- accepts the leadership role
- is able to delegate tasks appropriately (preferably before the event)
- is knowledgeable and has sufficient credibility to influence the team through role modelling and professionalism
- recognises their own limitations and asks for support from the team
- is a good communicator – not just good at giving instructions, but also a good listener and decisive in action
- stays calm, keeps everyone focused and controls distractions
- is empathetic towards the whole team
- is assertive and authoritative when required
- shows tolerance towards hesitancy or nervousness in the emergency setting
- has good situational awareness; able to constantly monitor the situation, with an up-to-date overview, listening and deciding on a course of action.

During an arrest, the role of team leader is not always immediately obvious. The leader should clarify early on that they are assuming the role of team leader.

Specifically, at a cardiorespiratory arrest the team leader should:

- Follow current resuscitation guidelines or explain a reason for any significant deviation from standard protocols.
- Consult with the team or call for senior advice and assistance if unsure about an intervention.

- Play to the strengths of team members and allow them some autonomy if their skills are adequate.
- Allocate roles and tasks throughout the resuscitation and be specific. This avoids several people or nobody attempting the task!
- Use the two-minute cycle of chest compressions to plan tasks and safety aspects of the resuscitation attempt with the team.
- Thank the team at the end of the resuscitation attempt and ensure that staff and relatives are being supported.
- Complete all documentation and ensure an adequate handover.

Task management

During the resuscitation of a child, either in full cardiorespiratory arrest or peri-arrest, there are numerous tasks to be carried out by the team members, either sequentially or simultaneously. Cognitive aids such as a checklist or easy access guidelines could be used as support, but will need a dedicated team member to read and check them. The coordination and control, or management, of these tasks, is the responsibility of the team leader (Figure 15.2). Tasks can include:

- identifying the resources required - ensuring that equipment is checked and specifics organised and delegated
- being inclusive of all team members
- being prepared for both the expected and the unexpected
- prioritising actions of the team
- watching out for fatigue, stress and distress amongst the team
- managing conflict
- communicating with relatives
- communicating with experts for safe handover both by telephone and in person
- debriefing the team
- reporting untoward incidents, particularly equipment or system failures
- participation in audit.

The importance of communication when managing a sick child

Communication problems are a factor in up to 80% of adverse incidents or near-miss reports in hospitals. This failure of communication is also evident when a medical emergency occurs on a ward and a doctor or nurse summons senior help. The call for help is often suboptimal, with failure by the caller to communicate the seriousness of the situation and to convey information in a way that informs the recipient of the urgency of the situation. The poor-quality information heightens the anxiety of the person responding to the call, who is then uncertain of the nature of the problem they are about to face. A well-structured process that is simple, reliable and dependable, will enable the caller to convey the important facts and urgency, and will help the recipient to plan ahead. It was for similar reasons that the ABCDE approach was developed as an aide memoire of the key technical skills required to manage seriously ill/deteriorating patients.

The use of the SBAR (Situation, Background, Assessment, Recommendation) or RSVP (Reason, Story, Vital signs, Plan) tool enables effective, timely communication between individuals from different clinical backgrounds and hierarchies (Table 15.1).

Resuscitation teams

The resuscitation team may take the form of a traditional cardiorespiratory arrest team which is called only when a cardiorespiratory arrest is recognised. Alternatively, hospitals may have strategies to recognise patients at risk of deterioration and to summon a team (e.g. medical emergency team) before a cardiorespiratory arrest occurs.

The term 'resuscitation team' reflects a range of immediate response teams. The resuscitation team may change daily or more frequently, and members may not know each other or the skill mix within the team. The team should, therefore, meet ('huddle') at the beginning of their period on duty to introduce themselves and allocate roles (Figure 15.3).

Preparation

During the 'huddle', the team will identify a team leader who will pre-allocate core tasks according to the number of team members available and the skill mix, these include:

- airway management and ventilation
- pulse check and chest compressions
- attaching monitoring and/or defibrillation
- obtaining IO/IV access, preparing and administering drugs
- recording events.

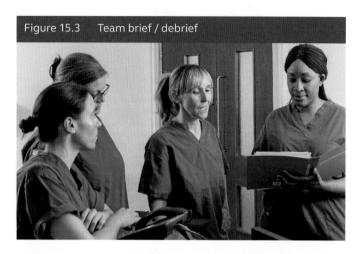

Figure 15.3 Team brief / debrief

Relatives can be looked after by another member of the team; this should not be the most junior member of staff as parents need a careful explanation of the events.

Clinical staff who participate as members of the resuscitation team must be up to date with advanced skills in paediatric life support and must be familiar with the local equipment.

It is also important that resuscitation teams practice skills together to try to avoid errors. This may involve high and low-fidelity scenarios on courses such as EPALS and involve on-site 'mock' clinical emergencies.

Team debrief

Every effort should be made to enable the team members to meet to debrief (e.g. difficulties or concerns about their performance, problems or concerns with equipment) and submit incident reports. Debriefing has been shown to enhance team performance. It may also be possible to carry out a formal handover to the incoming team.

Quality and Audit

The Institute of Medicine defines quality care as safe, effective, patient-centred, timely, efficient and equitable. Hospitals, resuscitation teams and EPALS providers should ensure they deliver these aspects of quality to improve the care of the deteriorating child and children in cardiorespiratory arrest. Two aspects of this are safety incident reporting (also called adverse or critical incident reporting) and collecting good quality data.

Audit and outcome after cardiorespiratory arrest

Most modern defibrillators allow the cardiorespiratory arrest management to be downloaded with a timeline of different rhythms and actions taken in terms of defibrillation, cardioversion and cardiopulmonary resuscitation; it also allows the quality of CPR delivered to be reviewed when a feedback device has been used.

Locally, this useful information can help teams use reflection and feedback to improve future performance,

Table 15.1 **SBAR** (Situation, Background, Assessment, Recommendation) **and RSVP** (Reason, Story, Vital signs, Plan)

SBAR	RSVP	Content	Example
Situation	**Reason**	Introduce yourself and check you are speaking to the correct person. Identify the patient you are calling about (who and where). Say what you think the current problem is, or appears to be. State what you need advice about. Useful phrases: • The problem appears to be cardiac/respiratory/neurological/sepsis. • I'm not sure what the problem is but the patient is deteriorating. • The patient is unstable, getting worse and I need help.	*Hi, I'm Dr Smith the paediatric F2.* *I am calling about Sam Brown on the paediatric ward who I think has a severe pneumonia and is septic.* *They have an oxygen saturation of 90% despite high-flow oxygen and I am very worried.*
Background	**Story**	Background information about the patient. Reason for admission. Relevant past medical history.	*They are 6 years old and previously fit and well.* *They have had a fever and a cough for 2 days.* *They were admitted yesterday.*
Assessment	**Vital signs**	Include specific observations and vital sign values based on ABCDE approach. • Airway • Breathing • Circulation • Disability • Exposure • The PEWS score is…	*They look very unwell and are tiring* *Airway – they can say a few words* *Breathing – their respiratory rate is 34, with widespread wheeze in both lung fields and has bronchial breathing on the left side. Their oxygen saturation is 90% on high-flow oxygen. I am getting a blood gas and chest X-ray* *Circulation – their pulse is 180, and blood pressure is 90/60* *Disability – they are drowsy and clinging onto their mum* *Exposure – there are no rashes*
Recommendation	**Plan**	State explicitly what you want the person you are calling to do. What by when? Useful phrases: • I am going to start the following treatment; is there anything else you can suggest? • I am going to do the following investigations; is there anything else you can suggest? • If they do not improve; when would you like to be called? • I don't think I can do anymore; I would like you to see the patient urgently.	*They are only on oral antibiotics so I am starting an IV* *I need help – please can you come straight away?*

especially in terms of adherence to resuscitation guidelines, the percentage of time CPR has been performed and 'hands-off' time.

National audit of resuscitation processes and outcomes provides information about whether interventions and changes made to resuscitation guidelines improve patient care. New interventions that improve survival rate even marginally are important because of the many individuals who have a cardiorespiratory arrest each year. Local hospitals or healthcare systems are unlikely to have sufficient patients to identify these effects or eliminate confounders.

Therefore, resuscitation outcome and processes should be reported in a standard manner to allow comparison between different areas of practice. The internationally agreed Utstein template is a standardised system of reporting that allows the comparison of resuscitation data across different countries and healthcare systems. This facilitates the use of large national and multi-national databases to evaluate the impact of new drugs or techniques.

National Cardiac Arrest Audit (NCAA)

In the UK, the National Cardiac Arrest Audit (NCAA) is an ongoing, national, comparative outcome audit of in-hospital cardiorespiratory arrests (Table 15.2). It is a joint initiative between Resuscitation Council UK and the Intensive Care National Audit & Research Centre (ICNARC) and is open to all acute hospitals in the UK and Ireland. The audit monitors and reports on the incidence of, and outcome from, in-hospital cardiorespiratory arrest in order to inform practice and policy. It aims to identify and foster improvements in the prevention, care delivery and outcomes from cardiorespiratory arrest. Data are collected according to standardised definitions and entered into the NCAA secure web-based system. Once data are validated, hospitals are provided with activity reports and comparative reports, allowing a comparison to be made, not only within, but also between hospitals locally, nationally and internationally. Furthermore, NCAA enables the monitoring of the effects of new guidelines, drugs, techniques etc. that would not be possible on a hospital-by-hospital basis.

Table 15.2   Outcomes following in-hospital cardiac arrest (UK) for children in participating hospitals January 2012 to December 2018 NCAA data. Total number Cardiac arrests = 1580

	VF/pVT	Asystole	PEA	Bradycardia
% of arrests	4.3%	22.2 %	30.3%	29.7%
% ROSC > 20 mins	75%	55.9%	55.9%	87%
% hospital discharge	63.9%	41%	41%	70.6%
Overall survival to hospital discharge (all events)	54.2 %	54.2 %	54.2 %	54.2 %

14: Summary learning

Non-technical skills are important during resuscitation.

Use SBAR or RSVP for effective communication.

My key take-home messages from this chapter are:

Further reading

Andersen PO, Jensen MK, Lippert A, et al.: Identifying non-technical skills and barriers for improvement of teamwork in cardiac arrest teams. Resuscitation 2010; 81:695–702.

Cooper S, Cant R, Porter J, et al.: Rating medical emergency teamwork performance: Development of the Team Emergency Assessment Measure (TEAM). Resuscitation 2010; 81:446–452.

Featherstone P, Chalmers T, Smith GB. RSVP: a system for communication of deterioration in hospital patients. Br J Nurs 2008;17:860-64.

Flin R, O'Connor P, Crichton M. Safety at the Sharp End: a Guide to Non- Technical Skills. Aldershot: Ashgate, 2008.

Peltonen V, Peltonen LM, Salantera S et al. An observational study of technical and non-technical skills in advanced life support in the clinical setting. Resuscitation 2020; 53:162-168

Yeung J, Ong G, Davies R, Gao F, Perkins GDP. Factors affecting team leadership skills and their relationship with quality of cardiopulmonary resuscitation. Crit Care Med 2012; 40:2617–2621.

Skellett S, Orzechowska I, Thomas K, Fortune PM. The Landscape of paediatric in-hospital cardiac arrest in the United Kingdom National Cardiac Arrest Audit. Resuscitation. 2020 Oct;155:165-171

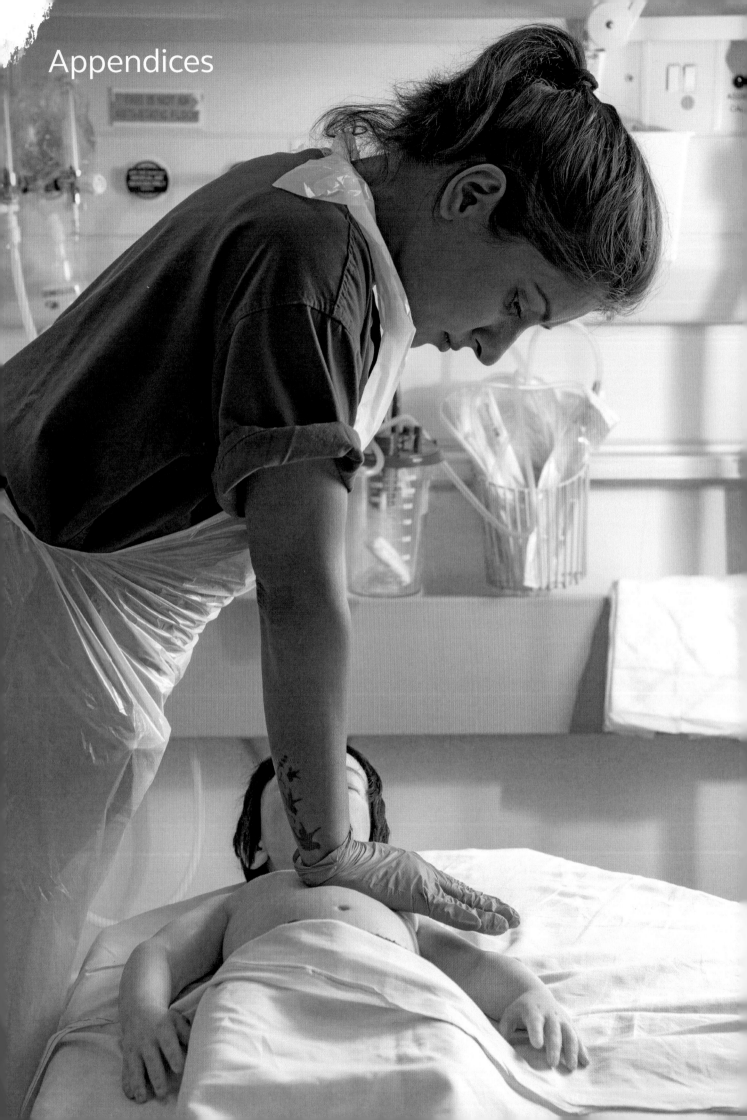

Resuscitation Council UK

Appendix A: Paediatric emergency drug chart

GUIDELINES 2021

		Adrenaline	Fluid bolus	Glucose	Sodium bicarbonate		Tracheal tube		Defibrillation
Strength		1:10 000	Balanced isotonic crystalloid OR, 0.9% Saline	10%	4.2%	8.4%	Uncuffed	Cuffed	4 joules kg⁻¹
Dose		10 mcg kg⁻¹	10 mL kg⁻¹	2 mL kg⁻¹	1 mmol kg⁻¹				Transthoracic
Route		IV, IO	IV, IO	IV, IO	IV, IO, UVC	IV, IO			Monophasic or biphasic
Notes			Consider warmed fluids	For known hypoglycaemia			Monitor cuff pressure		
Age	**Weight kg**	mL	mL	mL (recheck glucose after dose and repeat as required)	mL	mL	ID mm	ID mm	Manual
< 1 month	3.5	0.35	35	7	7	–	3.0	–	20
1 month	4	0.4	40	8	8	–	3.0–3.5	3.0	20
3 months	5	0.5	50	10	10	–	3.5	3.0	20
6 months	7	0.7	70	14	–	7	3.5	3.0	30
1 year	10	1.0	100	20	–	10	4.0	3.5	40
2 years	12	1.2	120	24	–	12	4.5	4.0	50
3 years	14	1.4	140	28	–	14	4.5–5.0	4.0–4.5	60
4 years	16	1.6	160	32	–	16	5.0	4.5	60
5 years	18	1.8	180	36	–	18	5.0–5.5	4.5–5.0	70
6 years	20	2.0	200	40	–	20	5.5	5.0	80
7 years	23	2.3	230	46	–	23	5.5–6.0	5.0–5.5	100
8 years	26	2.6	260	50	–	26	–	6.0–6.5	100
10 years	30	3.0	300	50	–	30	–	7.0	120
12 years	38	3.8	380	50	–	38	–	7–7.5	120
14 years	50	5.0	500	50	–	50	–	7–8	120–150
Adolescent	50	5.0	500	50	–	50	–	7–8	120–150
Adult	70	10.0	500	50	–	50	–	7–8	120–150

Cardioversion	Synchronised Shock, 1.0 joules kg⁻¹ escalating to 2.0 joules kg⁻¹ if unsuccessful.
Amiodarone	5 mg kg⁻¹ IV or IO bolus in arrest after 3rd and 5th shocks. Flush line with 0.9% saline or 5% glucose (max dose 300 mg).
Atropine	20 mcg kg⁻¹, maximum dose 600 mcg.
Calcium gluconate 10%	0.5 mL kg⁻¹ for hypocalcaemia, hyperkalaemia (max dose 20 mL); IV over 2–5 min if unstable, over 15–20 min if stable.
Lorazepam	100 mcg kg⁻¹ IV or IO for treatment of seizures. Can be repeated after 10 min. Maximum single dose 4 mg.
Adenosine	IV or IO for treatment of SVT: 150 mcg kg⁻¹ (0–11 months of age); 100 mcg kg⁻¹ (1–11 years of age) Increase dose in steps 50–100 mcg kg⁻¹ every 1–2 min for repeat doses. 12–17 years: 3 mg, followed by 6 mg after 1–2 min if required. Requires large saline flush and ECG monitoring.
Anaphylaxis	Adrenaline 1:1000 IM: < 6 months 100–150 mcg (0.1–0.15 mL), 6 months–6 years 150 mcg (0.15 mL), 6–12 years 300 mcg (0.3 mL), > 12 years 500 mcg (0.5 mL); can be repeated after 5 min. After 2 IM injections treat as refractory anaphylaxis and start low dose adrenaline infusion IV.

- Weights averaged on lean body mass from 50th centile weights for males and females.
- Drug doses based on Resuscitation Council UK Guidelines 2021 recommendations.
- Recommendations for tracheal tubes are based on full term neonates.
- For newborns glucose at 2.5 mL kg⁻¹ is recommended.

Useful links

The European Paediatric Advanced Life Support (EPALS) is an advanced course that trains healthcare professionals in the early recognition of the child in respiratory or circulatory failure and management of a cardiorespiratory arrest.

EPALS provides the knowledge and skills needed to prevent further deterioration and help to save young lives.

The EPALS course is a collaboration between Resuscitation Council UK and the European Resuscitation Council. It is approved by the Royal Colleges of Paediatric and Child Health (RCPCH), Emergency Medicine (RCEM), and Anaesthetics (RCoA), as well as the Association of Paediatric Anaesthetists (APAGBI).

Become an RCUK EPALS Instructor

The faculty may nominate exceptional candidates to become an EPALS instructor. The Course Director and faculty must support the nomination and provide a detailed statement of support to RCUK.

To be successfully put forward as an Instructor Potential (IP), the candidate must be a (statutory/voluntary) registered healthcare professional with significant/extensive clinical experience, work in an appropriate clinical setting, and be involved in acute clinical care involving resuscitation as part of their work.

Candidates must demonstrate excellent core knowledge of the course content, excellent and safe practical application of skills, and exceptional communication skills.

Potential instructors should be confident, flexible, adaptable, interactive, supportive and enthusiastic.

If successfully nominated, the candidate would need to undertake an RCUK Generic Instructor Course (GIC) and complete two supported supervised teaching practices as an Instructor Candidate (IC).

More information regarding the GIC can be accessed here: https://www.resus.org.uk/training-courses/instructor-courses/gic-generic-instructor-course.

Benefits of becoming an instructor for RCUK:

You will join the RCUK community of practice, with opportunities for portfolio development and ongoing access to the latest research and resuscitation practices.

You will become a subject matter expert, and your instructor qualification will be recognised throughout the UK and Europe. As an instructor, you'll be eligible to attend RCUK's popular Instructor Days, and you will also receive free RCUK Associate membership.

Being an active EPALS instructor means you are also an EPALS provider.

For more information on how you can become an RCUK EPALS instructor, please speak to the Course Director before or on the day of your course.

Resuscitation Council UK Guidelines
Read all of the 2021 guidelines:
resus.org.uk/rcukgl21
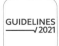

Lifesaver and Lifesaver VR apps
Teach your friends and family lifesaving skills anytime, anywhere:
resus.org.uk/rcuklifesaver

iResus app
Get RCUK guidelines on the go:
resus.org.uk/rcukiresus

e-Lifesaver
Bring lifesaving training to your non-clinical staff:
resus.org.uk/rcukworkplace

Resuscitation Council UK courses
See all of the courses available:
resus.org.uk/rcukcourses

Follow us on Twitter
@ResusCouncilUK
twitter.com/ResusCouncilUK

RCUK membership
Get involved and join our community:
resus.org.uk/rcukmembers

Like us on Facebook
facebook.com/ResuscitationCouncilUK

Notes

Notes